DIABETIC NEPHROPATHY

Edited by **John S. D. Chan**

Diabetic Nephropathy

Edited by John S. D. Chan

Published by InTech

Janeza Trdine 9, 51000 Rijeka, Croatia

Publishing Process Manager Vedran Greblo

Technical Editor Teodora Smiljanic

Cover Designer InTech Design Team

Additional hard copies can be obtained from orders@intechopen.com

Diabetic Nephropathy, Edited by John S. D. Chan
p. cm.
ISBN 978-953-51-0543-5

For EU product safety concerns:
IN TECH d.o.o., Prolaz Marije Krucifikse Kozulić 3, 51000 Rijeka, Croatia,
info@intechopen.com or visit our website at intechopen.com.

Meet the editor

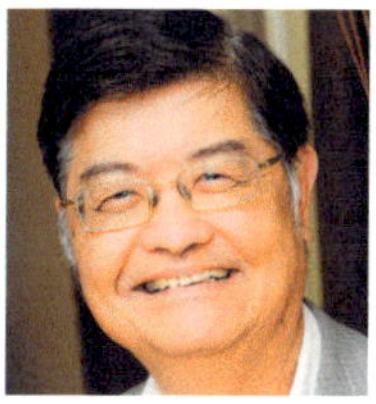

Dr. Chan is currently a Professor of Medicine at the Université de Montréal and the Chief of the Laboratory of Molecular Nephrology and Endocrinology at the Research Centre of Centre hospitalier de l'Université de Montréal (CRCHUM). Dr. Chan's research program seeks to understand the role(s) of intrarenal renin angiotensin system (RAS) and oxidative stress in the pathogenesis of diabetic nephropathy, with special emphasis on renal angiotensinogen gene expression and reactive oxygen species (ROS) generation on tubular apoptosis in diabetes. Dr. Chan has published over 100 papers in scientific journals and presented more than 250 abstracts in various scientific societies. Dr. Chan's research program is supported by several peer-reviewed granting agencies including the Canadian Institutes of Health Research, Kidney Foundation of Canada, Canadian Diabetes Association and Canadian Foundation of Innovation.

Contents

Preface

The idea for publishing a book on diabetic nephropathy has been developed during the last several years as my interest in studying diabetic complications has increased. The need for a book that described the various novel and old molecules involved in the development of diabetic nephropathy and the trend of future research became apparent. The book describes the important role of intrarenal renin-angiotensin-aldosterone system and immune system in the development of diabetic nephropathy as well as provided data on the biochemical and pathological changes in diabetic nephropathy. Relevant information on the treatments of diabetic nephropathy is also provided.

The authors are internationally known for their work in diabetic nephropathy. Each chapter has been peer-reviewed and edited and provide up-to-date information on the topic.

I hope that the book will be useful for researchers working in the field of diabetic nephropathy.

John S. D. Chan
Professor of Medicine at the Université de Montréal,
Chief of the Laboratory of Molecular Nephrology and Endocrinology,
Research Centre - Centre hospitalier de l'Université de Montréal (CRCHUM)
Montréal,
Canada

Section 1

Systemic and Local Intrarenal Renin-Angiotensin-Aldosterone System in the Development of Diabetic Nephropathy

Up-Regulation of Renin-Angiotensin System in Diabetes and Hypertension: Implications on the Development of Diabetic Nephropathy

Dulce Elena Casarini et al.*
Department of Medicine, Federal University of São Paulo, São Paulo Brazil

1. Introduction

The growing worldwide epidemic of metabolic syndrome and other chronic degenerative diseases continues to expand, with a rapid decrease in the age at which they are being diagnosed (Guarnieri et al.; 2010; Hsueh & Wyne, 2011). Metabolic syndrome is a multi-factorial disorder, strongly influenced by several lifestyle factors, with symptoms clustering on abnormalities that include obesity, hypertension, dyslipidemia, glucose intolerance and insulin resistance (Guarnieri et al.; 2010; Tanaka et al.; 2006). The syndrome is also referred to as "Diabesity" highlighting the incidence of diabetes mellitus (DM) in combination with obesity as a result of changes in human behavior (Astrup & Finer, 2000; Farag & Gaballa, 2011; Hu, 2011).

Obesity is considered an independent predictor of the development of hypertension and it has been estimated that about half of individuals with essential hypertension are considered insulin resistant (Hall et al.; 2010; Kotsis et al.; 2010). Likewise, insulin resistance and hyperinsulinemia increase the risk of hypertension, and it usually accompanies DM, early in type 2 (DM2) and delayed in type 1 (DM1). Moreover, among patients being treated for hypertension, the risk of new-onset diabetes is doubled in those with uncontrolled blood pressure (BP) (Gress et al.; 2000; Gupta et al.; 2008; Izzo et al.; 2009). Although effective antihypertensive agents are available, achieving adequate BP control remains difficult in hypertensive patients, particularly in the context of concomitant diabetes.

It is widely known that individuals with DM and/or hypertension are prone to develop a broad range of long term complications, including cardiovascular disease and nephropathy (Farag & Gaballa, 2011; Guarnieri et al.; 2010; Houston et al.; 2005; Handelsman, 2011; Tanaka et al.; 2006), and it has already been shown that several modifiable risk factors are associated with poor renal and cardiovascular outcome, including BP, plasma glucose and lipid concentrations, smoking, and body weight (Miao et al.; 2011). It is important to

* Danielle Yuri Arita[1], Tatiana Sousa Cunha[1,2], Fernanda Aparecida Ronchi[1], Danielle Sanches Aragão[1], Rodolfo Mattar Rosa[1], Nadia Sousa Cunha Bertoncello[1] and Fernanda Klein Marcondes[3]
[1]*Department of Medicine, Nephrology Division, Federal University of São Paulo, São Paulo, Brazil*
[2]*Science and Technology Institute, Federal University of São Paulo, São José dos Campos, Brazil*
[3]*Department of Physiological Sciences, Piracicaba Dental School, University of Campinas, Piracicaba, Brazil*

highlight that both DM and hypertension exacerbate each other in terms of subsequent complications (Cooper & Johnston, 2000) increasing the burden of social dysfunction and high risk of premature death.

DM is a chronic metabolic disorder characterized by hyperglycemia and insufficiency of secretion or action of endogenous insulin. Nowadays, diabetes afflicts around 6.6% of the global adult population, or approximately 285 million individuals, and this is projected to increase by more than 50% to a 7.8% worldwide prevalence in 20 years. Considering that DM is an important health problem and it has been recognized as a major risk factor for the development of complications in target organs, including retinopathy, neuropathy, nephropathy and cardiovascular disease, the comprehension of the mechanisms involved in the association among diabetes is the subject of many research groups (International Diabetes Federation, 2009).

Of these complications, diabetic nephropathy (DN), the most common etiology of chronic kidney disease (CKD) and common cause of end-stage renal disease (ESRD) in adults in the Western world (Choudhury et al.; 2010; Cooper, 1998; National Institute of Diabetes and Digestive and Kidney Diseases, 2010), is associated with the highest mortality (Cooper, 1998; Giacchetti et al.; 2005) making early diagnosis critical in preventing long term kidney loss. Approximately 30% of patients with either DM1 or DM2 develop DN (Dalla Vestra et al.; 2000), and in these patients, lowering of BP and of urinary albumin excretion significantly decrease the risk of progression to ESRD, myocardial infarction and stroke (Choudhury et al.; 2010; Cooper et al.; 2000; Gupta et al.; 2008; Handelsman, 2011; Keller et al.; 1996).

Approximately 80% of individuals with diabetic ESRD are affected by hypertension, which accelerates the progression rate of renal disease (Jandeleit-Dahm & Cooper, 2002). In DM1 the onset of hypertension appears to occur primarily as a consequence rather than as a primary cause of renal disease (Poulsen et al.; 1994). The link between glycemic control and the development of hypertension has been demonstrated in the follow-up of the landmark Diabetes Control and Complications Trial (DCCT), the Epidemiology of Diabetes Interventions and Complications (EDIC) study (Writing Team for the Diabetes Control and Complications Trial/Epidemiology of Diabetes Interventions and Complications Research Group [EDIC], 2003). It demonstrated that hypertension was developed in 40% of the patients in the conventionally treated group compared with 30% in the group treated with an intensified insulin regimen in year 8 of the EDIC follow-up. These beneficial effects were seen in the context of reduced renal disease consistent with the view that hypertension in DM1 is primarily a manifestation of DN in these subjects. Therefore, it appears likely that hyperglycemia or insulin plays a role in influencing BP in DM1 (Elliott et al.; 2001). Regarding DM2, the combination with hypertension appears to cluster clinically as part of a syndrome involving not only these two conditions but also insulin resistance, dyslipidemia, central obesity, hyperuricemia, and accelerated atherosclerosis (Eckel et al.; 2005; Sowers et al.; 2001; Williams, 1994). The underlying explanation for this cluster of clinical features remains unexplained but insulin resistance has been postulated by many investigators as playing a pivotal role (Isomaa et al.; 2001; Sowers et al.; 2001; Williams, 1994).

Clinical progression of DN can be characterized into 5 phases: 1) hyperfiltration with renal hypertrophy, increased renal plasma flow and glomerular filtration; 2) normoalbuminuria with early renal parenchymal changes of basement membrane thickening and mesangial expansion; 3) microalbuminuria with early hypertension; 4) overt proteinuria; and 5) ESRD (Mogensen, 1976). These factors collectively result in cell injury and apoptosis of podocytes, and an accumulation of extracellular matrix proteins in the glomerulus and in the tubule interstitium (Calcutt et al.; 2009; D'Agati & Schmidt, 2010; Decleves & Sharma, 2010; Ruggenenti et al.; 2010). In this process, the increasing severity of DN is rapid when there is progression from normoalbuminuria to macroalbuminuria, a transition which takes about ten years.

Pathogenesis of DN is strongly related to uncontrolled or chronic hyperglycemia, and various mechanisms that lead to pathological changes in the kidney, proteinuria, and decline in renal function seen in DN have been proposed (Calcutt et al.; 2009; Decleves & Sharma, 2010). Hyperglycemia can lead to the activation of oxidative stress and increased production of reactive oxygen species (ROS), increased formation of advanced glycation endproducts (AGEs), activation of the proinflammatory transcription factor NF-κB, activation of protein kinase C (PKC), transforming growth factor-β (TGF-β), and the renin angiotensin system (RAS) (Calcutt et al.; 2009; D'Agati & Schmidt, 2010; Decleves & Sharma, 2010; Ruggenenti et al.; 2010).

Apart from its importance in the regulation of arterial BP, salt balance and cardiovascular homeostasis, RAS is also involved in the control of almost every organ system and cell function. Recent advances in cellular and molecular biology, as well as cardiovascular and renal physiology, have provided a larger understanding of RAS involvement in many physiologic and pathophysiologic mechanisms and attesting to its importance in regulating the internal environment is the fact that overactivity of RAS can lead to arterial hypertension, congestive heart failure, and renal insufficiency (Kobori et al.; 2007; Navar et al.; 2011a; Navar et al.; 2011b; Ferrario, 2011; Unger et al.; 1998).

The RAS in diabetes has been studied in detail, including an assessment of the various components of this pathway in the kidney (Ferrario et al.; 2004; Ferrario & Varagic, 2010; Navar et al.; 2011a; Wehbi et al.; 2001; Zipelmann et al.; 2000). The system has been strongly implicated in the pathophysiology of diabetic renal disease on the basis of its ability to promote tissue remodeling (proliferation, hypertrophy and differentiation) and extracellular matrix remodeling repair and/or fibrosis (Hayden et al.; 2011) and of the therapeutic ability of angiotensin I-converting enzyme inhibitors (ACEi) and AT1 receptor blockers (ARB) to decrease microalbuminuria and the progression of DN to ESRD (Brenner et al.; 2001; Chan et al.; 2000; Heart Outcomes Prevention Evaluation [HOPE] Study Investigators; Lewis et al.; 2001; Parving et al.; 2001). Furthermore, it has been postulated that in diabetes there is a role for the RAS in mediating many of the functional effects, such as changes in intraglomerular hemodynamics as well as structural changes in the diabetic kidney at both glomerular and tubulointerstitial levels (Gilbert et al.; 1998). Based on these findings, pharmacologic interventions that inhibit production of angiotensin II (Ang II) or block angiotensin type-1 receptors (AT1R) that target the RAS are considered a cornerstone in the treatment of hypertension in patients with DN (Van Buren & Toto, 2011).

2. Circulanting and tissue renin-angiotensin systems

The RAS is a coordinated hormonal cascade initiated through biosynthesis of angiotensinogen (AGT), produced in the liver, that is cleaved by renin released from renal juxtaglomerular cells of the afferent arteriole. By this enzymatic cleavage, angiotensin I (Ang I)

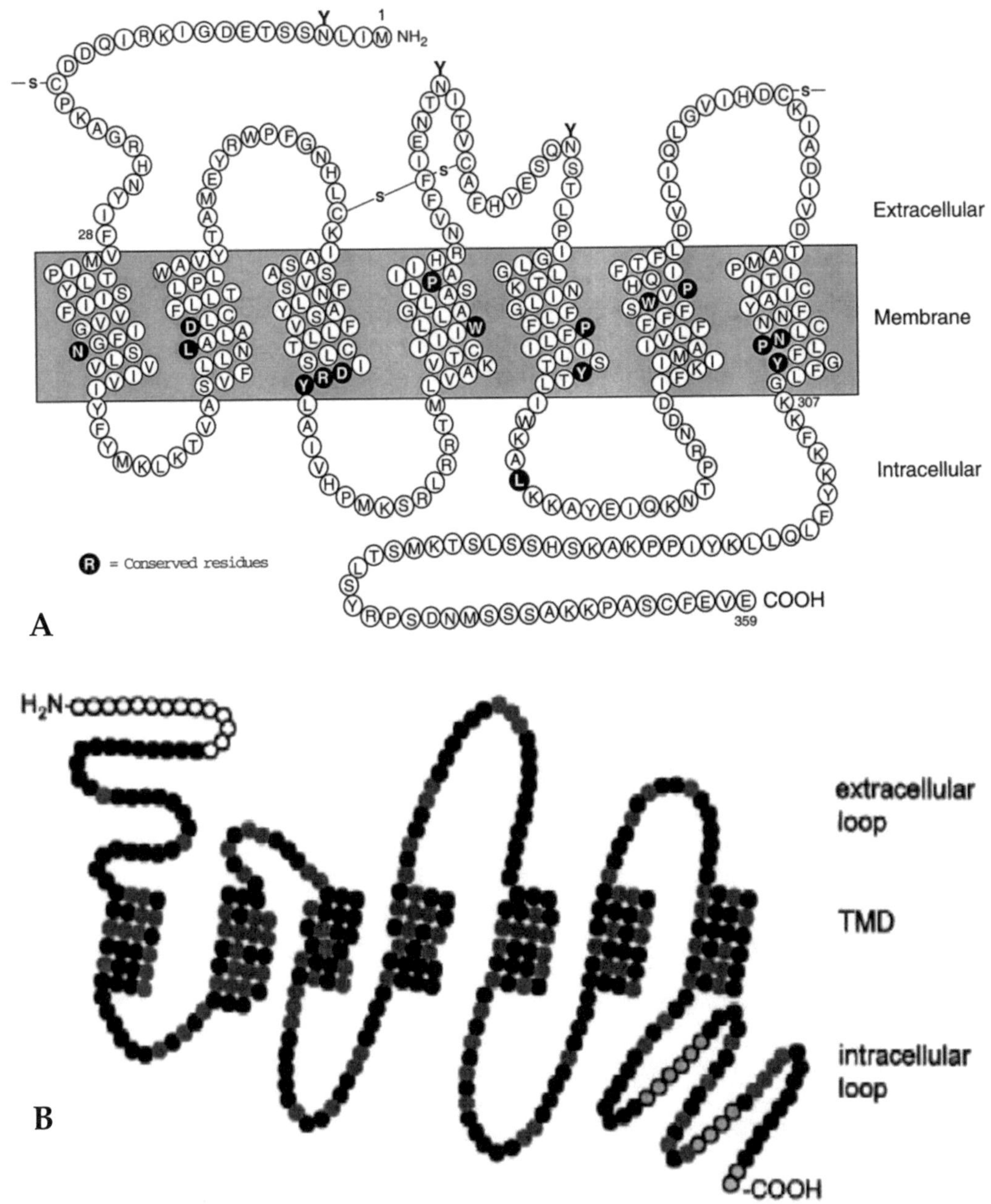

Fig. 1. (A) Secondary structure and consensus sequence of the mammalian angiotensin AT1 receptor. The amino acid residues that are highly conserved among G protein-coupled receptors are indicated in bold letters. The positions of the three extracellular carbohydrate chains, and of the two extracellular disulfide bonds, are also indicated (Adapted from de Gasparo et al.; 2000). (B) Comparison of the AT1 and AT2 receptors, sharing 33- 34% sequence homology. Grey circles indicate matching pairs of aminoacids. (TMD: transmembrane domain) (Adapted from de Gasparo & Siragy, 1999).

is generated, which, in turn is hydrolyzed by angiotensin I-converting enzyme (ACE) to produce Ang II. Over the last years, it has been established that most of the effects of Ang II are mediated through two distinct receptors, angiotensin type-1 receptors (AT1R) and angiotensin type-2 receptors (AT2R), acting antagonistically. AT2R shows only about 33-34% similarity to AT1R at the amino acid level (Figure 1A and 1B), which suggests that the two receptors derive from different ancestors (Mukoyama et al.; 1993; Kambayashi et al.; 1993; de Gasparo & Siragy, 1999; Unger & Sandmann, 2000; de Gasparo et al.; 2000).

Angiotensin actions via AT1R promotes vasoconstriction, inflammation, salt and water reabsorption and oxidative stress (Carey & Siragy, 2003). AT2R is generally associated with opposite actions to the AT1R, and it has already been shown that its activation induces bradykinin (BK) and nitric oxide formation, leading to natriuresis and vasodilatation. The AT2R is abundant in fetal tissue, decreasing after birth, with low amounts expressed in adult tissue such as kidney, adrenal and brain (Touys & Schiffrin, 2000; Carey & Padia, 2008; Rosivall, 2009) (Table 1A and 1B).

- Always expressed (Unger & Sandmann, 2000)
- Increased arterial pressure (Navar et al.; 2002)
- Aldosterone synthesis and secretion (Allen et al.; 2000; Navar et al.; 2002)
- Release of vasopressine (Unger & Sandmann, 2000)
- Decreased renal blood flow (Navar et al.; 2002)
- Renin secretion (Navar et al.; 2002)
- Cardiac contractility and hypertrophy (Allen et al.; 2000)
- Vascular smooth muscle cells proliferation (Touyz & Schiffrin, 2000)
- Mediates vasoconstriction, modulation of central sympathetic nervous system activity (Allen et al.; 2000; Unger & Sandmann, 2000)
- Mediates cell growth (Unger & Sandmann, 2000)
- Extracellular matrix formation (Touyz & Schiffrin, 2000)

Table 1A. Functions of AT1R

- Expressed during stress or injury (Unger & Sandmann, 2000)
- Fetal tissue development (Nakajima et al.; 1995; Stoll & Unger, 2001)
- Left ventricular hypertrophy (Senbonmatsu et al.; 2003)
- Mediates vasodilation (Unger & Sandmann, 2000)
- Neuronal regeneration (Stoll & Unger, 2001)
- Mediates cell differentiation (Unger & Sandmann, 2000)
- Inhibits cell growth (antiproliferation) (Unger & Sandmann, 2000)
- Cellular differentiation (Yamada et al.; 1999)
- Mediates tissue regeneration, apoptosis (Matsubara, 1998; Stoll & Unger, 2001; Unger & Sandmann, 2000)
- Modulation of extracellular matrix (Matsubara, 1998)

Table 1B. Functions of AT2R

The classical view of RAS cascade has been increasingly challenged with the discovery of new components such as the angiotensin converting enzyme 2 (ACE2). This enzyme with homology to ACE, is expressed in several tissues, including heart and kidney consistent with a role for this enzyme in renal and cardiovascular physiology (Burrell et al.; 2004; Crackower et al.; 2002; Danilczyk et al.; 2003; Donoghue et al.; 2000; Harmer et al.; 2002; Tipnis et al.; 2000). Both isoforms of ACE are type-I transmembrane glycoproteins with an extracellular amino-terminal ectodomain and short intracellular cytoplasmic tail (Figure 2). This membrane localization is ideally positioned it to hydrolyse peptides in the extracellular milieu.

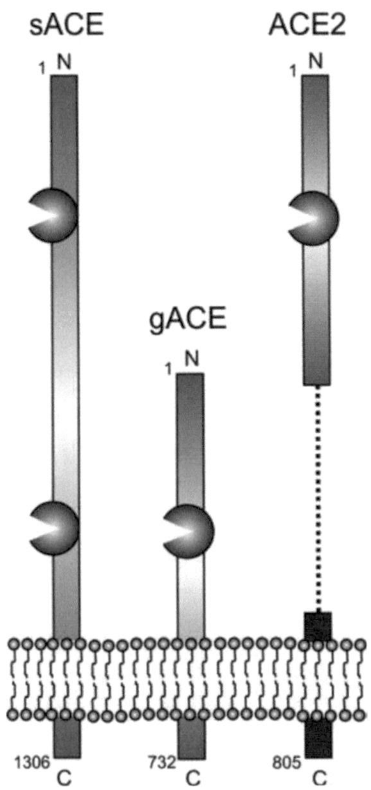

Fig. 2. Membrane topology and homology between ACE and ACE2. The ACE isoforms somatic ACE (sACE) and germinal ACE (gACE) and ACE2, are type I transmembrane proteins with an intracellular C-terminal domain and an extracellular N-terminal domain. In the case of the ACE isoforms and ACE2, the N-terminal extracellular domains contain HEMGH zinc-dependent catalytic domains (denoted as 'Pacman' symbols); two in ACE and one in both gACE and ACE2. Germinal ACE is entirely homologous to the C-terminal domain of sACE. ACE2 shares homology in its ectodomain with the N-terminal domain of sACE but has no homology with its C-terminal cytoplasmic domain (Adaptated from Lambert et al.; 2010).

ACE2 presents a single catalytic site and catalyzes the cleavage of Ang I to Ang 1-9, which can be further cleaved by ACE to Ang 1-7 (Burrell et al.; 2004; Donoghue et al.; 2000). Furthermore, Ang II can be converted directly by ACE2 to Ang 1-7. Ang 1-7 has been shown to exert vasodilatory properties and to antagonize the vasoconstriction mediated by Ang II, thereby contributing to the balance of vasodilators and vasoconstrictors generated by the various components of the RAS (Almeida et al.; 2000; Moriguchi et al.; 1995; Ferrario, 2006; Santos & Ferreira, 2007).

Another relevant change in our understanding of the classical endocrine RAS was the description of all components of the system in several tissues, including kidney, heart, brain, pancreas, adrenal, reproductive aparatus, retina, liver, gastrointestinal tract, lung and adipocytes, leading to the identification of new roles for angiotensins as paracrine and autocrine/intracrine function (Bataller et al.; 2003; Danser & Schalekamp, 1996; Lavoie & Sigmund, 2003; Navar et al.; 1994; Paul et al.; 2006; Ribeiro-Oliveira Jr et al.; 2008; Senanayake et al.; 2007; Tikellis et al.; 2003). RAS tissue appears to be regulated independently of the systemic one, and has been shown to contribute to a great number of homeostatic pathways, including cellular growth, vascular proliferation, extracellular formation and apoptosis (Paul et al.; 2006), via its specific receptors, such as AT1R, AT2R, prorenin/renin [(P)RR], Mas and also Ang III and IV receptors (Figure 3) (Nguyen et al. 2002; Santos et al.; 2003).

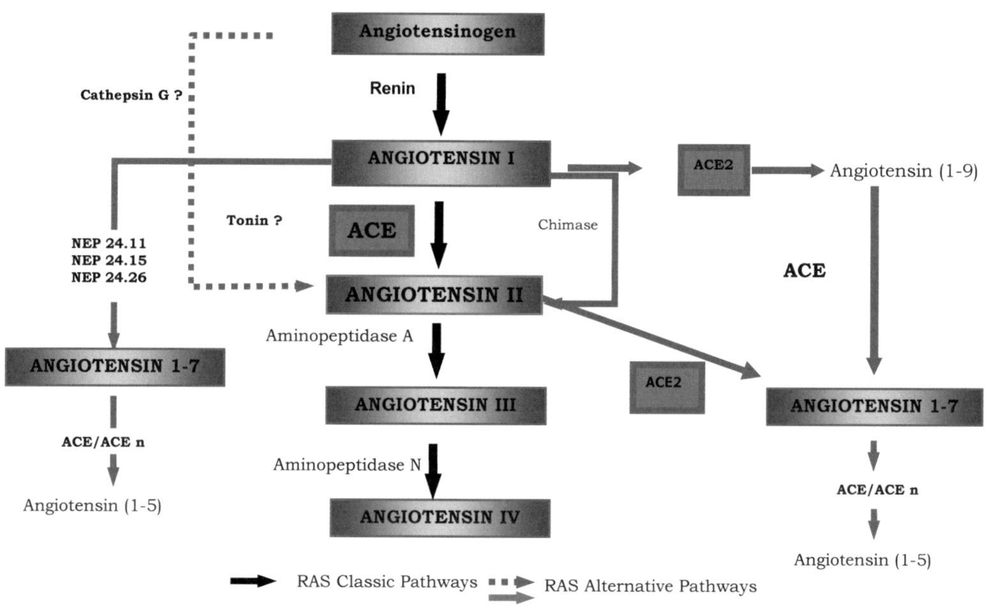

Fig. 3. Schematic representation of RAS. ACE, ACE 2, Neutral endopeptidase (NEP), N-domain ACE (ACEn).

3. The intrarenal RAS

3.1 Angiotensinogen

AGT is a glycoprotein produced in the liver, kidney, heart, vessels and adipose tissue, which circulates as an inactive protein. AGT is hydrolyzed by renin to generate Ang I, and both the peptide and renin are considered the rate-limiting steps in the formation of Ang II. Studies with mice harboring the gene for human AGT fused to the kidney-specific androgen regulated protein promoter demonstrated that AGT mRNA and the protein were localized in the proximal tubule cells, and urinary AGT was described as a product secreted by the proximal tubules and excreted in urine (Ding et al.; 1997; Kobori et al.; 2003). AGT synthesis is stimulated by inflammation, insulin, estrogen, glucorticoids (Kobori et al.; 2007; Prieto-Carrasquero et al.; 2004), and Kobori et al. (2001) described that Ang II can stimulate renal AGT mRNA and AGT protein synthesis, amplifying the activity of the intrarenal RAS (Kobori et al.; 2001).

3.2 Renin and prorenin

Renin is an aspartyl protease produced by the juxtaglomerular apparatus of the kidney. Its active form contains 339 amino acid residues after proteolytic cleavage at the N-terminus of prorenin, and in the circulation prorenin concentration is higher than that of renin. The activation of prorenin may occur by proteolytic or non proteolytic pathtways, both being able to generate Ang I from AGT. Circulating active renin and prorenin are originated mainly from the kidney, but other tissues are able to secrete both enzymes into the circulation, and therefore renin was also detected in urine suggesting its tubular formation, especially in the collecting duct (Prescott et al.; 2002; Prieto-Carrasquero et al.; 2004). As renin was also described in the collecting ducts, authors observed that Ang II is unable to inhibit renin secretion in this segment, the opposite to that which has been described in the juxtaglomerular apparatus (Kang et al.; 2008; Prieto-Carrasquero et al.; 2004; Rosivall, 2009).

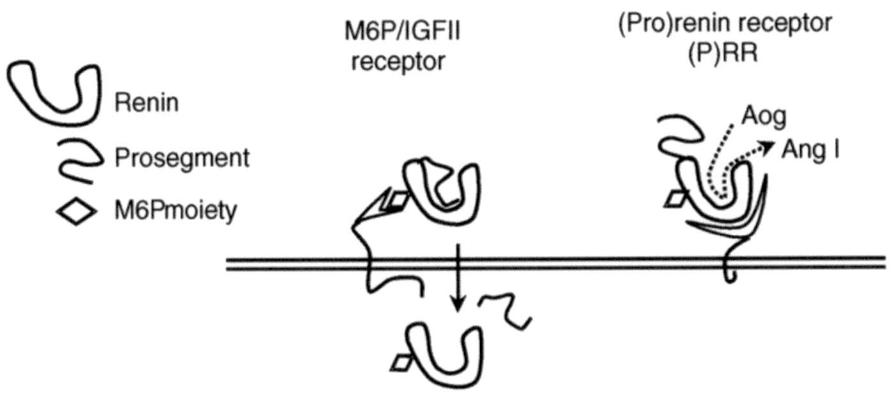

Binding of renin and prorenin:	*via* M6P residues	Specific, K_D nM
Angiotensin I generation:	Intracellular	Cell surface
Activation of prorenin:	Proteolytic	Non-proteolytic
Signalling:	No, Clearance receptor	MEK1/2, ERK1/2 P38, HSP70
Cellular effects:	None	Up-regulation of TGFβ, PAI1, collagens, fibronectin expression, Mesangial cells proliferation

Fig. 4. Principal characteristics of the two receptors for renin and prorenin, the mannose-6-phosphate receptor and the (pro)renin receptor ((P)RR) (Adapted from Nguyen & Contrepas, 2008).

The specific receptor for renin and for its inactive proenzyme form, prorenin, was cloned in 2002 and called (P)RR for (pro)renin receptor. The PRR gene is named ATP6ap2/PRR because a truncated form of (P)RR was previously described to coprecipitate with the vacuolar H+-proton adenosine triphosphatase (V-ATPase) (Nguyen et al.; 2002). The (P)RR is a single trans-membrane domain receptor that acts as co-factor for renin and prorenin by increasing their enzymatic activity on the cell-surface and mediating an intracellular signaling. It activates the mitogen activated protein kinases ERK1/2 cascade leading to cell proliferation and to up-regulation of profibrotic gene expression (Nguyen, 2011).

Two (P)RRs have been characterized to date, the functional receptor specific for renin and prorenin (Nguyen et al.; 2002) and the ubiquitous mannose-6-phosphate receptor (M6P-R) which is admitted to be a clearance receptor (Saris et al.; 2001) (Figure 4). It is known that the binding of renin with (P)RR increases its catalytic efficiency upon its substrate, a phenomena that may be implicated in target-organ lesion in the kidney and the development of DN (Ichihara et al.; 2006; Nguyen et al.; 2002). On the other hand, increases in prorenin concentration may decrease the (P)RR expression that can act as a negative feedback (Ichihara et al.; 2006; Nguyen et al.; 2002; Staessen et al.; 2006). Moreover, studies in genetically modified animals overexpressing (P)RR a role for (P)RR cardiovascular and renal pathologies since rats overexpressing (P)RR in vascular smooth-muscle cells develop high BP and those with an ubiquitous overexpression of (P)RR have glomerulosclerosis and proteinuria (Nguyen & Contrepas, 2008).

3.3 Angiotensin I-converting enzyme (ACE)

ACE is an ectoenzyme located in many vascular beds and also on cell surface of mesangial, proximal and collecting duct cells in the kidney and was described as a dipeptidyl carboxypeptidase (Camargo de Andrade et al.; 2006; Redublo Quinto et al.; 2008). It catalyzes the conversion of the decapeptide Ang I to the octapeptide Ang II, which is a potent vasoconstrictor, and in addition inactivates the vasodilator BK (Erdos, 1976).

The ACE gene encodes two enzymes: a somatic isozyme (150–180 kDa) and a germinal or testicular isozyme isozyme (90–100 kDa) identical to the C-terminal portion of endothelial ACE, only expressed in sperm (Hall, 2003; Lattion et al.; 1989). A soluble isoform of ACE, which is derived from the membrane bound isoform by the action of secretases, is also present in serum and other body fluids such as urine (Casarini et al.; 1995; Casarini et al.; 2001; Xiao et al.; 2004). ACE homologs have also been found in other animal species, including chimpanzee, cow, rabbit, mouse, chicken, goldfish, electric eel, house fly, mosquito, horn fly, silk worm, Drosophila melanogaster and Caenorhabditis elegans, and in the bacteria Xanthomonas spp. and Shewanella oneidensis (Corvol & Williams, 1998; Riordan, 2003). The cDNA of one form of D. melanogaster ACE (termed AnCE) encodes a protein of 615 amino acids that have a high degree of similarity to both domains of human sACE, indicating that the D. melanogaster protein is a single-domain enzyme (Williams et al.; 1996; Riordan, 2003) (Figure 5A). It contains a signal peptide but no carboxy-terminal membrane-anchoring hydrophobic sequence. A second ACE-related gene product, termed Acer, has also been identified in D. melanogaster. Selective inhibition by phosphinic peptides (containing -PO2-CH2- links instead of -CO-NH- links) indicates that Acer has active site features characteristic of the N - domain of sACE (Riordan, 2003).

ACE presents two distinct catalytic domains, called N- and C-terminus (Wei et al.; 1991) (Figure 5 A and B), and both sites hydrolyze Ang I. However, the N-domain has two specific physiological substratum, Ang 1-7 and N-acetyl-Seryl-Aspartyl-Lysyl-Proline, a hematopoietic peptide (Jaspard et al.; 1993; Rousseau et al.; 1995). ACE is distributed along human and rat kidney, and has already been described in glomeruli, mesangial cells and also in proximal and collecting duct cells (Camargo de Andrade et al.; 2006; Redublo Quinto et al.; 2008). Casarini et al. (1995 and 2001) observed two N-domain ACE isoforms (nACE)

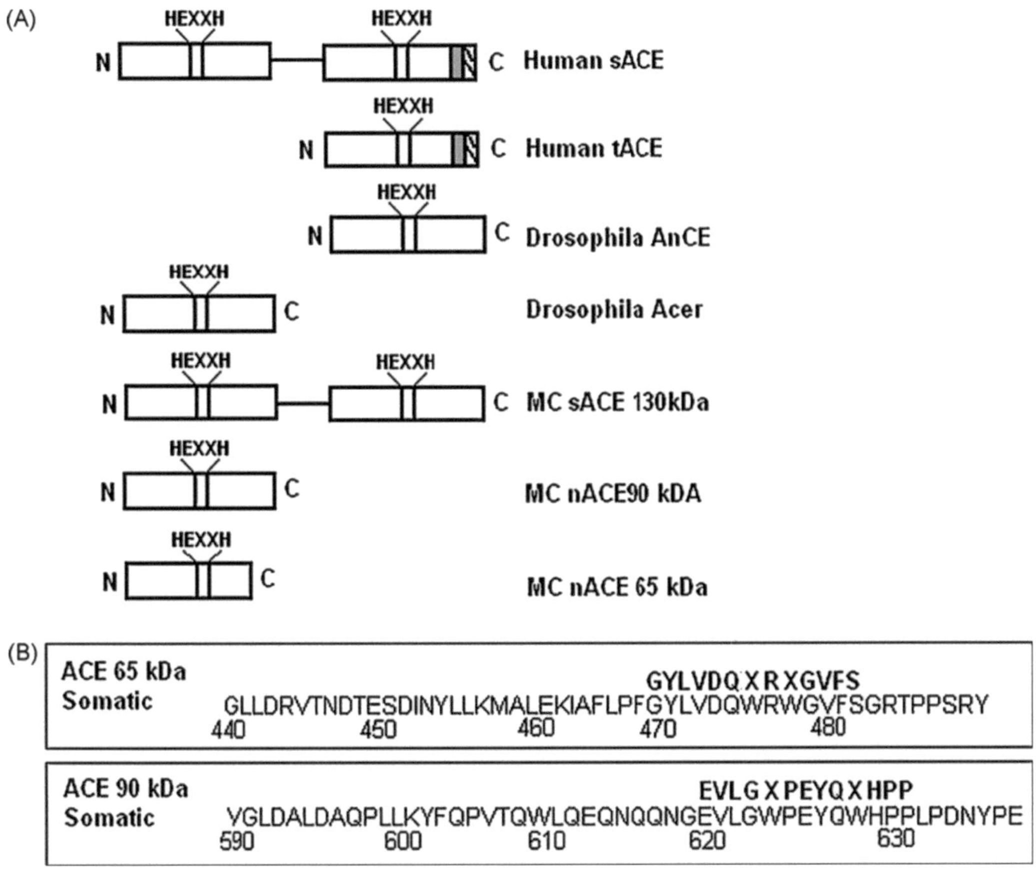

Fig. 5. Schematic representation of primary structure of several members of the ACE protein family. (A) Location of the active-site-zinc-binding motifs are indicated by HEXXH; transmembrane domains are in black. The sequence of testicular ACE (tACE) is identical to that of the C-domain of the sACE, except for its first 36 amino acids. Human tACE and sACE have the same carboxyl-terminal transmembrane and cytosolic sequence. Drosophila ACEs, cDNA of one form of D. melanogaster ACE (termed AnCE) and a second ACE-related gene product (termed Acer) lack a membrane-anchoring sequence. Dimensions are not to scale. N, amino terminus; C, carboxyl terminus (Adapted from Riordan, 2003). (B) The C-terminal alignment of 65 kDa nACE with rat ACE ended at Ser482. The same analysis for 90 kDa nACE evidenciated that the enzyme finished at Pro629 amino acid after their alignment with rat ACE. Both structures are similar for urine, tissue and mesangial cells (Adapted from de Andrade et al.; 2010).

with molecular weight of 190 and 65 kDa in the urine of healthy subjects, and two isoforms of 90 and 65 kDa, both nACE, in the urine of hypertensive patients (Casarini et al.; 1995, 2001). The same nACE enzymes were obtained by Marques et al. (2003) in the urine of Wistar-Kyoto and Spontaneously Hypertensive rats (SHR), and by Ronchi et al. (2005) in different tissues of SHR, suggesting that the 90/80 kDa ACE could be a possible biological marker of hypertension (Marques et al.; 2003; Ronchi et al.; 2005). Moreover, Deddish et al. (1994) described an active soluble form of nACE in human ileal fluid, with a molecular mass of 108 kDa, thereby differing from the enzymes described in human urine (Deddish et al.; 1994).

Apart from the classic actions of ACE, several groups have recently demonstrated that ACE presents novel actions, mainly related to cell signaling. As demonstrated by Kolstedt et al (2004), ACE also functions as a signal transduction molecule and binding of ACE substrates or inhibitors to the enzyme initiates a cascade of events, including the phosphorylation of its Ser1270 residue, increasing ACE and COX2 synthesis. Moreover, using *in vitro* models such as Chinese hamster ovary and melanoma cells, it was demonstrated that Ang II can also interact with ACE evoking calcium signaling and promoting an increase in the generation of ROS (Guimaraes et al.; 2011; Kohlstedt et al.; 2004).

3.4 ACE2

ACE2 is a new member of RAS, homologue of ACE, which acts as a monocarboxipeptidase. The enzyme consists of 805 amino acids and is a type I transmembrane glycoprotein with a single extracellular catalytic domain (Donoghue et al.; 2000; Tipnis et al.; 2000). Unlike somatic ACE, ACE2 removes a single C-terminal Leu residue from Ang I to generate Ang 1-9, a peptide with unknown function. Although ACE2 was described originally for its ability to generate Ang 1-9 from Ang I (Donoghue et al.; 2000), it also degrades Ang II to the biologically active peptide Ang 1-7 (Burrell L et al, ,2004; Vickers et al.; 2002). *In vitro* studies showed that the catalytic efficiency of ACE2 for Ang II is 400-fold greater than for Ang I (Vickers et al.; 2002), indicating that the major role for ACE2 is the convertion of Ang II to Ang 1-7.

The human ACE2 gene has been cloned and mapped to the X chromosome (Crackower et al.; 2002). This enzyme exists as a membrane-bound protein in the lungs, stomach, spleen, intestine, bone-marrow, kidney, liver, brain (Gembardt et al.; 2005) and the heart and is not inhibited by ACE inhibitors (Ribeiro-Oliveira Jr et al.; 2008). ACE2 is abundantly expressed in renal epithelial cells including proximal tubular cells (Danilczyk & Penninger, 2006; Donoghue et al.; 2000; Shaltout, et al.; 2007), and in the pancreas, ACE2 was found to be localized to acini and islets following a similar distribution to that of ACE (Tikellis et al.; 2004).

Several studies support a counter-regulatory role for Ang 1-7 by opposing many AT1R-mediated actions, especially regarding vasoconstriction and cellular proliferation (Ferrario, 2006, Santos et al.; 2005). Thus, Ang 1-7 has become a key component of the RAS system due to its beneficial effects in the cardiovascular system. Although the pathophysiological significance of ACE2 in renal injury remains to be established, emerging evidence suggests that ACE2 deficiency leads to increases in intrarenal Ang II levels (Ribeiro Oliveira Jr et al.; 2008; Ferrario, 2006; Oudit et al.; 2010; Wolf & Ritz, 2005; Ye et al.; 2006). Thus, recently ACE2 has also been proposed as an acute biomarker of renal disease, considering that upregulation of ACE2, and the subsequent increase in Ang 1-7 levels, may be a compensatory response to protect against tissue injury. In fact, in response to chronic injury, ACE2 protein levels are significantly downregulated in the kidneys of hypertensive (Crackower et al.; 2002), diabetic (Tikellis et al.; 2003) and pregnant rats (Brosnihan et al.; 2004; Brosnihan et al.; 2003) suggesting the potential role of the enzyme as a kidney disease biomarker.

3.5 Angiotensins and receptors

BP is modulated by changes in plasma concentrations of Ang II, due to an increase in total peripheral resistance to maintain arterial BP in face of an acute hypontesive modification as blood loss and/or vasodilation. Ang II causes a slow pressor response to stabilize the arterial BP mediated by a renal response, through mechanisms that include a direct effect to increase sodium reabsortion in proximal tubules, release of aldosterone from adrenal and altered renal hemodynamics (Carey et al.; 2000), including increased capillary glomerular pressure, hyperfiltration and proteinuria (Navar & Harrison-Bernard, 2000). Ang II also has important effects on cardiovascular system, stimulating migration, proliferation, hypertrophy, increased production of growth factors and extracellular matrix proteins such as collagen, fibronectin (Carey et al.; 2000).

Angiotensins have their actions exerted through AT1R and AT2R interaction, and Ang II, but not Ang I, has affinity to both of them. The actions of AT1R include vasoconstriction, aldosterone secretion, tubular sodium retention, release of vasopressin, increased sympathetic nervous activity and increased thirst. In the long term, actions of AT1R also include cell growth, organ hypertrophy, inflammation, remodeling and erythropoietic stimulation. On the other hand, AT2R mediates effects that are opposed to the actions of AT1R, and it has already been shown that AT2R is upregulated in response to tissue injury, suggesting its important role in the pathophysiology of several diseases (Hunyady & Catt, 2006).

Several studies demonstrated AT1R and AT2R expression in renal tissue, and their role in the development of renal disease. A study with SHR after 32 weeks of STZ-induced DM, suggested that hypertension, increased albuminuria and renal injury were resulted from the reduction of expression of enconding genes for AT1R, and treatment with ibersatan prevented the down regulation of the AT1R receptor, with no effect on AT2R expression (Bonnet et al.; 2002). Moreover, Velloso et al. (2006) also demonstrated an interaction between RAS and the insulin signaling pathways, through AT1R as a result of treatment with ARB (Velloso et al.; 2006).

Changes in the population of renal ATR can be involved in DN. Diabetes reduced gene and protein expression of AT1R but not AT2R in the kidneys of SHR rats, without changes in Wistar-Kyoto (WKY) strain. This reduction is supposed to be a protective mechanism against the intrarenal RAS activation by diabetes, and this effect was cancelled by the ARB ibersatan (Bonnet et al., 2002). Also, the cross-talk between AT1R and insulin receptor signaling pathways is related to the association between diabetes and hypertension, and may contribute to tissue damage (Velloso et al. 2006) induced by these pathologies.

4. RAS and diabetes

The activation of renal RAS, and the subsequent generation of Ang II, is the primary etiologic event in the development of hypertension in people with DM. Subsequently, the increase of Ang II is responsible for the development of DN, a major cause of ESRD, via several hemodynamic, tubular and growth-promoting actions, as evidenced by the fact that blockade of this system has a beneficial effect on the kidney (Lewis et al.; 1993, 2001).

RAS inhibition is important to prevent renal and cardiovascular complications of both DM1 and DM2, through mechanisms that include improvement in endothelial fuction (Mukai et al.; 2002), decrease in inflammatory response (Mervaala et al.; 1999), increase in BK and Ang 1-7 levels (Maia et al.; 2004). The initial studies with RAS inhibition in people with DN demonstrated that there was an effect beyond BP lowering. When compared with conventional antihypertensive therapy, those who received RAS blockade consistently had greater improvement in DN despite presenting similar BP control, through effects of RAS blockade on insulin resistance and glucose homeostasis (Gillespie et al.; 2005; Lewis et al.; 1993; Ravid et al.; 1998). Thus, it was suggested a role for ACE in mediating renal injury by increasing local Ang II formation, prevented by both ACEi and ARB in the kidney. ACEi reduce the production of Ang II, and decrease degradation of endothelial BK, resulting in vasodilatation by stimulating nitric oxide and prostacyclin production and BP reduction. Moreover, ACEi have been shown to decrease the rate of progression of diabetic and non-diabetic nephropathies, and improve insulin sensitivity, allowing better insulin action in patients with DM2 (Lewis et al.; 1993; Yusuf et al.; 2000). On the other hand, ARB have also been shown to decrease the risk of stroke in patients with hypertension and reduce the rate of progression of DN (Lewis et al.; 1993). ABR prevent the binding of Ang II to AT1R, leading to accumulation of Ang II, which in turn is converted to Ang 1-7 and increases the levels of this vasodilator peptide (Barra et al.; 2009; Ferrari, 2005; Maia et al.; 2004).

Several studies have demonstrated that activity of circulating (systemic) RAS is normal or suppressed in DM, as reflected by measurements of plasma renin activity and Ang II concentrations, while local renal tissue RAS (tRAS) has already been shown to be activated on cell culture, in response to high glucose exposure, and also on spontaneously or induced diabetic animals (Carey & Siragy.; 2003b).

During the activation of tRAS in DM, Ang II activates NADPH oxidase enzyme which contributes to the generation of ROS. This process may result from over production of precursors to reactive oxygen radicals and or decreased efficiency of inhibitory and scavenger systems. In DM, the additional AT1R activation results in a vicious cycle of ROS production which contributes to organ damage (Hayden et al.; 2011). The mechanisms that contribute to increased oxidative stress in diabetes may include not only increased non enzymatic glycosylation (glycation) and autoxidative glycosylation (Baynes, 1991), but it is also related to several abnormalities, including hyperglycemia, insulin resistance, hyperinsulinemia and dyslipidemia, each of which contributes to mitochondrial superoxide overproduction in endothelial cells in large and small vessels as well as the myocardium.

The pathophysiological mechanism that underlies diabetic complications could be explained by increased production of ROS via the polyol pathway flux, increased formation of advanced glycation end products, increased expression of the receptor for AGEs, activation of protein kinase C isoforms and overactivity of the hexosamine pathway. Furthermore, the effects of oxidative stress in individuals with DM2 are compounded by the inactivation of two critical anti-atherosclerotic enzymes: endothelial nitric oxide synthase and prostacyclin synthase (Folli et al.; 2011).

Increased AGT expression, in response to high glucose exposure, was also described to be involved in the development of DN, *in vitro* (Hsieh et al, 2003) and *in vivo.* Using an *in vitro* model, Vidotti et al. (2004) demonstrated that high glucose exposure increased Ang II generation, decreased prorenin secretion and induced an increase in intracellular renin activity of mesangial cells. In response to 72h of high glucose exposure, there was an increase in mRNA levels for AGT and ACE, while 24h of the stimulus increased mRNA levels of ACE, prorenin and cathepsin B. In this study, increased generation of Ang II, induced by high glucose exposure, was shown to be dependent on at least three factors: a time-dependent stimulation of (pro)renin gene transcription, a reduction in prorenin enzyme secretion, and an increased rate of conversion of prorenin to active renin, probably mediated by cathepsin B. Moreover, the consistent upregulation of ACE mRNA suggests that, along with renin, ACE is directly involved in the increased mesangial Ang II generation induced by high glucose (Vidotti et al.; 2004).

In the kidney of streptozotocin (STZ)-induced diabetic animals, an increase in intrarenal AGT mRNA is attributed to the proximal tubule, and it seems to be mediated by glucose response element located in the AGT promoter (Zimpelman et al.; 2000). Studies with Zucker obese rat, a model of DM2 with nephropathy and hypertension, is also associated with increased activation of RAS, as demonstrated by an increase in intrarenal Ang II generation, which was prevented by treatment with ACEi (Sharma et al.; 2006). Using Non-obese diabetic model (NOD) (Makino et al.; 1980), our group demonstrated that diabetes onset increases ACE activity and expression and decreases ACE2 expression in kidney, suggesting that the higher renal ACE/ACE2 ratio may contribute to renal injury leading to overt nephropathy (Colucci et al.; 2011).

Ronchi et al. (2007) studied the association between sACE with 136 kDa and nACE with 69 kDa from Wistar (W) rat tissue with DM. The authors analysed three groups: control (CT), insulin treated diabetic (DT) and untreated (D). In D group, urine ACE activity increased for both substrates, Hippuryl-His-Leu and Z-Phe-His-Leu, that distinguished nACE from somatic ACE when compared with CT and DT, despite the decreased activity in renal tissues. Immunostaining of renal tissue demonstrated that ACE is more strongly expressed in the proximal tubule of D than in the same nephron portion in the other groups. Ang I increased in the renal tissue of D and DT groups, but Ang II levels decreased in the D and DT groups when compared to the control. Ang 1-7 was detected in all studied groups with low levels in DT. These findings indicate that Ang I increase and Ang II decrease, as a result of renin and NEP simultaneous activation, increasing Ang 1-7. Since Ang 1-7 can counterbalance Ang II effects, this modulation of angiotensin peptides has a protective role against renal damage in DM (Ronchi et al., 2007).

Few studies were described using animal models with genetic alterations in the RAS in DN. Studies have suggested associations between incidence of DN and a variety of genetic polymorphisms. An association was identified between nephropathy in DM1 and the D allele of an insertion/deletion (I/D) polymorphism in intron 16 of ACE gene. Huang et al.; (2001) described that the induction of diabetes by SZT was not affected by ACE gene copy number. The authors compared the changes with the time of BP of one, two and three-copy mice with the pressures of untreated controls. The BPs of untreated mice were not affected by ACE gene copy, however the BP of the three-copy diabetic mice with genetically higher ACE activity increased with time, and 12 weeks after induction of diabetes were 10-20 mmHg higher than the BPs of the one and two copy diabetic mice (Huang et al.; 2001).

Regarding ACE2, differences in renal enzyme levels have been detected in hypertensive humans when compared with controls (Van Buren & Toto, 2011). Wong et al. (2002) have shown that pharmacological inhibition of ACE2 and genetic ablation in different rodent of models of diabetes, increased albuminuria and glomerular lesions. Furthermore, animals with STZ-induced DN have decreased renal expression of ACE2 (Tikellis et al.; 2003). In humans, biopsies from patients with DN showed a decrease in glomerular expression of ACE2, suggesting that a therapy increasing the activity of this enzyme can help in the future in the treatment of diabetic kidney disease (Wong et al.; 2007).

Aldosterone has been implicated in DM complications. Sato et al (2003) in a study in patients with DM2 described that patients with aldosterone escape of 40% have higher albumin excretion than those without. Treating these patients with spironolactone associated to ACEi, the authors detected reduction in urinary albumin excretion over a 24-week period. They conclude that RAS activation in DN could be related to an aldosterone-mediated increase in disease progression. (Sato et al.; 2003).

5. Conclusion

We reviewed the physiology of the RAS in DM and hypertension, highlighting the importance of this system in diabetic nephropathy. The RAS is up or down regulated in the kidney and Table 2 summarizes the role of components of the RAS in diabetic nephropathy. Figure 6 presents our understanding of the intrarenal RAS in diabetic nephropathy. Increased Ang II is responsible for both intrarenal insulin resistence and renal injury, as well as, decrease AT2R expression might contribute to accelerated renal injury (Carey and Siragy, 2003b). In addition to controling blood pressure, we evidenciated the importance of ACEi and ARB in protecting the kidney against injury. The newly discovered components of RAS, such as renin receptor, ACE2, Ang IV and also aliskeren, the renin inhibitor, represent that

Description	References
RAS up regulation	
• Renal Ang II increase	Lewis et al., 1993, 2001; Zimpelman et al., 2000
• AT1R activation - organ damage	
• Increased AGT expression – diabetic nephropathy	Hayden et al.., 2011. Hsieh et al, 2003.
• Increased mRNA levels of ACE, prorenin and cathepsin B.	Vidotti et al., 2004.
• Ang I increase and renin/neutral endopeptidase activation	Ronchi et al., 2007.
RAS down regulation	
• ACE inhibition – increase in BK and Ang 1-7, control of blood pressure	Maia et al., 2004.
• ACE inhibition, improve insulin sensitivity	Lewis et al., 1993; Yusuf et al., 2000.
• ACE2 decrease	Colucci et al., 2011; Wong et al., 2007
• ACE2 inhibition - increased albuminuria and glomerular lesions	Wong et al.,2002.

Table 2. RAS is up- or down-regulated in diabetic kidneys

research is open in this field. New pathways and signaling compounds can be discovered explaining the modulation of the RAS resulting in expression of other genes.

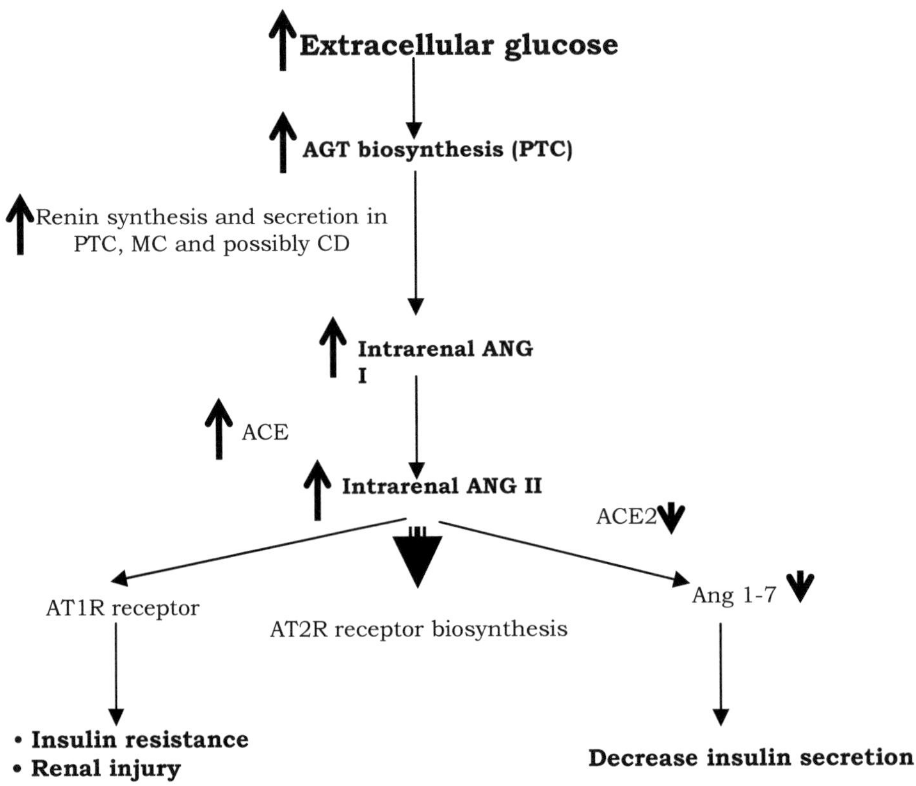

Fig. 6. Pathways through which the intrarenal renin–angiotensin system contributes to diabetic nephropathy based on current evidence. Solid arrows represents biochemical pathways or ligand–receptor interactions. The broken arrow indicates decreased ligand–receptor interaction owing to decreased AT2R synthesis. Abbreviations: ACE, angiotensin-converting enzyme; ACE2, angiotensin-converting enzyme2; AGT, angiotensinogen; ANG, angiotensin; AT1R, angiotensin II receptor; AT2R angiotensin II receptor; MC, glomerular mesangial cell; PTC, proximal tubule cell. Adapted from Carey and Siragy, 2003b.

6. References

Allen, A.M.; Zhuo, J.; Mendelsohn, F.A. (2000). Localization and function of angiotensin AT1 receptors. *American Journal of Hypertension*, Vol. 13, No. (1 Pt 2), (January 2000), pp. 31S-38S, ISSN 0895-7061.

Almeida, A.P.; Frabregas, B.C.; Madureira, M.M.; Santos, R.J.; Campagnole-Santos, M.J. & Santos, R.A. (2000). Angiotensin-(1-7) potentiates the coronary vasodilatatory effect of bradykinin in the isolated rat heart. *Brazilian Journal of Medical and Biological Research*, Vol.33, No.6, pp. 709-13, ISSN 0100-879X.

Astrup, A. & Finer, N. (2000). Redefining type 2 diabetes: 'diabesity' or 'obesity dependent diabetes mellitus'?. *Obesity Reviews,* Vol.1, No.2, (October 2000), pp. 57–59, ISSN 1467-7881.

Barra, S.; Vitagliano, A.; Cuomo, V.; Vitagliano, G. & Gaeta, G. (2009). Vascular and metabolic effects of angiotensin II receptor blockers. *Expert Opinion on Pharmacotherapy,* Vol.10, No.2, (February 2009), pp. 173-189, ISSN 1465-6566.

Bataller, R.; Sancho-bru, P.; Ginés, P.; Lora, J.M.; Al-garawi, A.; Solé, M.; Colmenero, J.; Nicolás, J.M.; Jiménez, W.; Wich, N.; Gutiérrez-Ramos, J.; Arroyo, V. & Rodés, J. (2003). Activated human hepatic stellate cells express the renin angiotensin system and synthetize angiotensin II. *Gastroenterology,* Vol.25, (July 2003), pp. 117-125, 2003, ISSN 0016-5085.

Baynes, J.W. (1991). Role of oxidative stress in development of complications in diabetes. *Diabetes,* Vol.40, No.4, (April 1991), pp. 405–412, ISSN 0012-1797.

Bonnet, F.; Candido, R.; Carey, R.M.; Casley, D.; Russo, L.M.; Osicka, T.M.; Cooper, M.E. & Cao, Z. (2002). Renal expression of angiotensin receptors in long-term diabetes and the effects of angiotensin type 1 receptor blockade. *Journal of Hypertension* Vol.20, No.8, (August 2002), pp. 1615-1624, ISSN 0263-6352.

Brenner, B.M.; Cooper, M.E.; de Zeeuw, D.; Keane, W.F.; Mitch, W.E.; Parving, H.H,, Remuzzi, G.; Snapinn, S.M.; Zhang, Z.; Shahinfar, S.& RENAAL Study Investigators. (2001). Effects of losartan on renal and cardiovascular outcomes in patients with type 2 diabetes mellitus and nephropathy. *The New England Journal of Medicine,* Vol. 345, No.12, (September 2001), pp. 861–869, ISSN 0028-4793

Brosnihan, K.B.; Neves, L.A.; Anton, L.; Joyner, J.; Valdes, G .& Merrill, D.C. (2004) Enhanced expression of Ang-(1-7) during pregnancy. *Brazilian Journal of Medical and Biological Research,* Vol.37, No.8, (August 2004), pp. 1255-1262, ISSN0100-879X.

Brosnihan, K.B.; Neves, L.A.; Joyner, J. Averill, D.B.; Chappell, M.C.; Sarao, R.; Penninger, J. & Ferrario, C.M. (2003). Enhanced renal immunocytochemical expression of ANG-(1-7) and ACE2 during pregnancy. *Hypertension,* Vol42, No.4, (October 2003), pp. 749-53), ISSN 0194-911X.

Burrell, L.M.; Johnston, C.I.; Tikellis, C. & Cooper, M.E. (2004). ACE2, a new regulator of the renin-angiotensin system. *Trends in Endocrinology and Metabolism,* Vol.15, No.4, (May-June 2004), pp. 166-169, ISSN 1043-2760.

Calcutt, N.A.; Cooper, M.E.; Kern, T.S. & Schmidt, A.M. (2009). Therapies for hyperglycaemia-induced diabetic complications: from animal models to clinical trials. *Nature Reviews Drug Discovery,* Vol.8, No.5, (May 2009), pp. :417-429. ISSN 1474-1776.

Camargo de Andrade, M.C.; Di Marco, G.S.; de Paulo Castro Teixeira, V.; Mortara, R. Sabatini, R.A.; Pesquero, J.B.; Boim, M.A.; Carmona, A.K.; Schor, N. & Casarini, D.E. (2006). Expression and localization of N-domain ANG I-converting enzymes in mesangial cells in culture from spontaneously hypertensive rats. *American Journal of Physiology. Renal Physiology,* Vol.290, No.2, (February 2006), pp. F364–F375, ISSN 1931-857X.

Carey, R.M. & Padia, S.H. (2008). Angiotensin AT2 receptors: control of renal sodium excretion and blood pressure. *Trends in Endocrinology and Metabolism.* Vol.19, No.3, (April 2008), pp. 84-87, ISSN 1043-2760.

Carey, R.M. & Siragy, H.M. (2003a). Newly recognized components of the renin-angiotensin system: potential roles in cardiovascular and renal regulation. *Endocrine Reviews*, Vol.24, No.3 (June 2003a), pp. 261–271, ISSN 0163-769X.

Carey, R.M. & Siragy, H.M. (2003b). The intrarenal rennin-angiotensin system and diabetic nephropathy. *Trends in Endocrinology and Metabolism*, Vol.14, No.6, (August 2003b), pp. 274-281, ISSN 1043-2760.

Carey, R.M.; Wang, Z.Q. & Siragy, H.M. (2000). Role of angiotensin type 2 receptor in the regulation of blood pressure and renal function. *Hypertension*, Vol.35, No.1 (Pt 2) , (January 2000), pp. 155-116, ISSN 0194-911X.

Casarini, D.E.; Carmona, A.K.; Plavnik, F.L.; Zanella, M.T.; Juliano, L. & Ribeiro, A.B. (1995). Calcium channel blockers as inhibitors of angiotensin I-converting enzyme. *Hypertension*, Vol.26, No.6(Pt 2), (Dcember 1995), pp. 1145-1148, ISSN 0194-911X.

Casarini, D.E.; Plavinik, F.L.; Zanella, M.T.; Marson, O.; Krieger, J.E.; Hirata, I.Y. & Stella, R.C. (2001). Angiotensin converting enzymes from human urine of mild hypertensive untreated patients resemble the N-terminal fragment of human angiotensin I-converting enzyme. *International Journal of Biochemistry and Cell Biology*, Vol.33, No.1, (January 2001), pp. 75-85, ISSN 1357-2725.

Chan, J.C.; Ko, G.T.; Leung, D.H.; Cheung, R.C.; Cheung, M.Y.; So, W.; Swaminathan, R.; Nicholls, M.G.; Critchley, J.A. & Cockram, C.S. (2000). Long-term effects of angiotensin-converting enzyme inhibition and metabolic control in hypertensive type 2 diabetic patients. *Kidney International*, Vol.57, No.2, (February 2000), pp. 590-600, ISSN 0085-2538.

Choudhury, D.; Tuncel, M. & Levi, M. (2010). Diabetic nephropathy -- a multifaceted target of new therapies. *Discovery Medicine*, (November 2010), Vol.10, No.54, pp. 406-415, ISSN 1539-6509.

Colucci J.A.; Arita D.Y.; Cunha T.S.; Di Marco G.S.; Vio C.P.; Silva Filho A.P. & Casarini D.E. (2011). Renin-angiotensin system may trigger kidney damage in NOD mice. *Journal of Renin-Angiotensin-Aldosterone System*, Vol.12, No.1, (March 2011), pp. 15-22, ISSN 1470-3203.

Cooper, M.E. & Johnston, C.I. (2000). Optimizing treatment of hypertension in patients with diabetes. *Journal of the American Medical Association*, Vol.283, No.24, (June 2000), pp. 3177–3179, ISSN 0098-7484.

Cooper, M.E. (1998). Pathogenesis, prevention, and treatment of diabetic nephropathy. *The Lancet*, Vol.352, No.9123, (July 1998), pp. 213-219, ISSN 0140-6736.

Corvol, P.; Williams, T.A. (1998). Peptidyl-dipeptidase A/angiotensin 1-converting enzyme. In: Handbook of Proteolytic Enzymes. A.J. Barrett, N.D. Rawlings, J.F Woessner (Ed.), 1066-1076, Academic Press, ISBN 978-0-12-079610-6, San Diego, CA, USA.

Crackower, M.A.; Sarao, R.; Oudi,t G.Y.; Yagil, C.; Kozieradzki, I.; Scanga, S.E.; Oliveira-dos-Santos, A.J.; da Costa, J.; Zhang, L.; Pei, Y.; Scholey, J.; Ferrario, C.M.; Manoukian, A.S.; Chappell, M.C.; Backx, P.H.;Yagil,Y. & Penninger JM.. (2002). Angiotensin-converting enzyme 2 is an essential regulator of heart function. *Nature*, Vol.417, No.6891, pp. 822-8, ISSN 0028-0836.

D'Agati, V. & Schmidt, A.M. (2010). RAGE and the pathogenesis of chronic kidney disease. *Nature Review Nephrology*, Vol.6, No.6, (Jun 2010), pp. 352-360, ISSN 1759-5061.

Dalla Vestra, M.; Saller, A.; Bortoloso, E.; Mauer, M. & Fioretto, P. (2000). Structural involvement in type 1 and type 2 diabetic nephropathy. *Diabetes & Metabolism*, Vol.26 (Suppl 4), (July 2000), pp. 8-14, ISSN 1262-3636.

Danilczyk, U. & Penninger, J.M. (2006). Angiotensin-converting enzyme II in the heart and the kidney. *Circulation Research*, Vol.98, No.98, (March 2006), pp. 463-471, ISSN 0009-7330.

Danilczyk, U.; Eriksson, U.; Crackower, MA. & Penninger, JM. (2003). A story of two ACEs. *Journal of Molecular Medicine*, Vol.81, No.4, (April 2003), pp. 227-34, ISSN 0946-2716.

Danser, A.H.J & Schalekamp, M.A.D.H. (1996). Is there an internal cardiac rennin-angiotensin system? *Heart*, Vol.76, No.3 (suppl 3), (November 1996), pp. 28-32, ISSN 1355-6037.

De Andrade, M.C.; Affonso, R.; Fernandes, F.B.; Febba, A.C.; da Silva, I.D.; Stella, R.C.; Marson, O.; Jubilut, G.N.; Hirata, I.Y.; Carmona, A.K.; Corradi, H.; Acharya, K.R.; Sturrock, E.D.; Casarini, D.E. (2010). Spectroscopic and structural analysis of somatic and N-domain angiotensin I-converting enzyme isoforms from mesangial cells from Wistar and spontaneously hypertensive rats. International Journal of Biological Macromolecules, Vol. 47, No. 2, (August 2010), pp. 238-43, ISSN 0141-8130.

De Gasparo, M. ; Catt, K.J. ; Inagami, T., Wright, J.W. ; Unger, T. (2000). International union of pharmacology. XXIII. The angiotensin II receptors. *Pharmacological Reviews*, Vol. 52, No. 3, (September 2000), pp. 415-472, ISSN 0031-6997.

De Gasparo, M.; Siragy, H.M.. (1999). The AT2 receptor: fact, fancy and fantasy. *Regulatory Peptides*, Vol. 81, No. (1-3), (May 1999), pp. 11-24, ISSN 0167-0115.

Declèves, A.E. & Sharma, K. (2010). New pharmacological treatments for improving renal outcomes in diabetes. *Nature Reviews Nephrology*, Vol.6, No.6, (June 2010), pp. 371-380, ISSN 1759-5061.

Deddish, P.A.; Wang, J.; Michel, B.; Morris, P.W.; Davidson, N.O.; Skidgel, R.A &, Erdös, E.G. (1994). Naturally occurring active N-domain of human angiotensin I-converting enzyme. *Proceedings of the national academy of sciences of the United States of America*, Vol.91, No.16, (August 1994), pp. 7807–7811, ISSN 0027-8424.

Ding, Y.; Davisson, R.L.; Hardy, D.O.; Zhu, L.J.; Merrill, D.C.; Catterall, J.F. & Sigmund, C.D. (1997). The kidney androgen-regulated protein promoter confers renal proximal tubule cell-specific and highly androgen-responsive expression on the human angiotensinogen gene in transgenic mice. *Journal of Biological Chemistry*, Vol.272, No.44, (October 1997), pp. 28142-28148, ISSN 0021-9258.

Donoghue, M.; Hsieh, F.; Baronas, E.; Godbout, K.; Gosselin, M.; Stagliano, N.; Donovan, M.; Woolf, B.; Robison, K.; Jeyaseelan, R.; Breitbart, R.E & Acton, S. (2000). A novel angiotensin-converting enzyme-related carboxypeptidase (ACE2) converts angiotensin I to angiotensin 1-9. *Circulation Research,* Vol.87, No.5, (September 2000), pp. E1-E9, ISSN 0009-7330.

Eckel, R.H.; Grundy, S.M. & Zimmet, P.Z. (2005). The metabolic syndrome. *The Lancet*,

Elliott, M.D.; Kapoor, A.; Parker, M.A.; Kaufman, D.B.; Bonow, R.O & Gheorghiade, M. (2001). Improvement in hypertension in patients with diabetes mellitus after kidney/pancreas transplantation. *Circulation*, Vol.104, No.5, (July 2001), pp. 563-569. ISSN 0009-7322.

Erdös, E.G. (1976). Conversion of angiotensin I to angiotensin II. *American Journal of Medicine,* Vol.60, No.6, (May 1976), pp. 749-759, ISSN 0002-9343.

Farag, Y.M. & Gaballa, M.R. (2011). Diabesity: an overview of a rising epidemic. *Nephrology Dialysis Transplantation*, Vol.26, No.1 (January 2011), pp. 28-35, ISSN 0931-0509.

Ferrari, R. (2005). Angiotensin-converting enzyme inhibition in cardiovascular disease: evidence with perindopril. *Expert Reviews of Cardiovascular Therapy*, Vol.3, No.1 (January 2005), pp. 15-29, ISSN: 1477-9072.

Ferrario, C.; Abdelhamed, A.I & Moore, M. (2004). Angiotensin antagonists in hypertension, heart failure, and diabetic nephropathy: focus in losartan. *Current Medical Research and Opinion*, Vol.20, No.3, (March 2004), pp. 279-93, ISSN 0300-7995.

Ferrario, C.M. (2006). Angiotensin-converting enzyme 2 and angiotensin-(1-7): an evolving story in cardiovascular regulation. *Hypertension*, Vol.47, No.3, (March 2006), pp. 515-21, ISSN 0194-911X.

Ferrario, CM. & Varagic, J. (2010). The ANG-(1-7)/ACE2/mas axis in the regulation of nephron function. *American Journal of Physiology Renal Physiology*, Vol.298, No.6, (June 2010), pp. F1297-1305. Epub 2010 Apr 7. Review. Erratum in: *American Journal of Physiology Renal Physiology*, Vol.299, No.6, (December 2010), pp. F1515, ISSN 0363-6127

Ferrario, CM. (2011). ACE2: more of Ang-(1-7) or less Ang II? *Current Opinion in Nephrology and Hypertension*, Vol.20, No.1, pp. 1-6, ISSN 1062-4821.

Folli, F.; Corradi, D.; Fanti, P.; Davalli, A.; Paez, A.; Giaccari, A.; Perego, C. & Muscogiuri, G. (2011). The Role of Oxidative Stress in the Pathogenesis of Type 2 Diabetes Mellitus Micro- and Macrovascular Complications: Avenues for a Mechanistic-Based Therapeutic Approach. *Current Diabetes Reviews*, (August 2011), [Epub ahead of print], ISSN 1573-399898

Gembardt, F.; Sterner-Kockm A.;Imboden, H.; Spalteholz, M.; Reibitz, F.; Schultheiss, H.P.; Siems, W.E. & Walther, T. (2005). Organ-specific distribution of ACE2 mRNA and correlating peptidase activity in rodents. *Peptides*, Vol.26, No.7, (July 2005), pp. 1270-1277, ISSN 0196-9781.

Giacchetti, G.; Sechi, L.A.; Rilli, S. & Carey, R.M. (2005). The renin-angiotensin-aldosterone system, glucose metabolism and diabetes. *Trends in Endocrinology and Metabolism*, Vol.16, No.3, (April 2005), pp. 120-126, ISSN 1043-2760.

Gilbert, RE.; Cox, A.; Wu, LL.; Allen, TJ.; Hulthen, L.; Jerums, G. & Cooper, M.E. (1998). Expression of transforming growth factor-1 and type IV collagen in the renal tubulointerstitium in experimental diabetes: effects of angiotensin converting enzyme inhibition. *Diabetes*, Vol.47, pp. 414–422, ISSN 0012-1797.

Gillespie, E.L.; White, C.M.; Kardas, M.; Lindberg, M. & Coleman, C.L. (2005). The impact of ACE inhibitors or angiotensin II type 1 receptor blockers on the development of new-onset type 2 diabetes. *Diabetes Care*, Vol.28, No.9 (September 2005), pp. 2261–2266, ISSN 0149-5992.

Gress, T.W.; Nieto, F.J.; Shahar, E.; Wofford, M.R. & Brancati, F.L. (2000). Hypertension and antihypertensive therapy as risk factors for type 2 diabetes mellitus. Atherosclerosis Risk in Communities Study. *The New England Journal of Medicine*, Vol.342, No.13, (March 2000), pp. 905-912, ISSN 0028-4793.

Guarnieri, G.; Zanetti, M.; Vinci, P.; Cattin, M.R.; Pirulli, A. & Barazzoni, R. (2010) Metabolic syndrome and chronic kidney disease. *Journal of Renal Nutrition*, Vol.20, Suppl.5, (September 2010), pp. S19-S23, ISSN 1051-2276.

Guimaraes, P.B.; Alvarenga, E.C.; Siqueira, P.D.; Paredes-Gamero, E.J.; Sabatini, R.A.; Morais, R.L.T.; Reis, R.I.; Santos, E.L.; Teixeira, L.G.D.; Casarini, D.E.; Martin, R.P.; Shimuta, S.I.; Carmona, A.K.; Nakaie, C.R.; Jasiulionis, M.G.; Ferreira, A.T.; Pesquero, J.L.; Oliveira, S.M.; Bader, M.; Costa-Neto, C.M. & Pesquero, J.B. (2011).

Angiotensin II Binding to Angiotensin I–Converting Enzyme Triggers Calcium Signaling. *Hypertension,* Vol.57, No.5, (May 2011), pp. 965-972, ISSN 0194-911X.

Gupta, A.K.; Dahlof, B.; Dobson, J.; Sever, P.S.; Wedel, H.; Poulter, N.R. & Anglo-Scandinavian Cardiac Outcomes Trial Investigators. (2008). Determinants of new-onset diabetes among 19,257 hypertensive patients randomized in the Anglo-Scandinavian Cardiac Outcomes Trial--Blood Pressure Lowering Arm and the relative influence of antihypertensive medication. *Diabetes Care,* Vol.31, No.5, (May 2008), pp. 982-988, ISSN 0149-5992.

Hall, J.E. (2003). Historical perspective of the renin-angiotensin system. *Molecular Biotechnology,* Vol.24, No.1, pp. 27-39, ISSN 1073-6085.

Hall, J.E.; da Silva, A.A.; do Carmo, J.M.; Dubinion, J.; Hamza, S.; Munusamy, S.; Smith, G. & Stec, D.E. (2010). Obesity-induced hypertension: role of sympathetic nervous system, leptin, and melanocortins. *The Journal of Biological Chemistry,* Vol.285, No.23, (June 2010), pp. 17271-17276, ISSN 0021-9258.

Handelsman, Y. (2011). Diabetes and hypertension: a comprehensive report on management and the prevention of cardiovascular and renal complications. *The Journal of Clinical Hypertension,* Vol.13, No.4, (April 2011), pp. 221-223, ISSN 1524-6175.

Harmer, D.; Gilbert, M.; Borman, R. & Clark, KL. (2002). Quantitative mRNA expression profiling of ACE 2, a novel homologue of angiotensin converting enzyme. *Federation of European Biochemical Societies Letters,* Vol.4, No.532, (December 2002), pp. 107-10, ISSN 0014-5793.

Hayden, M.R.; Sowers, K.M.; Pulakat, L.; Joginpally, T.; Krueger, B.; Whaley-Connell, A. & Sowers, J.R. (2011). Possible Mechanisms of Local Tissue Renin-Angiotensin System Activation in the Cardiorenal Metabolic Syndrome and Type 2 Diabetes Mellitus. *Cardiorenal Medicine,* Vol.1, No.3, (June 2011), pp. 193–210, ISSN 1664-3828.

Heart Outcomes Prevention Evaluation (HOPE) Study Investigators. (2000). Effects of ramipril on cardiovascular and microvascular outcomes in people with diabetes mellitus: results of the HOPE study and MICRO-HOPE substudy. *The Lancet,* Vol.355, No9200, (January 2000), pp. 253–269. ISSN 0140-6736. Erratum in *The Lancet,* Vol.356, No. 9232, (September 2000), pp. 860.

Houston, M.C.; Basile, J.; Bestermann, W.H.; Egan, B.; Lackland, D.; Hawkins, R.G.; Moore, M.A.; Reed, J.; Rogers, P.; Wise, D. & Ferrario, C.M. Addressing the global cardiovascular risk of hypertension, dyslipidemia, and insulin resistance in the southeastern United States. *American Journal of the Medical Sciences,* Vol.329, No.6, (June 2005), pp. 276-291, ISSN 0002-9629.

Hsieh, T.J.; Fustier, P.; Zhang, S.L.; Filep, J.G.; Tang, S.S.; Ingelfinger, J.R.; Fantus, I.G.; Hamet, P.; & Chan JS. (2003). High glucose stimulates angiotensinogen gene expression and cell hypertrophy via activation of the hexosamine biosynthesis pathway in rat kidney proximal tubular cells. *Endocrinology,* vol.144, No.10, (October 2003), pp. 4338-4349, ISSN 0013-7227.

Hsueh, W.A. & Wyne, K. (2011). Renin-Angiotensin-aldosterone system in diabetes and hypertension. *Journal of Clinical Hypertension (Greenwich),* Vol.13, No.4, (April 2011), pp. 224-37, ISSN 1524-6175.

Hu, F.B. (2011). Globalization of diabetes: the role of diet, lifestyle, and genes. *Diabetes Care,* Vol.34, No.6, (June 2011), pp. 1249-1257, ISSN 0149-5992.

Huang, W.; Gallois, Y.; Bouby, N.; Bruneval, P.; Heudes, D.; Belair, M.F.; Krege, J.H.; Meneton, P.; Marre, M.; Smithies, O. & Alhenc-Gelas, F. (2001). Genetically increased angiotensin I-converting enzyme level and renal complications in diabetic mouse. *Proceedings of the National Academy of Sciences of the United States of America,* Vol.98, No. 23, (November 2001), pp. 13330-13334, ISSN 0027-8424.

Hunyady, L. & Catt, K.J. (2006). Pleitropic AT1 receptor signaling pathways mediating physiological and pathogenic actions of angiotensin II. *Molecular Endocrinology,* Vol.20, No.5, (May 2006), pp. 953-970, ISSN 0888-8809.

Ichihara, A.; Suzuki, F.; Nakagawa, T.; Kaneshiro, Y.; Takemitsu, T.; Sakoda, M.; Nabi, A.H.; Nishiyama, A.; Sugaya, T.; Hayashi, M. & Inagami, T. (2006). Prorenin receptor blockade inhibits development of glomerulosclerose in diabetic angiotensin II type 1a receptor deficient mice. *Journal of the American Society of Nephrology.* Vol.17, No.7, (July 2006), pp. 1950-1961, ISSN 1046-6673.

International Diabetes Federation: The Diabetes Atlas, 4th Edition. International Diabetes Federation, 2009. Brussels, http://www.idf.org/diabetesatlas.

Isomaa, B.; Almgren, P.; Tuomi, T.; Forsén, B.; Lahti, K.; Nissén, M.; Taskinen, M.R. & Groop, L. (2001). Cardiovascular morbidity and mortality associated with the metabolic syndrome. Diabetes Care, Vol.24, No.4, (April 2001), pp. 683-689, ISSN 1062-4821.

Izzo, R.; de Simone, G.; Chinali, M.; Iaccarino, G.; Trimarco, V.; Rozza, F.; Giudice, R.; Trimarco, B. & De Luca, N.; (2009). Insufficient control of blood pressure and incident diabetes. *Diabetes Care,* Vol. 32, No.5, (May 2009), pp. 845–850, ISSN 0149-5992.

Jandeleit-Dahm, K. & Cooper, M.E. (2002). Hypertension and diabetes. *Current Opinion in Nephrology and Hypertension,* Vol.11, No.2, (March 2002), pp. 221-228, ISSN 1062-4821.

Jaspard, E.; Wei, L. & Alhenc-Gelas, F. (1993). Differences in the properties and enzymatic specificities of the two active sites of angiotensin I-converting enzyme (kininase II). Studies with bradykinin and other natural peptides. *Journal of Biological Chemistry,* Vol.268, No.13, (May 1993), pp. 9496–9503, ISSN 0021-9258.

Kambayashi, Y.; Bardhan, S.; Takahashi, K.; Tsuzuki, S.; Inui, H.; Hamakubo, T.; Inagami, T. (1993). Molecular cloning of a novel angiotensin II receptor isoform involved in phosphotyrosine phosphatase inhibition. *Journal of Biological Chemistry,* Vol. 268, No. 33, (November 1993), pp. 24543-24546, ISSN 0021-9258.

Kang, J.J.; Toma, I.; Sipos, A.; Meer, E.J.; Vrgas, S.L. & Peti-Pertedi J. (2008). The collecting duct is the major source of pro-renin in diabetes. *Hypertension,* Vol.51, No.6, (June 2008), pp. 1597-1604, ISSN 0194-911X.

Keller, C.K.; Bergis, K.H.; Fliser, D. & Ritz, E. (1996). Renal findings in patients with short-term type 2 diabetes. Journal of the American Society of Nephrology, Vol.7, No.12, (December 1996), pp. 2627-2635, ISSN 1046-6673.

Kobori, H.; Harrison-Bernard, L.M. & Navar, L.G. (2001). Enhancement of angiotensinogen expression in angiotensin II-dependent hypertension. *Hypertension,* Vol.37, No.5, (May 2001), pp. 1329-1335, ISSN 0194-911X.

Kobori, H.; Nangaku, M.; Navar, G. & Nishiyama, A. (2007). The intrarenal renin-angiotensin system: from physiology to the pathobiology of hypertension and kidney disease. *Pharmacological Reviews,* Vol.59, No.3, (September 2007), pp. 251-287, ISSN 0031-6997.

Kobori, H.; Nishiyama, A.; Harrison-Bernard, L.M. & Navar, L.G. (2003). Urinary angiotensinogen as an indicator of intrarenal angiotensin status in hypertension. *Hypertension,* Vol.41, No.1, (January 2003), pp. 42-49, ISSN 0194-911X.

Kohlstedt, K.; Brandes, R.P.; Muller-Esterl, W.; Busse, R. & Fleming, I. (2004). Angiotensin-converting enzyme is involved in outside-in signaling in endothelial cells. *Circulation Research,* Vol.94, No.1, (January 2004), pp. 60–67, ISSN 0009-7330.

Kotsis, V.; Stabouli, S.; Papakatsika, S.; Rizos, Z. & Parati, G. (2010) Mechanisms of obesity-induced hypertension. *Hypertension Research,* Vol.33, No.5, (May 2010), pp. 386-393, ISSN 0916-9636.

Lambert, D.W.; Clarke, N.E.; Turner, A.J. (2010). Not just angiotensinases: new roles for the angiotensin-converting enzymes. *Cellular and Molecular Life Sciences,* Vol. 67, No. 1, (January 2010), pp. 89-98, ISSN 1420-682X.

Lattion, A.L.; Soubrier, F.; Allegrini, J.; Hubert, C.; Corvol, P. & Alhenc-Gelas, F. (1989). The testicular transcript of the angiotensin Iconverting enzyme encodes for the ancestral, non-duplicated form of the enzyme. *FEBS Letters,* Vol.252, No(1-2), (July 1989), pp. 99-104, ISSN 0014-5793.

Lavoie, J.L. & Sigmund, C.D. (2003). Minireview: overview of the rennin-angiotensin system-an endocrine and paracrine system. *Endocrinology,* Vol144, (June 2003), pp. 2179-2183, ISSN 0013-7227.

Lewis, E.J.; Hunsicker, L.G.; Bain, R.P. & Rohde, R.D. (1993). The Collaborative Study Group. The effect of angiotensin-converting-enzyme inhibition on diabetic nephropathy. *The New England Journal of Medicine,* Vol.329, No.20, (November 1993), pp. 1456-1462, ISSN 0028-4793.

Lewis, E.J.; Hunsicker, L.G.; Clarke, W.R.; Berl, T.; Pohl, M.A.; Lewis, J.B.; Ritz, E.; Atkins, R.C.; Rohde, R. & Raz, I. (2001). Renoprotective effect of the angiotensin-receptor antagonist irbesartan in patients with nephropathy due to type 2 diabetes. *The New England Journal of Medicine,* Vol.345, No.12, (September 2001), pp. 851-860, ISSN 0028-4793.

Maia, L.G.; Ramos, M.C.; Fernandes, L.; de Carvalho, M.H.C.; Campagnole-Santos, M.J. & Souza dos Santos, R.A. (2004). Angiotensin –(1-7) antagonist A-779 attenuates the potentiation of bradykinin by captopril in rats. *Journal of Cardiovascular Pharmacology,* Vol.43, No.5, (May 2004), pp. 685-691, ISSN 0160-2446.

Makino, S.; Kunimoto, K.; Muraoka, Y.; Mizushima, Y.; Katagiri, K. & Tochino, Y. (1980). Breeding of a non-obese, diabetic strain of mice. *Jikken Dobutsu,* Vol.29, No.1, (January 1980), pp. 1–13, ISSN 0007-5124.

Marques, G.D.; Quinto, B.M.; Plavinik, F.L.; Krieger, J.E.; Marson, O. & Casarini, D.E. (2003). N-domain angiotensin I-converting enzyme with 80 kDa as a possible genetic marker of hypertension. *Hypertension,* Vol.42, No.4, (October 2003), pp. 693-701, ISSN 0194-911X.

Matsubara, H. (1998). Pathophysiological role of angiotensin II type 2 receptor in cardiovascular and renal diseases. *Circulation Research,* Vol. 83, (September 1998), pp. 1182-1191, ISSN 0009-7330.

Mervaala, E.M.; Müller, D.N.; Park, J.K.; Schmidt, F.; Löhn, M.; Breu, V.; Dragun, D.; Ganten, D.; Haller, H. & Luft, F.C. (1999). Monocyte infiltration and adhesion molecules in a rat model of high human renin hypertension. *Hypertension,* Vol.33, No.1, Pt 2, (January 1999), pp. 389-395, ISSN 0194911X.

Miao, Y.; Smink, P.A.; de Zeeuw, D. & Lambers Heerspink, H.J. (2011). Drug-induced changes in risk/biomarkers and their relationship with renal and cardiovascular long-term outcome in patients with diabetes. *Clinical Chemistry.* Vol.57, No.2, (February 2011), pp. 186-195, ISSN 0009-9147.

Mogensen, CE. (1976). Renal function changes in diabetes. Diabetes, Vol.25, (2 Suppl), (1976), pp. 872-9, ISSN 0012-1797.

Moriguchi, A.; Tallant, EA.; Matsumura, K.; Reilly, TM.; Walton, H.; Ganten, D. & Ferrario, C.M. (1995). Opposing actions of angiotensin-(1-7) and angiotensin II in the brain of transgenic hypertensive rats. *Hypertension*, Vol. 25, No.6, pp. 1260-5, ISSN 0194911X.

Mukai, Y.; Shimokawa, H.; Higashi, M.; Morikawa, K.; Matoba, T.; Hiroki, J.; Kunihiro, I.; Talukder, H.M. & Takeshita, A. (2002). Inhibition of renin-angiotensin system ameliorates endothelial dysfunction associated with aging in rats. *Arteriosclerosis, Thrombosis and Vascular Biology,* Vol.22 (September 2002), pp. 1445-1450, ISSN 1049-8834.

Mukoyama, M.; Nakajima, M.; Horiuchi, M.; Sasamura, H.; Pratt, R.E.; Dzau, V.J. (1993). Expression cloning of type-2 angiotensin II receptor reveals a unique class of seven-transmembrane receptors. *The Journal of Biological Chemistry* 1993;268:24539–42, ISSN 0021-9258.

Nakajima, M.; Hutchinson, H.G.; Fujinaga, M.; Hayashida, W.; Morishita R.; Zhang, L.; Horiuchi, M.; Pratt, R.E. & Dzau, V.J. (1995). The angiotensin II type 2 (AT2) receptor antagonizes the growth effects of the AT1 receptor: gain-of-function study using gene transfer. *Proceedings of the National Academy of Sciences of United States of America*, Vol. 10, No. 3, (June 1998), pp. 188-193. ISSN 0027-8424.

National Institute of Diabetes and Digestive and Kidney Diseases. US Renal Data Systems: *USRDS 2010 annual data report: Atlas of End Stage Renal Disease in the United States.* National Institues of Health, Bethesda, Maryland, USA, 2010.

Navar, L.G.; Harrison-Bernard, L.M.; Nishiyama, A.; Kobori, H. (2002). Regulation of intrarenal angiotensin II in hypertension. *Hypertension*, Vol., 39, No. (2 Pt 2), (February 2002), pp. 316-322, ISSN 0194-911X.

Navar, L.G. & Harrison-Bernard LM. (2000). Intrarenal angiotensin II augmentation in angiotensin II dependent hypertension. *Hypertension Research,* Vol.23, No.4, (July 2000), pp. 291-301, ISSN 0916-9636.

Navar, L.G.; Lewis, L.; Hymel, A.; Braan, B. & Mitchel, K.D. (1994). Tubular fluid concentrations and kidney contents of angiotensins I and II in anesthetized rats. *Journal of the American Society of Nephrology*, Vol.5, No.4, (October 1994), pp. 1153-1158, ISSN 1046-6673.

Navar, LG.; Kobori, H.; Prieto, MC. & Gonzalez-Villalobos, RA. (2011a). Intratubular renin-angiotensin system in hypertension. *Hypertension,* Vol.57, No.3, (March 2011a), pp. 355-62, ISSN 0194911X.

Navar, LG.; Prieto, MC.; Satou, R. & Kobori, H. (2011b). Intrarenal angiotensin II and its contribution to the genesis of chronic hypertension. *Current Opinion in Pharmacology,* Vol.11, No.2, (April 2011b), pp. 180-6, ISSN 1471-4892.

Nguyen, G.; Contrepas, A. (2008). Physiology and pharmacology of the (pro)renin receptor. *Current Opinion in Pharmacology,* Vol. 8, No. 2, (April 2008), pp. 127-132, ISSN 1471-4892.

Nguyen, G. (2011). Renin and prorenin receptor in hypertension: what's new? *Current Hypertension Reports*, Vol. 13, No. 1, (February 2011), pp. 79-85, ISSN 1522-6417.

Nguyen, G.; Delarue, F.; Burckle, C.; Bouzhir, L.; Giller, T. & Sraer, J.D. (2002). Pivotal role of the renin/prorenin receptor in angiotensin II production and cellular responses to renin. *Journal of Clinical Investigation*, Vol109, No.11, (June 2002), pp. 1417-1427, 2002, ISSN 0021-9738

Oudit, G.Y.; Liu, G.C.; Zhong, J.; Basu, R.; Chow, F.L.; Zhou, J.; Loibner, H.; Janzek, E.; Schuster, M.; Penninger, J.M.; Herzenberg, A.M.; Kassiri, Z. & Scholey, J.W. (2010). Human recombinant ACE2 reduces the progression of diabetic nephropathy. *Diabetes*, Vol.59, No.2, (February 2010), pp. 29-38, ISSN 0012-1797.

Parving, H.H.; Lehnert, H.; Bröchner-Mortensen, J.; Gomis, R.; Andersen, S. & Arner, P. (2001). Irbesartan in Patients with Type 2 Diabetes and Microalbuminuria Study Group.The effect of irbesartan on the development of diabetic nephropathy in patients with type 2 diabetes. *The New England Journal of Medicine*. Vol.345, No.12, (September 2001), pp. 870-878, ISSN 0028-4793.

Paul, M.; Mehr, A.P. & Kreutz, R. (2006). Physiology of local angiotensin systems. *Physiological Reviews*, Vol.86, (July 2006), pp. 747-781, ISSN 0031-9333.

Poulsen, P.L.; Hansen, K.W. & Mogensen, C.E. (1994). Ambulatory blood pressure in the transition from normo- to microalbuminuria. A longitudinal study in IDDM patients. *Diabetes*, Vol.43, No.10, (October 1994), pp. 1248-1253, ISSN 0012-1797.

Prescott, G.; Silversides, D.W. & Reudelhuber, T.L. (2002). Tissue activity of circulanting prorenin. *American Journal of Hypertension*, Vol.15, No.3, (March 2002), pp. 280-285, ISSN 0895-7061.

Prieto-Carrasquero, M.C.; Harrison-Bernard, L.M.; Kobori, H.; Ozawa, Y.; Hering-Smith, K.S.; Hamm, L.L. & Navar, L.G. (2004). Enhancement of collecting duct rennin in angiotensin II-dependent hypertensive rats. *Hypertension*, Vol.44, No.2, (August 2004), pp. 223-229, ISSN 0194-911X.

Ravid, M.; Brosh, D.; Levi, Z.; Bar-Dayan, Y.; Ravid, D. & Rachmani, R. (1998). Use of enalapril to attenuate decline in renal function in normotensive, normoalbuminuric patients with type 2 diabetes mellitus. A randomized, controlled trial. *Annals of Internal Medicine*, Vol. 128, No.12, Pt 1, (June 1998), pp. 982–988, ISSN 0003-4819.

Redublo Quinto, B.M, Camargo de Andrade, M.C.; Ronchi, F.A.; Santos, E.L.; Correa, S.A.A.; Shimuta, S.I.; Pesquero, J.B.; Mortara, R.A. & Casarini, D.E. (2008). Expression of angiotensin I-converting enzymes and bradykinin B2 receptors in mouse inner medullary-collecting duct cells. *International Immunopharmacology*, Vol.8, No.2, (February 2008), pp. 254–260, ISSN 1567-5769.

Ribeiro-Oliveira Jr, A.; Nogueira, A.I.; Pereira, R.M.; Boas, W.W.V.; Santos, R.A.S. & Simoes e Silva, A.C. (2008). The renin-angiotensin system and diabetes: an update. *Vascular Health and Risk Management*, Vol.4, No.4, (2008), pp. 787-803, ISSN 1176-6344.

Riordan, J.F. (2003). Angiotensin-I-converting enzyme and its relatives. *Genome Biology*, Vol. 4, No. 8, (2003), pp. 225, ISSN 1465-6906.

Ronchi, F.A.; Andrade, M.C.; Carmona, A.K.; Krieger, J.E. & Casarini, D.E. (2005). N-domain angiotensin-converting enzyme isoform expression in tissues of Wistar and spontaneously hypertensive rats. *Journal of Hypertension*, Vol.23, No.10, (October 2005), pp. 1869-78, ISSN 0263-6352.

Ronchi, F.A.; Irigoyen, M.C. & Casarini DE. Association of somatic and N-domain angiotensin-converting enzymes from Wistar rat tissue with renal dysfunction in diabetes mellitus. *Journal of the Renin-Angiotensin-Aldosterone System*, Vol.8, No.1, (March 2007), pp. 34-41, ISSN 1470-3203.

Rosivall, L. (2009). Intrarenal renin-angiotensin system. *Molecular and cellular Endocrinology*, Vol.302, No. 2, (April 2009), pp. 185-192, ISSN 0303-7207.

Rousseau, A.; Michaud, A.; Chauvet, M.T.; Lenfant, M. & Corvol, P. (1995). The hemoregulatory peptide N-acetyl-Ser-Asp-Lys-Pro is a natural and specific substrate of the N-terminal active site of human angiotensin-converting enzyme. *Journal of Biological Chemistry*, Vol.270, No.8, (February 1995), pp. 3656–3661, ISSN 0021-9258.

Ruggenenti, P.; Cravedi, P. & Remuzzi, G. (2010). The RAAS in the pathogenesis and treatment of diabetic nephropathy. *Nature Reviews Nephrology*, Vol.6, No.6, (June 2010), pp. 319-330, ISSN 1759-5061.

Santos, R.A. & Ferreira, A.J. (2007). Angiotensin 1-7 and renin-angiotensin system. *Current Opinion Nephrology and Hypertension*, Vol.16, No.2, (March 2007), pp. 122-128, ISSN 1062-4821.

Santos, R.A.; Frezard, F. & Ferreira, A.J. (2005). Angiotensin-(1-7): blood, heart, and blood vessels. *Current Medicinal Chemistry - Cardiovascular & Hematological Agents*, Vol.3, No.4, (October 2005), pp. 383-91, ISSN 1568-0169.

Santos, R.A.; Simoes e Silva, A.C.; Maric, C.; Silva, D.M.; Machado, R.P.; de Buhr, I.; Heringer-Walther, S.; Pinheiro, S.V.; Lopes, M.T.; Bader, M.; Mendes, E.P.; Lemos, V.S.; Campagnole-Santos, M.J.; Schultheiss, H.P.; Speth, R. & Walther, T. (2003). Angiotensin –(1-7) is an endogenous ligand for the G protein-coupled receptor Mas. *Proceedings of the National Academy of Sciences of the United States of America*, Vol.100, No.14, (July 2003) pp. 8258-8263, ISSN 0027-8424.

Saris, J.J.; Derkx, F.H.; De Bruin, R.J.; Dekkers, D.H.; Lamers, J.M.; Saxena, P.R.; Schalekamp, M.A.; Jan Danser, A.H. High-affinity prorenin binding to cardiac man-6-P/IGF-II receptors precedes proteolytic activation to renin. *American Journal of Physiology*, Vol. 280, No. 4, (April 2001), pp. H1706-H1715. ISSN 1040-0605.

Sato, A.; Hayashi, K.; Naruse, M. & Saruta, T. (2003). Effectiveness of aldosterone blockade in patients with diabetic nephropathy. *Hypertension*, Vol.41, No.1, (November 2003), pp. 64-68, ISSN 0194-911X.

Senanayake, P.; Drazba, J.; Shadrach. K.; Milsted, A.; Rungger-Brandle, E.; Nishiyama, K.; Miura, S.; Karnik. S.; Sears, J.E. & Hollyfield, J.G. (2007). Angiotensin II and its receptor subtypes in the human retina. *Investigative Ophthalmology & Visual Science*, Vol.48, No.7, (July 2007), pp. 3301-3311, ISSN 0146-0404.

Senbonmatsu, T.; Saito, T.; Landon, E.J.; Watanabe, O.; Price Jr, E.; Roberts, R.L.; Imboden, H.; Fitzgerald, T.G, Gaffney, F.A & Inagami. (2003). A novel angiotensin II type 2 receptor signaling pathway: possible role in cardiac hypertrophy. *The European Molecular Biology Organization Journal (EMBO)*. Vol 22, No. 24, (December 2003), pp. 6471-6482, ISSN 0261-4189.

Shaltout, H.A.; Westwood, B.M.; Averil,l D.B.; Ferrario, C.M.; Figueroa, J.P.; Diz, D.I.; Rose, J.C. & Chappell, M.C. (2007). Angiotensin metabolism in renal proximal tubules, urine, and serum of sheep: evidence for ACE2-dependent processing of angiotensin II. *American Journal of Physiology Renal Physiology*, Vol.292, No.1, (January 2007), pp. F82-F91, ISSN 1931-857X

Sharma, R.; Sharma, M.; Reddy, S.; Savin, V.J.; Nagaria, A.M. & Wiegmann, T.B. (2006). Chronically increased intrarenal angiotensin II causes nephropathy in an animal model of type 2 diabetes. *Frontiers in Bioscience*, Vol.11, (January 2006), pp. 968-976, ISSN 1093-4715.

Touyz, R.M.; Schiffrin, E.L. (2000). Signal transduction mechanisms mediating the physiological and pathophysiological actions of angiotensin II in vascular smooth muscle cells. *Pharmacological Reviews*, Vol. 52, No. 4, (December 2000), pp. 639-672, ISSN 0031-6997.

Sowers, J.R.; Epstein, M. & Frohlich, E.D. (2001). Diabetes, hypertension, and cardiovascular disease: an update. *Hypertension,* Vol.37, No.4, (April 2001), pp. 1053-1059, ISSN 0194911X

Staessen, J.A.; Li Y. & Richard, T. (2006). Oral renin inhibitors. *Lancet,* Vol.368, No.9545, (October 2006), pp. 1449-56, ISSN 0140-6736.

Stoll, M. & Unger, T. Angiotensin and its AT2 receptor: new insights into an old system. *Regulatory Peptides.* Vol. 99, No. (2-3), (June 2001), pp. 175-182, ISSN 0167-0115.

Tanaka, H.; Shiohira, Y.; Uezu, Y.; Higa, A. & Iseki, K. (2006). Metabolic syndrome and chronic kidney disease in Okinawa, Japan. *Kidney International,* Vol.69, No.2, (January 2006), pp. 369–374. ISSN 0085-2538

Tikellis, C.; Johnston, C.I.; Forbes, J.M.; Burns, W.C.; Burrell, L.M.; Risvanis, J. & Cooper, M.E. (2003). Characterization of renal angiotensin-converting enzyme 2 in diabetic nephropathy. *Hypertension,* (Vol.41, No.3, (March 2003), pp. 392-7, ISSN 0194-911X.

Tikellis, C.; Wookey, P.J.; Candido, R.; Andrikopoulos, S.; Thomas, M.C & Cooper, M.E. (2004). Improved islet morphology after blockade of the renin-angiotensin system in the ZDF rat. *Diabetes,* Vol.53, No.4, (April 2004), pp. 989-997, ISSN 0012-1797.

Tipnis, S.R.; Hooper, N.M.; Hyde, R.; Karran, E.; Christie, G. & Turner, A.J. (2000). A human homolog of angiotensin-converting enzyme. Cloning and functional expression as a captopril-insensitive carboxypeptidase. *Journal of Biological Chemistry,* Vol.275, No.43, (October 2000), pp. 33238-33243), ISSN 0021-9258.

Touys & Schiffrin. (2000). Signal transduction mechanisms mediating the physiological and pathophysiological actions of angiotensin II in vascular smooth muscle cells. *Pharmacological Reviews,* Vol.52, (December 2000), pp. 639-72, ISSN 0031-6997.

Unger, T. & Sandmann, S. (2000). Angiotensin receptor blocker selectivity at the AT1- and AT2-receptors: conceptual and clinical effects. *Journal of Renin-Angiotensin-Aldosterone System,* Vol. 1, (suppl 2), (December 2000), pp. S6-S9, ISSN 1470-3203.

Unger, T.; Culman, J. & Gohlke, P. (1998). Angiotensin II receptor blockade and end-organ protection: pharmacological rationale and evidence. *Journal of Hypertension,* Vol.16, (suppl7), pp. S3–9, ISSN 0263-6352.

Van Buren, P.N. & Toto, R. (2011). Hypertension in diabetic nephropathy: epidemiology, mechanisms, and management. *Advances in chronic kidney disease,* Vol.18, No.1, (January 2011), pp. 28-41, ISSN 1548-5595.

Velloso, L.A.; Folli, F.; Perego, L. & Saad, M.J. (2006). The multi-faceted cross-talk between the insulin and angiotensin II signaling systems. *Diabetes/metabolism Research and Reviews,* Vol.22, No.2, (March 2006), pp. 98-107, ISSN 1520-7552.

Vickers, C.; Hales, P.; Kaushik, V.; Dick, L.; Gavin, J.; Tang, J.; Godbout, K.; Parsons, T.; Baronas, E.; Hsieh, F.; Acton, S.; Patane, M.; Nichols, A. & Tummino, P. (2002). Hydrolysis of biological peptides by human angiotensin-converting enzyme-related carboxypeptidase. *Journal of Biological Chemistry,* Vol.277, No.17, (April 2002), pp. 14838-43, ISSN 0021-9258.

Vidotti, D.B.; Casarini, D.E.; Cristovam, P.C.; Leite, C.A.; Schor, N. & Boim, M.A. (2004). High glucose concentration stimulates intracellular renin activity and angiotensin II generation in rat mesangial cells. *American Journal of Physiology - Renal Physiology,* Vol.286, No.6, (June 2004), pp. F1039-1045, ISSN 0363-6127..

Wehbi, GJ.; Zimpelmann, J.; Carey, RM.; Levine, DZ. & Burns, KD. (2001). Early streptozotocin–diabetes mellitus downregulates rat kidney AT(2) receptors.

American Journal Physiology Renal Physiology, Vol.280, No.2, (February 2001), pp. F254–65, ISSN 1931-857X

Wei, L.; Alhenc-Gelas, F.; Corvol, P. & Clauser, E. (1991). The two homologous domains of human angiotensin I-converting enzyme are both catalytically active. *Journal of Biological Chemistry*, Vol.266, No.14, (May 1991), pp. 9002–9008, ISSN 0021-9258.

Williams, T.A.; Michaud, A.; Houard, X.; Chauvet, M.T.; Soubrier, F.; Corvol, P. (1996) Drosophila melanogaster angiotensin I-converting enzyme expressed in Pichia pastoris resembles the C domain of the mammalian homologue and does not require glycosylation for secretion and enzymatic activity. *Biochemical Journal,* Vol. 318, (Pt 1), (August 1996), pp. 125-131, ISSN 0264-6021

Williams, B. (1994). Insulin resistance: the shape of things to come. *The Lancet,* Vol.344, No.8921, (August 1994), pp. 521-524, ISSN 0140-6736.

Wolf, G. & Ritz, E. (2005). Combination therapy with ACE inhibitors and angiotensin II receptor blockers to halt progression of chronic renal disease: pathophysiology and indications. Kidney international, Vol.67, No.3, (March 2005), pp. 799-812, ISSN 0085-2538.

Wong, D.W.; Oudit, G.Y.; Relcd, H.; Kassiri, Z.; Zhou, J.; Liu, Q.C.; Backx, P.H.; Penninger, J.M.; Herzenberg, A.M. & Scholey, J.W. (2007). Loss of angitensin converting enzyme-2 (ACE2) accelerates diabetic kidney injury. *American Journal of Pathology,* Vol.171, No.2, (August 2007) pp. 438-451, ISSN 0002-9440.

Xiao, H.D.; Fuchs, S.; Frenzel, K.; Teng, L. & Bernstein, K.E. (2004). Circulating versus local angiotensin II in blood pressure control: lessons from tissue-specific expression of angiotensin-converting enzyme (ACE). *Critical Reviews in Eukaryotic Gene Expression,* Vol.14, No.(1-2), (2004), pp. 137-45, ISSN 1045-4403.

Yamada, H.; Akishita, M.; Ito, M.; Tamura, K.; Daviet, L.; Lehtonen, J.Y.; Dzau, V.J.; Horiuchi, M. (1999). AT2 receptor and vascular smooth muscle cell differentiation in vascular development. *Hypertension.* Vol. 33, No. 6, (June 1999), pp. 1414-1419, ISSN 0194-911X.

Ye, M.; Wysocki, J.; William, J.; Soler, M.J.; Cokic, I. & Batlle, D. (2006). Glomerular localization and expression of Angiotensin-converting enzyme 2 and Angiotensin-converting enzyme: implications for albuminuria in diabetes. *Journal of the American Society of Nephrology,* Vol.17, No.11, (November 2006), pp. 3067-3075.

Yusuf, S.; Sleight, P.; Pogue, J.; Bosch, J.; Davies, R. & Dagenais, G. (2000). Effects of an angiotensin converting-enzyme inhibitor, ramipril, on cardiovascular events in high-risk patients. The Heart Outcomes Prevention Evaluation Study Investigators. *New England Journal of Medicine,* Vol.342, No.3, (January 2000), pp. 145-153, ISSN 0028-4793.

Zimpelmann, J.; Kumar, D.; Levine, D.Z.; Wehbi, G.; Imig, J.D.; Navar, L.G. & Burns, K.D. (2000). Early diabetes mellitus stimulates proximal tubule renin mRNA expression in the rat. *Kidney International,* Vol.58, No.6, (December 2000), pp. 2320-2330, ISSN 0085-2538.

2

Renal Angiotensinogen Gene Expression and Tubular Atrophy in Diabetic Nephropathy

Brice E. T. Nouthe[1], Maya Saleh[2], Shao-Ling Zhang[1] and John S. D. Chan[1,*]
[1]*Université de Montréal, Centre de Recherche du Centre Hospitalier de l'Université de Montréal (CRCHUM), Hôtel-Dieu Hospital, Pavillon Masson, Montreal, QC*
[2]*McGill University, Department of Medicine, Centre for the Study of Host Resistance and Complex Trait Group, Montreal, QC*
Canada

1. Introduction

The growing incidence of diabetes mellitus, with predicted rises in prevalence from 285 to 380 million cases in 2025, then 438 million by 2030, is a major public health burden in both developing and developed countries. Type 1 and type 2 diabetes increase the risk of microvascular complications, which cause significant morbidity and mortality. Diabetic nephropathy (DN) and retinopathy represent the major causes of end-stage renal disease and blindness (1-2) in developed countries. DN is associated with an increased risk of hypertension, adverse cardiovascular events (3), chronic kidney diseases and haemodialysis (4). Efforts are therefore being made to find ways of preventing and/or slowing down the progression of DN worldwide.

DN is initiated by glomerular changes, namely hypertrophy, then thickening of the basement membrane with subsequent expansion of the mesangial matrix and glomerulosclerosis (5). This is associated not only with microalbuminuria, an early clinically detectable lesion, but also with tubulointerstitial fibrosis and tubular atrophy (5-6). Oxidative stress, hyperglycemia and renin-angiotensin system (RAS) dysfunction have been linked to the development of these lesions (5-6). Although albuminuria is a useful clinical marker, tubulointerstitial fibrosis and tubular atrophy represent a better predictor of nephropathy progression because of their close association with declining renal function (5). Many randomized controlled trials have shown the efficacy of optimal glycemic control and RAS blockade in the primary and secondary prevention of DN (4, 7-9). The former is easily understood, as decreased "glucotoxicity" reduces end-organ damage. However, the mechanisms underlying the protective action of RAS inhibition, notably angiotensin II (Ang II) receptor blockade, are not well understood. In this review, we present the recent results of studies aiming to understand the consequences of RAS blockade at the molecular level, with an emphasis on tubular lesions in DN.

---

* Corresponding Author

2. The renin-angiotensin system in diabetic nephropathy

2.1 Clinical findings on the implications of RAS blockade in diabetic nephropathy

The benefits of RAS inhibition on end-organ protection in diabetic patients are well established. One of the early clinical trials on diabetic patients was performed with captopril, an angiotensin-converting enzyme inhibitor (ACE-I), and showed a reduction in the risks of death, dialysis and transplantation (10). Other trials initially used monotherapy with ACE-I, but also angiotensin receptor blockers (ARB) (11-12). Dual blockade was proposed after one of the largest clinical trials, the Candesartan And Lisinopril Microalbuminuria (CALM) Study, showed reduced albuminuria with dual therapy compared to monotherapy (13). Further clinical trials with larger sample sizes, however, have failed to confirm the superiority of dual RAS blockade compared to monotherapy; multicentric clinical trials are ongoing to resolve this issue (14).

2.2 Background on the roles of angiotensin II in the kidney

Despite controversies over the efficacy of dual or simple RAS blockade, the importance of Ang II in diabetic nephropathy development is well accepted. Ang II, an octapeptide discovered in the 1930s in the United States and characterized in Switzerland, was initially named for its first-known function: contraction of blood vessels (15). It is the most powerful biologically active peptide of the RAS, with vasoconstriction but also nonhemodynamic effects, such as electrolyte reabsorption, renal hypertrophy and tubular apoptosis in the kidneys (15).

2.2.1 Receptors

It is well established that Ang II mediates its effects mainly via binding to two G protein-coupled receptors: AT_1R (which has 2 subtypes in rodents, namely AT_{1a} and AT_{1b}) and AT_2R. AT_1R, a seven-transmembrane domain receptor, is the main known mediator of Ang II actions (16); its action is summarized in **Table 1**. Ang II stimulation leads to upregulation of AT_1R in the tubular compartment but downregulation of the same receptors in the glomerular compartment (17). The role of AT_2R in kidneys is still not fully understood: upon stimulation by Ang II, it can counteract the effects of AT_1R (18) but also activate inflammation (cf **Table 1**). In animal models of kidney damage, de novo expression of AT_2R in glomeruli and vessels was induced by Ang II together with upregulation of AT_2R in tubular cells (19).

Recent studies have shown the importance of 2 other receptors, the Ang1-7 or Mas receptors and the AT4 receptor (20). The latter is still under investigation and has been proven to be linked to memory. However, it is also present in vessels and kidneys (proximal and distal tubules); it increases intracellular Ca^{2+} levels and activates Erk and MAPK signalling (21).

2.2.2 Actions

Ang II stimulates glomerular cell proliferation and causes accumulation of extracellular matrix material by stimulating transforming growth factor β_1 (TGF-β_1), which leads to increased protein synthesis. TGF-β_1 decreases protein degradation by stimulating matrix metalloproteinases, mainly MMP-2, but also plasminogen activators inhibitor-1 (PAI-1) (22-23).

AT_1 R		AT_2 R		Mas receptors	
Activation	Inhibition	Activation	Inhibition	Activation	Inhibition
Phospholipase A2 Phospholipase C Jak/STAT ITP Ca^{2+} p21ras, C-Src PKC (MAPK&TGF-β_1) NADPH (ROS)	Adenyl cyclase	iNOs/L-arginine/O_2 +NADPH (NO&cGMP) NF-kappa B	PKC (MAPK)	p38MAPK, SHIP-1 (PI3K) Erk 1/2 Bradykinines COX (Prostaglandins), NO	TGF-β_1

Table 1. Signalling pathways stimulated by AT_1, AT_2 and Mas receptors

It has been demonstrated that high glucose, together with Ang II, is involved in tubular lesions seen in DN (5, 24). Indeed, high glucose and Ang II enhance angiotensinogen (Agt, the sole precursor of all angiotensins) gene expression, both in vitro in rat immortalized renal proximal tubular cells (iRPTC) (25, 26) and in vivo in streptozotocin-treated mice (a model of diabetic mice) proximal tubules (5, 24). This turns into a vicious circle, increasing tubular atrophy, as Agt is the sole substrate of the RAS and is used for synthesis of Ang II.

2.3 From angiotensinogen to angiotensin II

The importance of the systemic RAS in blood pressure control and sodium homeostasis has been well accepted and Ang II has been recognized as a cardinal parameter in the development of both hypertension and kidney injury (5, 13, 15, 27). Overactivation of AT_1 R by Ang II therefore represents a target for treatment, but as Ang II has many other paracrine effects (induction of inflammation, mitogenesis, cell growth, apoptosis, differentiation, migration, etc.), current therapies are not sufficient to reverse the consequences of Ang II hyperaction. Of note, local RAS have been unravelled in some organs, notably the kidneys, with luminal fluid levels of Ang II being at least 1,000-fold higher than in the plasma (28). This local RAS could also play an important role in sodium retention and blood pressure regulation and hypertension, representing both a cause and a consequence of kidney injury. Complex interactions between diabetes and hypertension due to similar etiologies of both conditions, together with the stimulating effect of hyperglycemia on Ang II production in vitro, point to an important role for local RAS in DN.

2.3.1 Synthesis and degradation of angiotensin II

The classic components of the RAS are all found in renal proximal tubules, including Agt and the enzymes (prorenin/renin, ACE, angiotensin-converting enzyme 2 (Ace2), aminopeptidases and carboxy peptidases). Upon cleavage of the prorenin into a proteolytic enzyme, renin will cleave Agt into a decapeptide: angiotensin I (Ang I). Then the dipeptidyl peptidase ACE will remove 2 amino acids from the latter and generate Ang II. Ang II is further metabolized into smaller fragments, such as Ang 1-7 and Ang III, Ang IV and Ang V, by various peptidases. Among those peptidases, Ace2 is a human homologue to ACE (42% similarity) that was discovered in 2000; it cleaves Ang I into Ang 1-9 / Ang II to Ang 1-7, both having hemodynamic properties (29). While ACE is present in most tissues, Ace2 is specifically expressed in the kidney, and less in the testes and heart ,with neither ARB nor

ACE-I, which can inhibit its activities (29). Ace2 levels in glomerules and proximal tubules are decreased in patients with chronic kidney disease and DN (30).

The following diagram illustrates the pathway for the synthesis and degradation of Ang II.

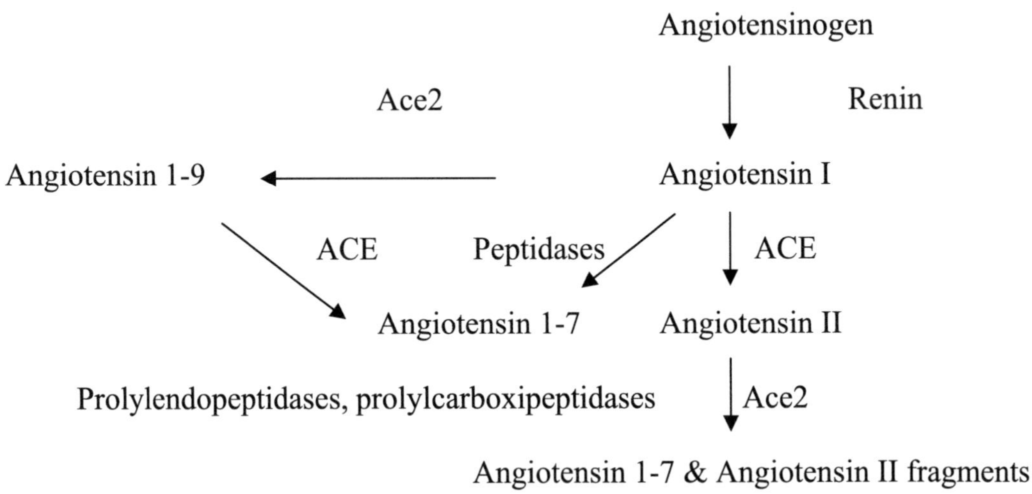

Fig. 1. Synthesis and degradation of Ang II

When Ace2 null mice were bred with the Akita model of type 1 diabetes, the obtained Ace2(-/y) Ins2(WT/C96Y) mice exhibited increased mesangial matrix scores, urinary albumin excretion rates and glomerular basement membrane thicknesses compared to Ace2(+/y)Ins2(WT/C96Y) with the same blood glucose levels (31). This highlights once more the role of RAS in the development of kidney injury in cases of chronic hyperglycemia.

2.3.2 Importance of angiotensinogen in diabetic nephropathy

Our laboratory has previously demonstrated that both ARB and ACE-I block Agt gene expression and induction of hypertrophy stimulated by high glucose levels in immortalized rat RPTCs and that renal Ang II acts in an autocrine manner to stimulate TGF-ß1 expression and, subsequently, TGF-ß1 enhances cellular hypertrophy and collagen α_1 (type IV) expression in RPTCs (32). Our experiments on RPTCs have shown that high glucose stimulates Agt gene expression via at least 4 pathways:

- Protein Kinase C via de novo synthesis of diacylglycerol;
- p38 MAP Kinase;
- Hexosamine biosynthesis;
- ROS.

The latter have been extensively studied within the frame of elucidating the molecular mechanisms of hyperglycemia action in DN. It is now accepted that elevated glucose levels enhance PKC activation, augment membrane lipid peroxidation in glomeruli and induce Agt gene expression in rat RPTCs via ROS generation (25). Excessive intracellular accumulation of glucose (seen in chronic hyperglycemia) leads to disturbances at the level of the TriCarboxylic Acid (TCA) pathway, followed by the formation of high quantities of electron donors (NADH, H^+ and $FADH_2$) and mitochondrial superoxide overproduction (33). Increased mitochondrial superoxide production activates three main pathways: the polyol/protein kinase C pathway, the hexosamine biosynthesis pathway, and increased production of advanced glycated end products (AGE) and its receptor, RAGE (33). Our transgenic (Tg) mice overexpressing rat catalase (CAT) in their RPTCs exhibit attenuated ROS generation, Agt gene expression and RPTC injury in streptozotocin (STZ)-induced diabetes in vivo (5), unequivocally demonstrating the importance of ROS in mediating Agt gene expression and in the development of DN.

2.4 Recent findings on diabetic nephropathy using transgenic mouse models

In order to elucidate in vivo the importance of local intrarenal RAS, at least two systems could be used: targeted renal expression of RAS in knock out mice for any component of RAS and targeted renal overexpression of one component of the RAS in wild type mice. Our laboratory has been using the latter approach to elucidate the role of intrarenal RAS in DN.

2.4.1 The angiotensinogen transgenic mouse model

To obtain specific overexpression of the rat Agt gene (rAgt) in RPTC, our laboratory used the Kidney-specific Androgen regulated Promoter 2 (KAP2) (34, 35). The cDNA encoding full-length rAgt fused with HA-tag at the carboxyl terminal and NotI restriction enzyme site attached at both 5′- and 3′-termini was thus inserted into the KAP2 promoter and thereafter microinjected into one-cell fertilized mouse embryos as shown below:

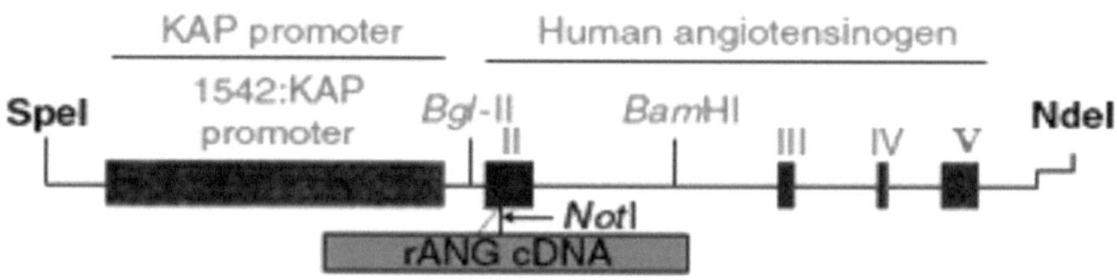

Fig. 2. Schematic map of the kidney androgen-regulated promoter (KAP2)-rat Agt construct

Studies using this rAgt-transgenic (Tg) mice model have demonstrated that overexpression of renal rAgt alone induces hypertension and albuminuria and that RAS blockade reverses these abnormalities (34). Thereafter the same model was used to assess a possible synergic deleterious action of local RAS overactivity and high glucose on RPTCs, which could contribute to the pathophysiology of DN and help unravel new protective mechanisms.

2.4.2 Tubular apoptosis in diabetic angiotensinogen transgenic mice

STZ was used to induce diabetes in non-transgenic (non-Tg) and Tg mice. As far as systemic hypertension is concerned, neither STZ-induced diabetes nor insulin treatment changed the blood pressure levels of Tg mice or non-Tg mice. STZ administration led, four weeks later, to diabetes, increased kidney/body weight and albuminuria, and were normalized by insulin treatment. RAS blockers did not affect glucose levels but reversed the deleterious effects of rAgt-overexpression in diabetic mice. Renal injury found in Tg mice was more severe in STZ-treated Tg mice, with loss of brush borders in RPTC and marked tubular luminal dilatation. In addition, glomerular and RPTC hypertrophy and increased tubular luminal area were markedly attenuated by insulin and RAS blockers in Tg and non-Tg STZ-treated mice, while a combination of both treatments completely reversed these abnormalities. Apoptotic assays (TUNEL) and immunohistochemistry using caspase-3 antibody showed increased levels of apoptosis in RPTC of Tg mice compared to non-Tg, the latter having higher levels than non-STZ treated mice. Investigations of the molecular pathways involved reveal an increased level of Bax and concomitant downregulation of Bcl-xL. One hypothesis could therefore be that hyperglycemia enhanced tubular apoptosis by increasing the Bax/Bcl-xL ratio, thus having a pro-poptotic effect. STZ-induced diabetes leads to apoptosis in RPTCs and to a lesser degree in distal tubules, but not in the glomeruli, confirming previous findings of a pro-apoptotic effect of diabetes on RPTCs (36). Treatment with insulin and/or RAS blockers leads to an almost complete absence of apoptosis in kidneys of non Tg and Tg mice. Another salient finding in Agt-Tg mice is the persistent kidney injury despite hydralazine treatment. In fact, hydralazine treatment markedly reduced systemic blood pressure but did not affect albuminuria and tubular apoptosis. Further investigations into the underlying mechanism of high glucose and Ang II action were performed on Tg mice overexpressing catalase (CAT-Tg) in their RPTCs. STZ-induced diabetic CAT-Tg mice exhibited attenuated ROS generation and tubular apoptosis (5). Furthermore, in double Tg mice having Agt and CAT specifically expressed in their RPTCs, ROS generation, NADPH activity and levels of hemoxygenase 1 (HO-1) were significantly lowered by CAT overactivity compared to Agt-Tg mice. Levels of collagen type IV, monocyte chemotactic protein-1 (MCP-1), TGF-β_1 and plasminogen activator inhibitor-1 were also lowered by CAT overexpression in double Tg mice compared to Agt Tg mice (37). Thus, CAT overexpression alleviates oxidative stress in RPTC and reduces the toxicity of Ang II and chronic hyperglycemia on the kidneys.

3. Conclusion and perspectives

Agt and chronic hyperglycemia act together at the level of the RPTC, leading to tubular atrophy due to pro-apoptotic activities and interstitial fibrosis. This unravels the importance of the local RAS in the development of DN. Both *in vitro* and *in vivo* experiments of overexpression of Agt indicate that the latter stimulates RPTC hypertrophy and apoptosis, but significant effects on the glomeruli remain to be determined. However, because tubular atrophy seems to be a better predictor of disease progression than glomeruli lesions, this finding may be considered of significant clinical importance, as therapeutics reproducing the effects of CAT may be specifically developed to impede or even stop the progression of DN.

Further directions include studying the effect of the local RAS on glomeruli and deciphering the molecular pathways by which Agt and chronic hyperglycemia induce RPTC apoptosis. One important clue is the role of ROS, which is induced by both intrarenal RAS overactivity and chronic hyperglycemia. Indeed, we have reported an increase of apoptotic cells in RPTCs of db/db mice (type II diabetic mouse model) and normalization by overexpression of catalase (CAT) in their RPTCs (db/db CAT-Tg mice) (38) as shown below:

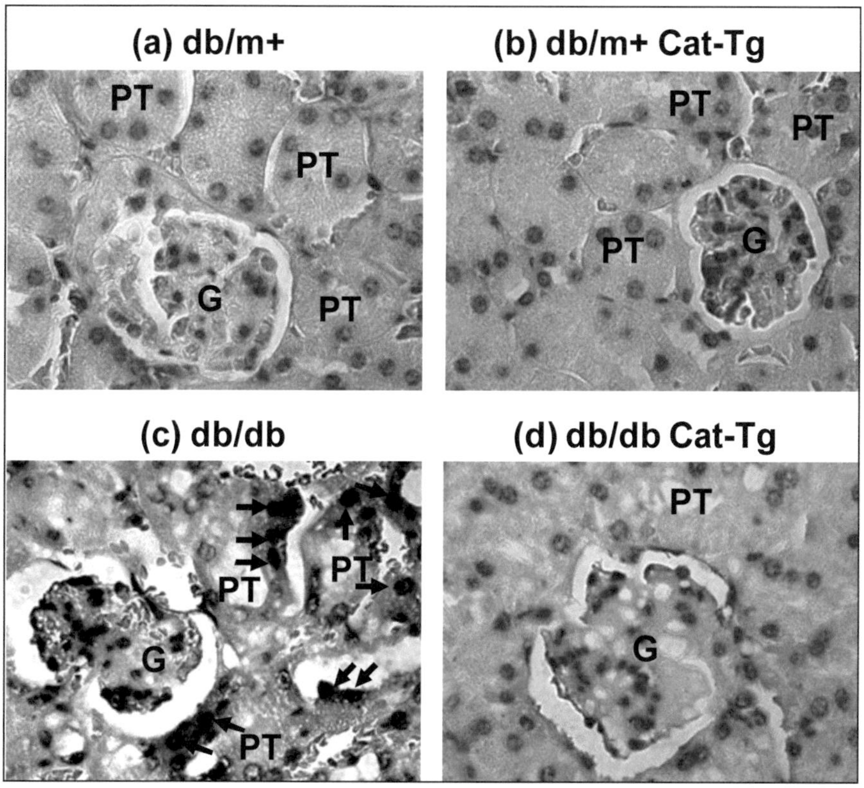

Fig. 3. Apoptosis in male non-Tg and Tg mouse kidneys at week 20, analyzed by TUNEL staining. Arrows indicate apoptotic cells. G, glomerulus; PT, proximal tubule. Magnification x600.

Using DNA chip microarrays technology, our laboratory recently identified 2 pro-apoptotic genes, Bcl-2 modifying factor (*Bmf*) and *Caspase-12,* which are differentially upregulated in renal proximal tubules of db/db mice but normalized in db/db CAT-Tg mice (39) as shown below:

Probe Set ID	Gene Title	Fold-change (db/db vs db/m+)	p-value (db/db vs db/m+)	Fold-change (db/db vs db/db-CAT Tg)	p-value (db/db vs db/db-CAT Tg)
1450231_a_at	baculoviral IAP repeat-containing 4	1.28	0.0039	1.29	0.0038
1454880_s_at	Bcl2-modifying factor	3.07	0.0099	3.07	0.0098
1449297_at	caspase 12	1.82	0.0069	1.81	0.0070
1431875_a_at	E2F transcription factor 1	1.19	0.0065	1.19	0.0064
1423602_at 1445452_at	Tnf receptor-associated factor 1	1.99	0.0073	1.97	0.0074

Fig. 4. List of genes up-regulated in microarray chips of db/db vs db/m+ and db/db vs db/db CAT-Tg mice

One hypothesis that needs further examination is whether intrarenal RAS overactivation and chronic hyperglycemia may act synergistically to induce ROS generation and subsequently induce endoplasmic reticulum (ER) stress in RPTCs and enhance ER-stress gene expression such as caspase-12, glucose-regulated protein 78 (GRP78)/ immunoglobulin-heavy-chain-binding protein (BiP), and CCAAT/enhancer-binding protein homologous protein (CHOP) expression and activation, triggering the initiation and amplification of the apoptotic cascade leading to tubular apoptosis.

4. References

[1] Kaul K, Hodgkinson A, Tarr J, Kohner EM, Chibber R. Is Inflammation a Common Retinal-Renal-Nerve Pathogenic Link in Diabetes? *Curr Diabetes Rev.* 2010; 6:294-303.

[2] Marcovecchio ML, Chiarelli F. Microvascular disease in children and adolescents with type 1 diabetes and obesity. *Pediatr Nephrol.* 2010; 26: 365-375.

[3] Jensen T, Borch-Johnsen K, Kofoed-Enevoldsen A, Deckert T. Coronary artery disease in young type 1 (insulin-dependent) diabetic patients with and without diabetic nephropathy: incidence and risk factors. *Diabetologia* 1987; 30:144-148

[4] Bello AK, Thadhani R, Hemmelgarn B, Klarenbach S, Gill J, Chan C, Zimmerman D, Holmes D, Cembrowski G, Opgenorth D, Sibrian R, Karkhaneh M, Tiv S, Wiebe N, Tonelli M. Design and implementation of the canadian kidney disease cohort study (CKDCS): A prospective observational study of incident hemodialysis patients. *BMC Nephrol.* 2011; 12:10.

[5] Dalla Vestra M, Saller A, Bortoloso E, Mauer M, Fioretto P. Structural involvement in type 1 and type 2 diabetic nephropathy. *Diabetes Metab.* 2000; 26 (Suppl 4):8-14.

[6] Brezniceanu ML, Liu F, Wei CC, Tran S, Sachetelli S, Zhang SL, Guo DF, Filep JG, Ingelfinger JR, Chan JSD. Catalase overexpression attenuates angiotensinogen expression and apoptosis in diabetic mice. *Kidney Int.* 2007; 71:912-23.

[7] National Kidney Foundation . KDOQI clinical practice guidelines and clinical practice recommendations for diabetes and chronic kidney disease. *Am J Kidney Dis.* 2007; 49 (suppl 2):S12–S154.

[8] Patel A; ADVANCE Collaborative Group, MacMahon S, Chalmers J, Neal B, Woodward M, Billot L, Harrap S, Poulter N, Marre M, Cooper M, Glasziou P, Grobbee DE, Hamet P, Heller S, Liu LS, Mancia G, Mogensen CE, Pan CY, Rodgers A, Williams B. Effects of a fixed combination of perindopril and indapamide on macrovascular and microvascular outcomes in patients with type 2 diabetes mellitus (the ADVANCE trial): a randomised controlled trial. *Lancet.* 2007; 370:829-840

[9] Yusuf S, Sleight P, Pogue J, Bosch J, Davies R, Dagenais G. Effects of an angiotensin-converting-enzyme inhibitor, ramipril, on cardiovascular events in high-risk patients. The Heart Outcomes Prevention Evaluation Study Investigators. N Engl J Med. 2000; 342:145-153.

[10] Lewis EJ, Hunsicker LG, Bain RP, Rohde RD, for the Collaborative Study Group. The effect of angiotensin-converting-enzyme inhibition on diabetic nephropathy. *N Engld Med.* 1993;329:1456-1462.

[11] Heart Outcomes Prevention Evaluation Study Investigators. Effects of ramipril on cardiovascular and microvascular outcomes in people with diabetes mellitus. Results of the HOPE Study and MICRO-HOPE Sub-Study. *Lancet* 2000; 355: 253–259.

[12] Brenner BM, Cooper ME, de Zeeuw D, for the RENAAL Study Investigators. Effects of losartan on renal and cardiovascular outcomes in patients with type 2 diabetes and nephropathy. *N Engl J Med* 2001; 345: 861–869.
[13] Mogensen CE, Neldam S, Tikkanen I, for the CALM Study group. Randomised controlled trial of dual blockade of renin-angiotensin system in patients with hypertension, microalbuminuria, and non-insulin dependent diabetes: the Candesartan and Lisinopril Microalbuminuria (CALM) study. *BMJ* 2000; 321: 1440–1444.
[14] Krause MW, Fonseca VA, Shah SV. Combination inhibition of the renin-angiotensin system: is more better? *Kidney Int.* 2011; 80:245-55.
[15] Basso N, Terragno NA. History about the discovery of the renin-angiotensin system. *Hypertension.* 2001; 38: 1246–1249.
[16] Murphy TJ, Alexander RW, Griendling KK, Runge MS, Bernstein KE. Isolation of a cDNA encoding the vascular type-1 angiotensin II receptor. *Nature* 1991; 351:233–236
[17] Cheng H-F, Becker BN, Burns KD, Harris RC. Angiotensin II upregulates type-1 angiotensin II receptors in renal proximal tubule. *J Clin Invest* 1995; 77:1993–2000.
[18] Burns KD. Angiotensin II and its receptors in the diabetic kidney. *Am J Kidney Dis* 2000; 36:449–467.
[19] Ruiz-Ortega M, Esteban V, Suzuki Y, Ruperez M, Mezzano S, Ardiles L, Justo P, Ortiz A, Egido J. Renal expression of angiotensin type 2 (AT2) receptors during kidney damage. *Kidney Int Suppl.* 2003 Oct;(86):S21-6.
[20] Zhuo JL, Li XC. New insights and perspectives on intrarenal renin-angiotensin system: focus on intracrine-intracellular angiotensin II. *Peptides* 2011; 32:1551-1565.
[21] Handa RK. Characterization and signaling of the AT4 receptor in human proximal tubule epithelial (HK-2) cells. *JASN* 2011; 12:440-449.
[22] Kagami S, Border WA, Miller DE, Noble NA. Angiotensin II stimulated extracellular matrix protein synthesis through induction of transforming growth factor-β expression in rat glomerular cells. *J Clin Invest* 1994; 93:2431–2437.
[23] Leehey DJ, Song RH, Alavi N, Singh AK. Decreased degradative enzymes in mesangial cells cultured in high glucose media. *Diabetes* 1995; 44:929–935.
[24] Liu F, Brezniceanu ML, Wei CC, Chénier I, Sachetelli S, Zhang SL, Filep JG, Ingelfinger JR, Chan JSD. Overexpression of angiotensinogen increases tubular apoptosis in diabetes. *J Am Soc Nephrol.* 2008;19: 269-80.
[25] Hsieh TJ, Zhang SL, Filep JG, Tang SS, Ingelfinger JR, Chan JSD. High glucose stimulates angiotensinogen gene expression via reactive oxygen species generation in rat kidney proximal tubular cells. *Endocrinology.* 2002; 143:2975-2985.
[26] Hsieh T-J, Fustier P, Wei C-C, Zhang S-L, Filep JG, Tang S-S, Ingelfinger JR, Fantus IG, Hamet P, Chan JSD. Reactive oxygen species blockade and action of insulin on the expression of angiotensinogen in proximal tubular cells. J Endocrinology 2004; 183:535-550.
[27] Li H, Weatherford ET, Davis DR, Keen HL, Grobe JL, Daugherty A, Cassis LA, Allen AM, Sigmund CD. Renal Proximal Tubule Angiotensin AT1A Receptors Regulate Blood Pressure. Am J Physiol Regul Integr Comp Physiol. 2011; 301: R1067-1077.
[28] Seikaly MG, Arant BS, Seney FD *et al*: Endogenous angiotensin concentrations in specific intrarenal fluid compartments of the rat. *J Clin Invest* 1990; 86: 1352-1357.
[29] Donoghue M, Hsieh F, Baronas E, Godbout K, Gosselin M, Stagliano N, Donovan M, Woolf B, Robison K, Jeyaseelan R, Breitbart RE, Acton S. A novel angiotensin-

converting enzyme-related carboxypeptidase (ACE2) converts angiotensin I to angiotensin 1-9. Circ Res. 2000; 87:E1-9.

[30] Reich HN, Oudit GY, Penninger JM, Scholey JW, Herzenberg AM. Decreased glomerular and tubular expression of ACE2 in patients with type 2 diabetes and kidney disease. *Kidney Int.* 2008; 74: 1610–6.

[31] Shiota A, Yamamoto K, Ohishi M, Tatara Y, Ohnishi M, Maekawa Y, Iwamoto Y, Takeda M, Rakugi H. Loss of ACE2 accelerates time-dependent glomerular and tubulointerstitial damage in streptozotocin-induced diabetic mice. *Hypertens Res.* 2010; 33:298-307.

[32] Zhang SL, To C, Chen X, Filep JG, Tang SS, Ingelfinger JR, Chan JSD. Essential role(s) of the intrarenal renin-angiotensin system in transforming growth factor-beta1 gene expression and induction of hypertrophy of rat kidney proximal tubular cells in high glucose. J Am Soc Nephrol. 2002; 13:302-12.

[33] Giacco F, Brownlee M. Oxidative stress and diabetic complications. *Circ Res.* 2010; 107: 1058-1070.

[34] Sachetelli S, Liu Q, Zhang SL, Liu F, Hsieh TJ, Brezniceanu ML, Guo DF, Filep JG, Ingelfinger JR, Sigmund CD, Hamet P, Chan JSD. RAS blockade decreases blood pressure and proteinuria in transgenic mice overexpressing rat angiotensinogen gene in the kidney. *Kidney Int.* 2006; 69:1016-1023.

[35] Ding Y, Davisson RL, Hardy DO, Zhu LJ, Merrill DC, Catterall JF, Sigmund CD. The kidney androgen-regulated protein promoter confers renal proximal tubule cell-specific and highly androgen-responsive expression on the human angiotensinogen gene in transgenic mice. *J Biol Chem.* 1997; 272: 28142-28148.

[36] Sugaru E, Nakagawa T, Ono-Kishino M, Nagamine J, Tikunaga T, Kitoh M, Hume WE, Nagata R, Taiji M: Amelioration of established diabetic nephropathy by combined treatment with SMP-534 (antifibrotic agent) and losartan in db/db mice. *Nephron Exp Nephrol.* 2006; 105: 45-52.

[37] Godin N, Liu F, Lau GJ, Brezniceanu ML, Chénier I, Filep JG, Ingelfinger JR, Zhang SL, Chan JSD. Catalase overexpression prevents hypertension and tubular apoptosis in angiotensinogen transgenic mice. *Kidney Int.* 2010; 77:1086-1097.

[38] Brezniceanu ML, Liu F, Wei C-C, Chénier I, Godin N, Zhang SL, Filep JG, Ingelfinger JR, Chan JSD. Attenuation of interstitial fibrosis and tubular apoptosis in db/db transgenic mice overexpressing catalase in renal proximal tubular cells. *Diabetes* 2008; 57:451-459

[39] Brezniceanu ML, Lau CJ, Godin N, Chénier I, Duclos A, Ethier J, Filep JG, Ingelfinger JR, Zhang SL, Chan JSD. Reactive oxygen species promote caspase-12 expression and tubular apoptosis in diabetic nephropathy. *J Am Soc Nephrol.* 2010; 21:943-954.

3

Diabetic Nephropathy: Role of Aldosterone and Benefits of Therapy with Aldosterone Receptor Blocker

Jayson Yap and Mohammad G. Saklayen
VA Medical Center and Wright State University Boonshoft School of Medicine, Dayton, OH USA

1. Introduction

ACE-inhibitor and angiotensin receptor blocker (ARB) have been shown to reduce proteinuria and progression of renal dysfunction in both type 1 and type 2 diabetics (1-11). However, even with optimal use of ACE-Inhibitor or ARB, the progression of renal dysfunction is not completely stopped. Even in studies where ACEI or ARB therapy showed improved outcome, a very high percentage of patients still progress. This scenario is now highlighted in a recent study published in JAMA, which shows the incidence of diabetic nephropathy increasing in USA in excess of what can be accounted for by the increased incidence of type 2 DM in the population (12). The present treatment strategy is therefore not adequate and other additional effective treatment strategies are urgently needed.

Since the publication of the landmark RALES study (13) showing a significant survival benefit in patients with systolic heart failure when treated with aldosterone inhibition in addition to ACEI and beta-blockers, the interest in the vasculotoxic effect of aldosterone and the beneficial therapeutic effects of aldosterone receptor blocker drugs like spironolactone has been steadily increasing (14).

2. Aldosterone biology and lessons learnt from animal models

In addition to its classical action in the distal nephron, aldosterone is now known to exert many other effects on other areas of kidneys as well as in cardiovascular tissues. (14)

Aldosterone is now known to have a significant role in renal hemodynamics, independent of Angiotensin II. In a remnant kidney model in the rat Greene et al showed that there was >10-fold rise in aldosterone in the remnant kidney rats (REM) compared to sham operated ones (15). As expected, proteinuria, hypertension and glomerulosclerosis in the REM rats were attenuated with treatment using ACE-inhibitor or angiotensin receptor blockers. However, when these treated rats (REM AIIA) were given an aldosterone infusion the extent of proteinuria, hypertension and glomerulosclerosis were similar to untreated (REM) rats, suggesting deleterious renal hemodynamic effects of aldosterone independent of angiotensin II. Use of spironolactone in these rats transiently reduced proteinuria and lowered arterial pressure.

In rats with 5/6th nephrectomy, adrenalectomy and protein restriction independently ameliorated the ablative nephropathy independent of the corticosterone maintenance level (16). In stroke-prone spontaneously hypertensive rats (SHRSP), renal vascular injury causing proteinuria and malignant nephrosclerotic lesions were markedly reduced by treatment with spironolactone (17). The effect of spironolactone alone was comparable to the effect of treatment with captopril. In another study the ameliorating effect of ACE-inhibition in the SHRSP rats could be fully reversed by infusion of aldosterone, suggesting a major additive role for aldosterone in the vascular injury in these rats(18). Importantly, the deleterious effects of aldosterone and the protective effects of spironolactone against renal damage in SHRSP rats appeared to be independent of the blood pressure.

Renal damage, as evidenced by albuminuria and glomerulosclerosis, in response to 5/6 nephrectomy was markedly less in mineralocorticoid resistant Wistar-Furth rats compared to Wistar rats. Treatment of hypertension in the nephrectomized Wistar rats did not protect them from renal injury(19), suggesting again that mineralocorticoid mediated deleterious effect was independent of the blood pressure.

Hyperaldosteronism has been noted as a component of clinical chronic renal insufficiency of various etiologies including diabetic nephropathy (20-21). In a cross sectional study of patients with mild to moderate renal insufficiency, Hene et al observed that the level of serum aldosterone increased several fold as creatinine clearance fell below 50% of normal (22). The significance of this hyperaldosteronism to the progression of the renal insufficiency has not been studied systematically, but in one longitudinal study Walker noted a significant correlation between aldosterone level and rate of progression of renal failure (23). In this longitudinal cohort study of 131 diabetics, Walker noted that hypertension, plasma angiotensin II and aldosterone were independent predictors of accelerated loss of renal function.

In vitro studies of cultured mesangial cells revealed increased production of type IV collagen after incubation with aldosterone (24-25). In addition to the classical genomic action through the type 1 mineralocorticoid receptor, aldosterone is now known to have significant non-genomic actions in many different tissues including kidney tubules, mesangial cells, podocytes and vascular smooth muscle cells. Aldosterone also up-regulates angiotensin II membrane receptors thereby multiplying the vascular effect of Ang II. This up-regulation is inhibited by treatment with spironolactone (26-30).

The renoprotective effects of MR blockers have been demonstrated in a variety of animal models. While the benefits were seen in most of these models , mechanism of the beneficial actions were deemed different in different models, depending on the primary focus of the investigators. One area of interest was ACE2 generation. Angiotensin II (which comes from angiotensinogen released by the liver which is converted to inactive Ang I by ACE and then to biologically active Ang II) acts mainly through the AT1 receptor to mediate vasoconstriction/proliferation and the AT2 receptor which mediates vasodilatation and antiproliferation. Ang(1-7) is generated from Ang II by ACE2 and counteracts some of the biologic effects of Ang II. In the Dahl-sensitive hypertensive rat fed a high salt diet, treatment with epleronone normalized blood pressure and decreased the levels of type IV collagen mRNA, angiotensinogen and ACE mRNA, but did not affect ACE2mRNA expression and is possibly protective by decreasing the formation of angiotensin II but not vasodilatory Ang (1-7). On the other hand, candesartan increased ACE 2 mRNA expression, suggesting that aldosterone blockade and angiotensin receptor blockade may be complimentary (31). Treatment with epleronone also reduced urinary protein excretion, renal injury scores and decreased (pro)renin receptor protein expression, angiotensinogen and AT1R mRNA levels and kidney Ang II content in the same rat model. (32)

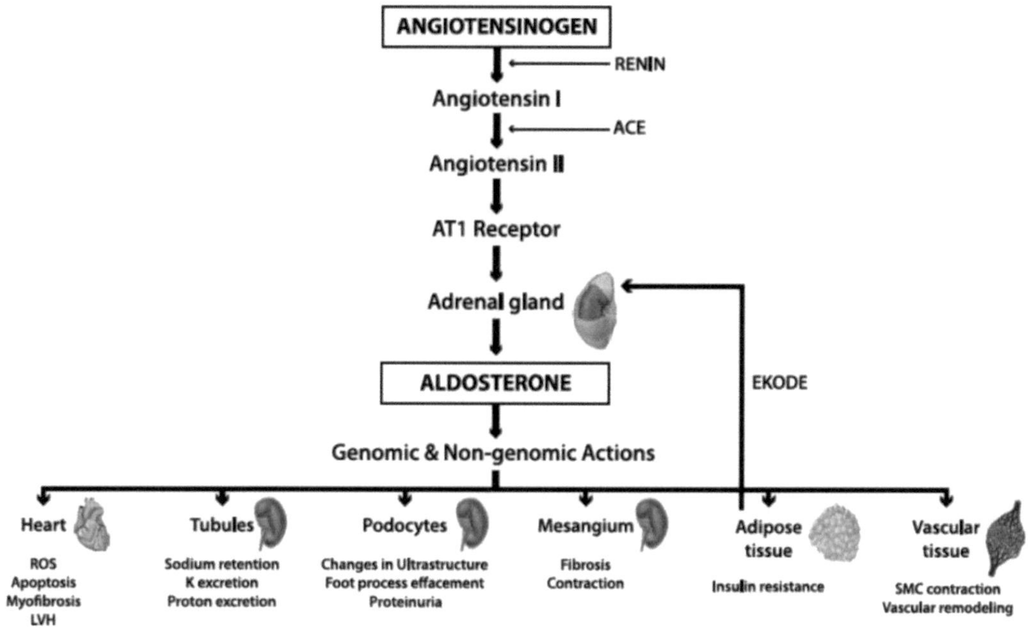

Fig. 1. Angiotensin-Aldosterone Axis and the Physiologic Effects of Aldosterone
ROS Reactive Oxygen Species, *AT1* Angiotensin I, *EKODE* epoxy-9keto-10trans-octadecenoic acid, *SMC* smooth muscle cell

In the diabetic rat model, spironolactone treatment was associated with a reduction in urinary albumin excretion and amelioration of glomerulosclerosis despite no change in blood pressure. In various organs including the kidney, there is a local system for aldosterone generation. High glucose stimulates the expression of CYP 11B2 and mineralocorticoid receptor. Spironolactone in addition to blockade of the aldosterone receptor, was also able to reduce intrinsic renal ACE and also aldosterone synthase gene (CYP 11B2) expression in the streptozotocin-induced diabetic mice without affecting blood sugar or blood pressure (33).

Monocyte chemotactic protein (MCP-1) synthesis and nuclear factor-kB are markers of inflammation increased in renal tissue and in urine of diabetic rats and patients. In the cultured mesangial and proximal tubular cells there was inhibition of urinary excretion of MCP-1 (MCP-1) and its upstream transcription factor NF-kB suggesting that aldosterone mediated activation of proinflammatory cytokines was blocked (34).

Transforming growth factor –B1 is a cytokine involved in ECM deposition, proliferation and fibrosis. Some of its tissue effects are mediated by connective tissue growth factor (CTGF). Aldosterone increases expression of TGF-1 and may directly induce CTGF. Spironolactone reduced TGF-B1 expression and CTGF and renal collagen synthesis through a TGF-B1 independent pathway (not inhibited by prior TGF-B1 neutralization). (35)

Plasminogen Activator inhibitor (PAI-1) inhibits fibrinolysis and mediates ECM accumulation in mesangial and fibroblast cells and glomerulosclerosis. Its synthesis is induced by aldosterone and potentiated by the presence of TGF-B1. Spironolactone treatment reduced expression of PAI-1 and TGF-b in streptozotocin-induced diabetic rats and improves the antioxidant environment by reducing the fall in superoxide dismutase and glutathione peroxidase that accompanies diabetes induction resulting in reduced malondialdehyde levels (lipid oxidation byproduct) (36).

VEGF is a cytokine involved in the early development of diabetic nephropathy and its expression is increased by glucose, AGE, TGF-B1 and IGF-1. Aldosterone infusion increases renal VEGF synthesis. Spironolactone alone and in combination with losartan reduced VEGF, MCP-1 and malondialdehyde expression resulting in reduced mesangial expansion and sclerosis in an OLETF model. (37)

Aldosterone inhibition was also useful in reducing blood pressure and renal injury in diabetic mice which had impaired endothelial nitric oxide response induced by eNOS knockout. These mice did not have good response to ACE or ARB therapy. (38).

Recent studies have also investigated the effects of epleronone alone or in addition to ACE or ARB therapy in the diabetic rat. Mineralocorticoid receptor (MR) expression is increased in diabetic rats (OLETF) and epleronone reduced cortical levels of MR protein, MR RNA, TGF–b mRNA and osteopontin mRNA and improved various histological measures of renal injury along with albuminuria (39). The combination of epleronone and enalapril resulted in greatest decrease in TGF-b, Type IV collagen and TPA-1 expression both in the whole kidney and in cultured mesangial cells accompanied by an improvement in albuminuria, GFR and glomerulosclerosis compared to either agent alone. (40). In streptozotocin diabetic rats, the addition of epleronone with ramipril prevented glomerular hyperfiltration but did not have an additive effect on proteinuria or glomerular hypertrophy (41). Again in OLETF diabetic rats, epleronone added to telmisartan did not alter systolic blood pressure but resulted in greater reduction in proteinuria and podocyte injury and a greater increase in nephrin and podocin mRNA levels. Hydralazine decreased SBP but did not alter any of the renal parameters. (42)

Epleronone protected against podocyte damage in the hypertensive rat model as evidenced by reduced expression of podocyte injury markers desmin and B7-1. Mechanisms involved include inhibition of NADPH oxidase (p22phox and gp91phox), which is induced by aldosterone and generates reactive oxygen species , and reduced aldosterone effector kinase Sgk1, which is involved in diabetes stimulated matrix deposition. Unlike epleronone, hydralazine did not improve proteinuria or marker expression despite equivalent BP control. Local expression of apoptosis related molecules (caspase-3 and Bax) as well as reduction of BCl-2 (apoptosis regulatory protein) in podocytes of diabetic rats was prevented by treatment with spironolactone. Based on these studies, Shibata et al surmised that it is possible that Sgk1 plays a key role as the common effector molecule of the MR signaling in podocytes. (43-45)

During the progression of renal damage, aldosterone might be involved in injury to the glomerular podocytes, mesangium, tubulointerstitium and tubules through locally expressed Mineralocorticoid receptor (MR).(46-48) However, the precise molecular mechanisms responsible for aldosterone and MR-induced cell injury are unclear. In the kidney, aldosterone activates multiple intracellular mechanisms including reactive oxygen species, mitogen-activated protein kinases (MAPKs) and Rho-kinase etc. by activating MR(49-50). These molecular mechanisms have been reviewed recently(51-52).

The renoprotective effects of spironolactone or epleronone had been seen in many other animal models of renal injury not limited to diabetic nephropathy, as noted in a recent review by Nishiyama et al. (46) These models included streptozotocin-induced and other forms of diabetic rats and mice, obese SHR rats, murine lupus nephritis, unilateral ureteral obstruction, ischemia reperfusion injury, 5/6th nephrectomised rats and rats treated with AngII infusion, NO synthase inhibitor or cyclosporine(53-66). In these animal models, treatment with aldosterone blockers had no effect on systemic blood pressure. Thus, these observations are consistent with the concept that aldosterone and MR-dependent renal injury is not dependent on blood pressure changes but on their local actions.

Metabolic syndrome with or without diabetes causes podocyte injury and progressive nephropathy. In type 2 diabetes, coexistent metabolic syndrome plays a synergistic role in progressive renal injury. Nagase et al investigated the role of aldosterone signaling in rats with metabolic syndrome(67). Proteinuria was prominent in SHR/NDmcr-cp compared with nonobese SHR, which was accompanied by podocyte injury as evidenced by foot process effacement, induction of desmin and attenuation of nephrin. Serum aldosterone level, renal and glomerular expression of aldosterone effector kinase Sgk1, and oxidative stress markers all were elevated in SHR/NDmcr-cp. Mineralocorticoid receptors were expressed in glomerular podocytes. Eplerenone treatment effectively reduced podocyte damage, proteinuria, Sgk1, and oxidant stress. Pretreatment with antioxidant tempol also alleviated podocyte impairment and proteinuria, along with inhibition of Sgk1.

When these investigators looked for the source of the excess aldosterone , it was found that visceral adipocytes, isolated from SHR/NDmcr-cp, secreted substances that stimulated aldosterone production in adrenocortical cells. The aldosterone-releasing activity of adipocytes was not inhibited by candesartan. Adipocytes from nonobese SHR did not show such activity. That visceral adipocytes may be the source of factors causing excess aldosterone was , however, first noted by Ehrhart-Bornstein et al (68) and later the secreted factor was further characterized as EKODE (12,13-epoxy-9keto-10(trans)-octadecenoic acid) by Goodfriend et al. (69) These are mainly oxidized polyunsaturated fatty acids produced by adipocytes. One of the most potent one is an oxidized product of linoleic acid (EKODE). EKODE stimulated aldosteronogenesis at concentrations from 0.5 to 5 micromol/L but inhibited it at higher dose. In samples from 24 adults levels of EKODE correlated directly with aldosterone level and in a subsample of 12 blacks in the cohort it correlated with body mass index and systolic blood pressure. The resistant hypertension seen in patients with abdominal obesity is partly due to these autacoids secreted by visceral adipocytes, and BP in these patients respond very well to the use of spironolactone. This may explain the observation in the Framingham study that plasma aldosterone concentration was significantly correlated with the risk of onset of the metabolic syndrome.

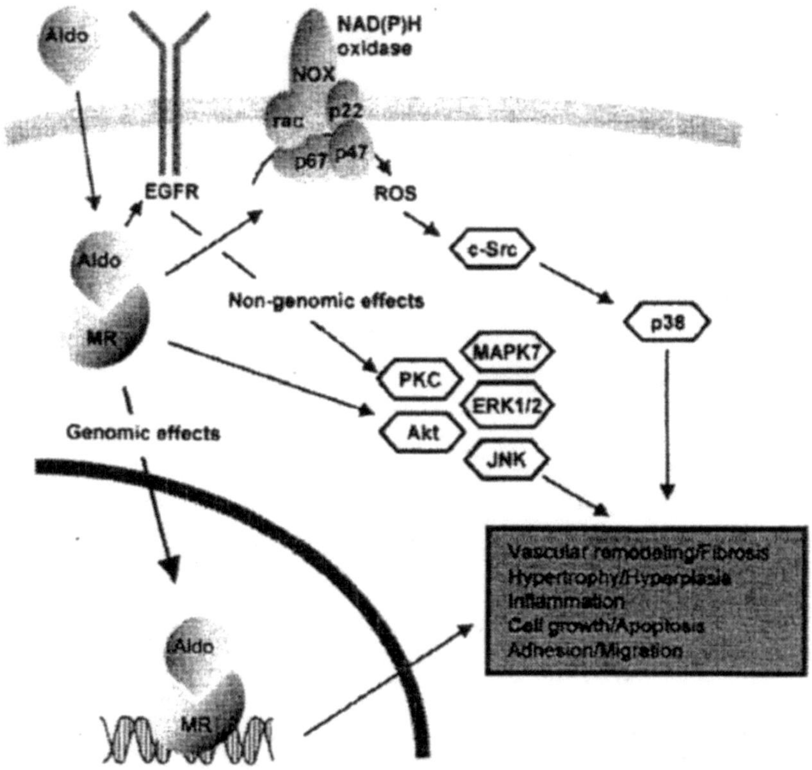

Fig. 2. Mechanisms of genomic (long term) and nongenomic (rapid) effects of aldosterone. Aldosterone activates the tyrosine kinase c-Src through the production of ROS, leading to the activation of p38MAPK and also various signalling molecules like PKC, Akt, ERK ½, ERK5, Mapk7, and JNK. Aldosterone also mediates the activation of EGFR. Genomic and rapid effects of aldosterone lead to vascularremodeling, hypertrophy, inflammation, cell growth, apoptosis, adhesion, and migration. *Aldo* aldosterone, *EGFR* epidermal growth factor, *MR* mineralocorticoid receptor, *ROS* reactive oxygen species. Other abbreviations as in Fig. 1. (Ref. 93)

2.1 Human studies using aldosterone receptor blockers

Within the past decade, several human studies have been conducted exploring the effects of spironolactone and epleronone on patients with chronic kidney disease with or without diabetes between which we shall be concentrating on the latter.

Since ACE-I/ARB therapy had been generally accepted as standard therapy for patients with diabetic nephropathy, most studies conducted with aldosterone receptor blocker drug like spironolactone involved the addition of this agent to either single agent ACE-I or ARB (referred hence to as single- drug add-on) (70-74) or to combined ACE-I/ARB therapy (dual-drug add-on) (75-76). Epleronone likewise has been tested as add-on therapy to enalapril (77-78).

In one study (79), albeit in non-diabetic patients, where spironolactone was compared head-to-head to the ACE-I drug cilazapril along with the combination, it was found that spironolactone was slightly better at reducing albuminuria than cilazapril, but the combination resulted in a further reduction. The blood pressure reduction was the same among the three groups.

A review of the studies where spironolactone was used as single-drug or dual-drug add-on, the degree of albuminuria or proteinuria reduction was about 30-35% with a trend towards a further reduction in studies that had an extended period of observation of up to a year (76). The reduction in albuminuria was greater when spironolactone was used as single-drug add on compared to dual-drug add on (although one study (80) reported an impressive 58% reduction). The addition of spironolactone to baseline ACE-I (lisinopril) therapy resulted in greater reduction in albuminuria compared to the addition of an ARB agent (losartan) to baseline ACE-I (74). This was confirmed in another study that demonstrated that the addition of spironolactone to either single-drug (ramipril) or dual-drug (ramipril + irbesartan) baseline therapy resulted in further reduction in albuminuria but the addition of ARB alone to the ACE-I did not further reduce albuminuria. (75). Several studies correlated the degree of proteinuria reduction to a drop in GFR and to the preexisting serum aldosterone level. Urinary type IV collagen, which is stimulated by aldosterone and is a reflection of renal fibrosis, was also decreased. (73,80)

The efficacy of spironolactone as add-on agent in patients with uncontrolled hypertension specifically those with features of aldosterone excess, such as obesity and low serum potassium levels, has been demonstrated in several studies . The reduction of systolic BP in these studies exceeds 20 mmHg. In the studies we are reviewing on diabetic nephropathy, most of whom again, were already on preexisting ACE-I and ARB therapy, the focus of the aldosterone antagonist add-on was on proteinuria and renal function. The reduction in BP was more modest. When used as single-agent add-on, several studies show a drop of 6-8 mmHg in systolic BP or ABPM with an additional smaller reduction with longer followup. One study showed no further drop in blood pressure, but this group of patients had overall a very high GFR (73). Addition of epleronone to enalapril produced only a non-significant change in BP (22). Spironolactone used as dual-drug add-on generally did not further reduce BP (75). There has been controversy among researchers in the field as to whether the reduction in proteinuria with aldosterone antagonists is a result purely of further BP lowering, but these studies demonstrate that it is much easier to show a reduction of proteinuria that is statistically significant compared to a reduction in blood pressure.

The study results regarding the effects of aldosterone antagonists on renal function must be interpreted with caution. First of all, most of the studies followed renal function through measurement of serum creatinine or an estimation of GFR mathematically derived from creatinine levels, and it is well recognized that this is an insensitive marker to small changes in renal function. One exception are the studies from Denmark (26) which actually measured GFR directly. Secondly, the studies all excluded patients with Stage 4 and 5 CKD., and in fact the mean baseline GFR in most studies exceeded 60 ml/minute, and there are not enough patients in Stage 3 CKD to really draw any meaningful conclusions as to the effects of aldosterone antagonists on patients with more advanced CKD. With these caveats, the published studies indicate that the effect of spironolactone or epleronone on GFR is comparable to the effect of initiation of ACE-I or ARB agents . Single-drug add-on in most studies resulted in a 3-5 ml/min drop in GFR, while dual-agent add-on caused no further drop in GFR. The effects are most prominent in the first month or two after initiation, and drop in GFR is greater in those with baseline impaired function. One study in particular showed a sharp 13 ml/min decrease in GFR with spironolactone compared to baseline ACE-I or ARB therapy, but this decrease occurred early and eventually leveled off. Associated with this was a sharp drop in albuminuria of 40%. Many studies confirm that the reduction in proteinuria correlates well with the degree in reduction of GFR.

Most of the adverse effects noted includes the known incidence of anti-androgenic effects of spironolactone and hyperkalemia which correlates with the dosage used. Epleronone is of course, free of the first set of side effects and generally results in less hyperkalemia, but this may be a function of the dosages currently being studied . Most studies excluded patients with baseline potassium exceeding 4.5 or 5.0 mmol/L. The trend of the results show that while dual-agent therapy had a greater tendency towards hyperkalemia when compared to single agent therapy, the addition of spironolactone to either ACE-I or ARB resulted in the highest risk of hyperkalemia. This complication may be more frequent among diabetics who tend to have hyporeninemic hypoaldosteronism and is definitely more prevalent in patients with lower baseline GFR, higher baseline potassium, and preexisting metabolic acidosis. With the background of the experience after publication of the RALES study, when practitioners promoted the use of spironolactone for heart failure in patients outside the inclusion criteria of the study, resulting in the appearance of several near fatal hyperkalemic episodes, it behooves us to follow the patients with more advanced CKD more closely and to check serum potassium agents earlier if we choose to use these agents for diabetic nephropathy. There was a suggestion that glucose tolerance worsened after spironolactone with a rise in Hba1c (70,81)), but this was not seen in other studies (78). Spironolactone may also decrease BNP over that achieved by ACE-I (84).

A small study conducted by these authors(82) using a randomized double-blind crossover design to study the effects of spironolactone when added to ACE-I or ARB shows similar results to the studies quoted above, in that spironolactone produced a 57% reduction in proteinuria along with a 7mmHg drop in systolic BP. This was accompanied by a rise in creatinine of about 0.2 mg/dl and serum potassium of 0.3 mEq/L.

The role of aldosterone antagonists in the treatment of diabetic nephropathy may lie in the group of patients whose blood pressure or proteinuria are uncontrolled despite ACE-I or ARB therapy, or who manifest so-called 'aldosterone escape" when aldosterone levels increase after long-term RAAS blockade. (83-84)). Table 1 lists all the clinical trials using Aldosterone receptor blockers in proteinuric patients. As shown in the table the range of proteinuria reduction with additional use of aldosterone receptor blocker was 19% to 58%.(70-87) Aldosterone antagonists seem to be more effective and more economical when added to ACE-I compared to ARBs at this time, albeit at the price of greater risk for acute GFR drop and hyperkalemia. Unfortunately, no long term studies are available at this time to demonstrate that renal function decline is slowed by this approach, and proteinuria is taken as a marker of disease progression, as was with ACE-I/ARB therapy at an earlier time point.

3. Future direction

The beneficial effects of mineralocorticoid/aldosterone receptor blockers in ameliorating or stopping the progression of diabetic nephropathy is impressive in in-vitro studies using mesangial, podocytes or endothelial cell culture system. These studies also help us understand the molecular mechanism by which these agents ameliorate the pathologic process. In-vivo animal model studies also showed encouraging results as elaborated in preceding pages. Similar benefits have been seen in human studies as summarized in the table 1. However most of the human studies were of relative short duration. Longest study

Author/Year	No. of Patients/ Design of Study	Drugs/Dose/ Duration (Weeks)	Reduction in Proteinuria (%)	△ In Sys.BPmmHg/ GFRml/min/ Kmeq/L
Chrysostomou / 2001	8 / Uncontrolled	SP / 25 / 4	54%	
Epstein / 2002	141/(74 + 67) RCT–Parallel	EP / 200 / 12	19%	3/ - / -
Rachmani /2004	60/RCT-Parallel	SP / 100 / 24	19%	--
Sato / 2005	32 / Uncontrolled	SP / 25 / 12	38%	- / - / ↑0·1
Bianchi / 2005	42 / Uncontrolled	SP / 25 / 8	37%	- / - / ↑0·4
Schjoedt / 2005	20 / RCT-Crossover	SP / 25 / 8	30%	↓8 / - / -
Rossing / 2005	21 / RCT-Crossover	SP / 25 / 8	33%	↓6 / ↓ 3 / -
Van den Meiracker / 2006	59 (29 + 30) RCT-Parallel	SP / 25-50 / 8	41%	↓7 / ↓ 8 / -
Schjoedt / 2006	20 / RCT-Crossover	SP / 25 / 8	32%	↓6 / ↓ 3 /↑0·2
Chrysostomou /2006	41 / RCT-Parallel	SP / 25 / 12 (4 group)	14%	↓9/ - /↑0·2
Bianchi / 2006	165 (82 + 83) RCT–Parallel	SP / 25 / 52	58%	- / ↑ ↓/↑ 0·8
Epstein/2006	268/RCT-Parallel	Ep/50-100/12	41%(high dose) 34%(low dose)	↓4 / ↓ 6 / -
Ogawa 2006	30/RCT	SP / 25 / 52	47%	↓11/ - / -
Furumatsu 2008	25/RCT	SP / 25 / 52	58%	/ - / -
Saklayen 2008	24/RCT-Crossover	SP / 25 / 12	57%	↓12 / ↓8 / ↑0.3
Davidson 2008	24/Uncontrol	SP / 25 / 4	26%	↓9 / - / -
Mehdi 2009	81/ RCT	SP/ 25 / 52	52%	/ - / ↑

Legend: Table showing summaries of the clinical studies done with aldosterone receptor blocker in addition to ACE inhibitor or ARB use in proteinuric patients.

Table 1.

follow up was 1 year. And none of these studies examined the long term renal outcomes, especially progression to ESRD, need for dialysis or overall mortality. This paucity of clinical outcome studies is of major concern. Of note, when clinical studies of short duration showed additional lowering of microalbuminuria/proteinuria in diabetic nephropathy as well as in other proteinuric renal diseases, nephrologists became enthusiastic about dual use of ACEI and ARB in patients with diabetic nephropathy. When the large international

ONTARGET study showed that renal outcomes (GFR deterioration, incidence of ESRD, need for dialysis and incidence of hyperkalemia) in diabetic nephropathy of patients on dual therapy was worse than on single agent therapy (ACEI or ARB alone), that initial enthusiasm was checked. (88) Dual ACEI and ARB use is no longer recommended in patients with diabetic nephropathy except in extraordinary situations.

However, the long term outcomes of MR/aldo blocker therapy with ACEI or ARB in diabetic nephropathy need not be similarly detrimental or non-beneficial. Of note while ONTARGET failed to show cardiovascular benefits with dual ACEI and ARB use and other studies showed lack of mortality benefits in dual use of ACEI and ARB in systolic heart failure(89), RALES and other studies (90) showed significant mortality benefit of adding spironolactone or epleronone to ACE or ARB in systolic heart failure patients. However, unless large clinical outcome studies confirm that adding aldosterone blockade to ACEI or ARB actually results in reduction of ESRD incidence, such therapy cannot be recommended without some caution.

When we did our small cross over study in a single institute, we selected patients carefully. Those patients who had hyperkalemia , even remotely, were excluded from participation. Most of our patients also were using high dose thiazide or loop diuretics. Our study, like many other similar studies, were of few weeks duration. As shown in POST RALES study, the incidence of hyperkalemia in Ontario was much higher than seen in the RALES study itself , when spironolactone use became widespread for systolic heart failure. (91)

Questions often arise if one were to use an aldosterone receptor blocker, which one to choose. Spironolactone is the first mineralocorticoid receptor antagonist (MRA) which has been in clinical use for over half a century. Epleronone is a relatively new mineralocorticoid receptor blocker and is still under patent protection. Compared to the latter, spironolactone blocks the androgen and progesterone receptors in addition to its primary blocking effects on mineralocorticoid receptors. This leads to some unpleasant problem of gynecomastia in male patients, the incidence of which is about 10%. Epleronone is much less likely to cause gynecomastia. But binding affinity of epleronone for MR is much lower than that of spironolactone. Spironolactone also has 3 active metabolites all of which have prolonged half life. Epleronone has half life of4-6 hours and its metabolites are not active. Because of these pharmacological and pharmacodynamic differences, spironolactone seems to be a clinically more effective MR blocking agent than epleronone. One recent comparison of treatment with spironolactone (75 to 225 mg daily) vs epleronone (100 to 300 mg daily) in patients with primary hyperaldosteronism showed better blood pressure lowering by spironolactone (diastolic BP reduction 12.5 mmHg in former vs 5.6 mmHg in later group). There has not been a head to head comparison of the two MR blockers in trials looking for a reduction of proteinuria or improvement in survival in patients with systolic dysfunction. (92)

4. References

[1] Lewis EJ, Hunsicker LG, Bain RP, et al. The effect of angiotensin-converting-enzyme inhibition on diabetic nephropathy.The Collaborative Study Group. N Engl J Med.1993;329(20):1456-1462.

[2] Viberti G, Mogensen CE, Groop LC, et al. Effect ofcaptopril on progression to clinical proteinuria in patientswith insulin-dependent diabetes mellitus and microalbuminuria. European Microalbuminuria Captopril Study Group. JAMA. 1994;271(4):275-279.

[3] Ravid M, Savin H, Jutrin I, et al. Long-term stabilizing effect of angiotensin-converting enzyme inhibition on plasma creatinine and on proteinuria in normotensive type II diabetic patients. Ann Intern Med. 1993;118(8):577-581.
[4] The Microalbuminuria Captopril Study Group. Captopril reduces the risk of nephropathy in IDDM patients with microalbuminuria. Diabetologia. 1996;39(5):587-593.
[5] Parving H-H, Lehnert H, Bro¨chner-Mortensen J, et al. The effects of Irbesartan on the development of diabetic nephropathy in patients with type 2 diabetes. N Engl JMed. 2001;345:870-878.
[6] Brenner BM, Cooper ME, de Zeeuw D, et al. Effects of losartan on renal and cardiovascular outcomes in patients with type 2 diabetes and nephropathy. N Engl J Med.2001;345:861-869.
[7] Rossing K, Jacobsen P, Pietraszek L, et al. Reno protective effects of adding angiotensin II receptor blocker to maximal recommended doses of ACE inhibitor in diabetic nephropathy: a randomized double-blind crossover trial. Diabetes Care. 2003;26:2268-2274.
[8] Andersen S, Tarnow L, Rossing P, et al. Reno protective effects of angiotensin II receptor blockade in type 1 diabetic patients with diabetic nephropathy. Kidney Int. 2000;57:601-606.
[9] Jacobsen P, Andersen S, Rossing K, et al. Dual blockade of the rennin-angiotensin system versus maximal recommended dose of ACE inhibition in diabetic nephropathy. Kidney Int. 2003;63:1874-1880.
[10] Sarafidis PA, Stafylas PC, Kanaki AI et al. Effects of renin-angiotensin system blockers on renal outcomes and all cause mortality in patients with diabetic nephropathy: an updated meta-analysis. Am J. Hypertens 2008; 21;922-9.
[11] Casas JP, Chua W, Loukogeorgakis S et al. Effects of inhibitors of the renin-angiotensin system and other antihypertensive drugs on renal outcomes: systemic review and met-analysis. Lancet 2005; 10:366:2026-33.
[12] De Boer IH, Rue TC , Hall YN et al. Temporal trends in the prevalence of Diabetic Kidney diseases in the United States. JAMA 2011; 305:2532-2539.
[13] Pitt B, Zannad F, Remme WJ, et al. The effect of spironolactone on morbidity and mortality in patients with severe heart failure. N Engl J Med. 1999;341:709-717.
[14] Ritz E and Tomaschitz A. Aldosterone, a vasculotoxic agent0 novel functions for an old hormone. Nephrol Dial Transplant 2009; 24:2302-2305.
[15] Greene EL, Kren S, Hostetter TH. Role of aldosterone in the remnant kidney model in the rat. J Clin Invest. 1996;98(4):1063-1068.
[16] Quan ZY, Walser M, Hill GS. Adrenalectomy ameliorates ablative nephropathy in the rat independently of corticosterone maintenance level. Kidney Int. 1992;41:326-33.
[17] Rocha R, Chander PN, Khanna K, et al. Mineralocorticoid blockade reduces vascular injury in stroke-prone hypertensive rats. Hypertension. 1998; 31:451-58.
[18] Rocha R, Chander PN, Zuckerman A, et al. Role of aldosterone in renal vascular injury in stroke-prone hypertensive rats. Hypertension. 1999; 33:232-37.
[19] Fitzgibbon WR, Greene EL, Grewal JS, Hutchison FN, Self SE, Latten SY, Ulian ME: Resistance to remnant nephropathy in the Wistar-Furth rat. J Am Soc Nephrol 1999 Apr;10(4):814-21
[20] Ferriss JB, Sullivan PA, Gonggrijp H, Cole M, O'Sullivan DJ: Plasma angiotensin II and aldosterone in unselected diabetic patients. Clin Endocrinol (Oxf) 1982 Sep;17(3):261-9

[21] Sugiyama H, Uchimura I, Odakura T, Maezawa H: Plasma renin and aldosterone in adult-onset diabetics with persistent proteinuria. Jpn J Med 1981 Jul;20(3):194-201

[22] Hene RJ, Boer P, Koomans HA, Mees EJ: Plasma aldosterone concentrations in chronic renal disease. Kidney Int 1982 Jan;21(1):98-101

[23] Walker WG: Hypertension-related renal injury: a major contributor to end-stage renal disease. Am J Kidney Dis 1993 Jul;22:164-73

[24] Wakisaka M, Spiro Mj, Spiro RG: Synthesis of type VI collagen by cultured glomerular cells and comparison of its regulation by glucose and other factors with that of type IV collagen. Diabetes 1994 Jan;43:95-103

[25] Wehling M: Aldosterone specific membrane receptors rapid activation of the sodium-hydrogen exchanger, and cardiovascular implications. Cardiovasc Res 1995 Feb;29(2):167-71

[26] Funder JW. Mini review: aldosterone and the cardiovascularsystem: genomic and nongenomic effects. Endocrinology.2006;147:5564-5567.

[27] Chun TY, Pratt JH. Non genomic renal effects of aldosterone. Dependency on NO and genomic actions. Hypertension. 2006;47:636-637.

[28] Arima S, Kohagura K, Xu HL, et al. Endothelium-derived nitric oxide modulates vascular action of aldosterone in renal arteriole. Hypertension. 2004;43:352-357.

[29] Arima S, Kohagura K, Xu HL, et al. Non genomic vascular action of aldosterone in the glomerular microcirculation. J Am Soc Nephrol. 2003;14:2255-2263.

[30] Ponda M, Hostetter T. Aldosterone antagonism in chronic Kidney disease. Clin J Am Soc Nephrol. 2006;1:668-677.

[31] Takeda Y, Zhu A, Yoneda T, Usukura M, Takata H, Yamagishi M. Effects of aldosterone and angiotensin II receptor blockade on cardiac angiotensinogen and angiotensin-converting enzyme 2 expression in Dahl salt-sensitive hypertensive rats. *Am J Hypertens* 2007 October;20(10):1119-24.

[32] Zhu A, Yoneda T, Demura M, Karashima S, Usukura M, Yamagishi M, Takeda Y. Effect of mineralocorticoid receptor blockade on the renal renin-angiotensin system in Dahl salt-sensitive hypertensive rats. *J Hypertens* 2009 April;27(4):800-5.

[33] Taira, Masateru1; Toba, Hiroe1 ; Murakami, Masafumi1; Iga, Ikumi1; Serizawa, Ryoko1; Murata, Shoko1; Kobara, Miyuki1; Nakata, Tetsuo1. Spironolactone exhibits direct renoprotective effects and inhibits renal renin–angiotensin–aldosterone system in diabetic rats. *European Journal of Pharmacology* . 2008 Jul 28: 589 (1-3) : 264-271

[34] Sang-Youb Han, Cy-Hyun Kim, Han-Seong Kim, Yi-Hwa Jee, Hye-Kyoung Song, Mi-Hwa Lee, Kum-Hyun Han, Hyoung-Kyu Kim, Young-Sun Kang, Jee-Young Han, Young-Sik Kim, and Dae-Ryong Cha. Spironolactone Prevents Diabetic Nephropathy through an Anti-Inflammatory Mechanism in Type 2 Diabetic Rats *JASN* May 1, 2006 17: 1362-1372

[35] K H Han1, Y S Kang1, S-Y Han2, Y H Jee1, M H Lee1, J Y Han3, H K Kim1, Y S Kim4 and D R Cha1. Spironolactone ameliorates renal injury and connective tissue growth factor expression in type II diabetic rats. *Kidney International (2006)* 70, 111–120. doi:10.1038/sj.ki.5000438; published online 24 May 2006.

[36] Jun Yuan; Ruhan Jia; Yan Bao. Beneficial effects of spironolactone on glomerular injury in streptozotocin-induced diabetic rats. *Journal of Renin-Angiotensin-Aldosterone System* September 2007 vol. 8 no. 3 118-126

[37] Lee MY, Shim MS, Kim BH, Hong SW, Choi R, Lee EY, Nam SM, Kim GW, Shin JY, Shin YG, Chung CH. Effects of Spironolactone and losartan on diabetic nephropathy in type 2 diabetic rat model. *Diabetes Metab J*. 2011 Apr;35(2):130-7.

[38] Kosugi, Tomoki1,2; Heinig, Marcelo1; Nakayama, Takahiro1; Matsuo, Seiichi3; Nakagawa, Takahiko1,2 . eNOS Knockout Mice with Advanced Diabetic Nephropathy Have Less Benefit from Renin-Angiotensin Blockade than from Aldosterone Receptor Antagonists. *The American Journal of Pathology*, Vol. 176, No. 2, February 2010

[39] Christine Guo, Diego Martinez-Vasquez, Gonzalo P. Mendez, Maria F. Toniolo, Tham M. Yao, Eveline M. Oestreicher, Taisuke Kikuchi, Nathalie Lapointe, Luminita Pojoga, Gordon H. Williams, Vincent Ricchiuti, and Gail K. Adler. Mineralocorticoid Receptor Antagonist Reduces Renal Injury in Rodent Models of Types 1 and 2 Diabetes Mellitus. *Endocrinology* 2006 147: 5363-5373;

[40] Kang, Young Sun1; Ko, Gang Jee2; Lee, Mi Hwa3; Song, Hye Kyoung1; Han, Sang Youb1; Han, Kum Hyun1; Kim, Hyoung Kyu1; Han, Jee Young1; Cha, Dae Ryong1. Effect of eplerenone, enalapril and their combination treatment on diabetic nephropathy in type II diabetic rats. *Nephrol Dial Transplant* (2009) 24: 73–84.

[41] Thomas A. Mavrakanasa, Angeliki Chevab, Konstantinos Kallarasc, Georgios Karkavelasb, Maria Mironidou-Tzouvelekia. Effect of Ramipril Alone Compared to Ramipril with Eplerenone on Diabetic Nephropathy in Streptozocin-Induced Diabetic Rats. *Pharmacology* 2010;86:85-91 (DOI: 10.1159/000316113)

[42] Akira Nishiyama, Hiroyuki Kobori, Yoshio Konishi, Takashi Morikawa, Isseki Maeda, Michiaki Okumura, Masatsugu Kishida, Masahiro Hamada, Yukiko Nagai, Toshitaka Nakagawa, Naro Ohashi, Daisuke Nakano, Hirofumi Hitomi, and Masahito Imanishi. Mineralocorticoid Receptor Blockade Enhances the Antiproteinuric Effect of an Angiotensin II Blocker through Inhibiting Podocyte Injury in Type 2 Diabetic Rats. *J Pharmacol Exp Ther* March 2010 332:1072-1080.

[43] Nagase M, Shibata S, Yoshida S, Nagase T, Gotoda T, Fujita T. Podocyte injury underlies the glomerulopathy of Dahl salt-hypertensive rats and is reversed by aldosterone blocker. *Hypertension* 2006 June;47(6):1084-93.

[44] Sun Ha Lee1,*, Tae-Hyun Yoo1,*, Bo-Young Nam1,*, Dong Ki Kim1, Jin Ji Li1,2, Dong-Sub Jung1, Seung-Jae Kwak1, Dong-Ryeol Ryu3, Seung Hyeok Han1, Jung Eun Lee1, Sung Jin Moon1, Dae Suk Han1, and Shin-Wook Kang1. Activation of local aldosterone system within podocytes is involved in apoptosis under diabetic conditions. *Am J Physiol Renal Physiol* November 2009 297:(5) F1381-F1390;

[45] Shibata S, Nagase M, Yoshida S, Kawachi H, Fujita T. Podocytes as the target for aldosterone: roles of oxidative stress and sgk1 Hypertension. 2007 Feb;49(2):355-64

[46] Nishiyama A, Hitomi H, Rahman A, Kiyomoto H. Drug discovery for overcoming chronic kidney disease (CKD): pharmacological effects of mineralocorticoid-receptor blockers.J Pharmacol Sci. 2009 Jan;109(1):1-6

[47] Nagai Y, Miyata K, Sun GP, Rahman M, Kimura S, Miyatake A,et al. Aldosterone stimulates collagen gene expression andsynthesis via activation of ERK1/2 in rat renal fibroblasts. Hypertension. 2005;46:1039–1045

[48] Miyata K, Rahman M, Shokoji T, Nagai Y, Zhang GX, Sun GP, et al. Aldosterone stimulates reactive oxygen species production through activation of NADPH oxidase in rat mesangial cells. J Am Soc Nephrol. 2005;16:2906–2912.

[49] Terada Y, Kobayashi T, Kuwana H, Tanaka H, Inoshita S, Kuwahara M, et al. Aldosterone stimulates proliferation of mesangial cells by activating mitogen-activated protein kinase 1/2, cyclin D1, and cyclin A. J Am Soc Nephrol. 2005;16:2296–2305.

[50] Sun GP, Kohno M, Guo P, Nagai Y, Miyata K, Fan YY, et al. Involvements of Rho-kinase and TGF-beta pathways in aldosterone-induced renal injury. J Am Soc Nephrol. 2006;17: 2193–2201.

[51] Nishiyama A, Abe Y. Molecular mechanisms and therapeutic strategies of chronic renal injury: renoprotective effects of aldosterone blockade. J Pharmacol Sci. 2006;100:9–16.

[52] Kiyomoto H, Rafiq K, Mostofa M, Nishiyama A. Possibleunderlying mechanisms responsible for aldosterone and mineralocorticoid receptor-dependent renal injury. J Pharmacol Sci.2008:108;399–405.

[53] Fujisawa G, Okada K, Muto S, Fujita N, Itabashi N, Kusano E, et al. Spironolactone prevents early renal injury in streptozotocin induceddiabetic rats. Kidney Int. 2004;66:1493–1502.

[54] Liu YJ, Nakagawa Y, Toya K, Wang Y, Saegusa H, Nakanishi T,et al. Effects of spironolactone on systolic blood pressure in experimental diabetic rats. Kidney Int. 2000;57:2064–2071.

[55] Han KH, Kang YS, Han SY, Jee YH, Lee MH, Han JY, et al. Spironolactone ameliorates renal injury and connective tissue growth factor expression in type II diabetic rats. Kidney Int.2006;70:111–120.

[56] Guo C, Martinez-Vasquez D, Mendez GP, Toniolo MF, Yao TM,Oestreicher EM, et al. Mineralocorticoid receptor antagonist reduces renal injury in rodent models of types 1 and 2 diabetes mellitus. Endocrinology. 2006;147:5363–5373.

[57] Nagase M, Matsui H, Shibata S, Gotoda T, Fujita T. Salt-induced nephropathy in obese spontaneously hypertensive rats via paradoxical activation of the mineralocorticoid receptor: roleof oxidative stress. Hypertension. 2007;50:877–883.

[58] Monrad SU, Killen PD, Anderson MR, Bradke A, Kaplan MJ. The role of aldosterone blockade in murine lupus nephritis. Arthritis Res Ther. 2008;10:R5.

[59] Rocha R, Stier CT Jr, Kifor I, Ochoa-Maya MR, Rennke HG, Williams GH, et al. Aldosterone: a mediator of myocardial necrosis and renal arteriopathy. Endocrinology. 2000;141:3871–78.

[60] Bobadilla NA, Gamba G. New insights into the pathophysiology of cyclosporine nephrotoxicity: a role of aldosterone. Am J Physiol Renal Physiol. 2007;293:F2–F9.

[61] Perez-Rojas J, Blanco JA, Cruz C, Trujillo J, Vaidya VS, Uribe N, et al. Mineralocorticoid receptor blockade confers renoprotection in preexisting chronic cyclosporine nephrotoxicity. Am J Physiol Renal Physiol. 2007;292:F131–F139.

[62] Feria I, Pichardo I, Juarez P, Ramirez V, Gonzalez MA, Uribe N, et al. Therapeutic benefit of spironolactone in experimental chronic cyclosporine A nephrotoxicity. Kidney Int. 2003;63:43-52.

[63] Brown NJ, Nakamura S, Ma L, Nakamura I, Donnert E, Freeman M, et al. Aldosterone modulates plasminogen activator inhibitor- 1 and glomerulosclerosis in vivo. Kidney Int. 2000;58:1219–27

[64] Trachtman H, Weiser AC, Valderrama E, Morgado M, Palmer LS. Prevention of renal fibrosis by spironolactone in mice with complete unilateral ureteral obstruction. J Urol. 2004;172:1590–1594.

[65] Mejia-Vilet JM, Ramirez V, Cruz C, Uribe N, Gamba G, Bobadilla NA. Renal ischemia-reperfusion injury is prevented by the mineralocorticoid receptor blocker spironolactone. Am J Physiol Renal Physiol. 2007;293:F78–F86.

[66] Aldigier JC, Kanjanbuch T, Ma LJ, Brown NJ, Fogo AB. Regression of existing glomerulosclerosis by inhibition of aldosterone. J Am Soc Nephrol. 2005;16:3306–3314.

[67] Nagase M, Yoshida S and Shibat S etal.Enhanced aldosterone signaling in the early nephropathy of rats with metabolic syndrome: possible contribution of fat-derived factor . JASN 2006 Dec;17(12):3438-46.

[68] Ehrhart-Bornstein M, Lamounier-Zepter V, Schraven A et al. Human adipocytes secrete mineraloc-orticoid-releasing factors. Proc Natl Acad Sci U S A 2003;100:14211-14216.

[69] Goodfriend TL, Ball DL, Egan BM, Campbell WB, Nithipatikom K. Epoxy- keto Derivative of Linoleic acid stimulates Aldosterone secretion.Hypertension. 2004 Feb;43(2):358-63.

[70] Schjoedt KJ, Rossing K, Juhl TR, et al. Beneficial impact of spironolactone in diabetic nephropathy. Kidney Int. 2005; 68:2829-2836.

[71] Rossing K, Schjoedt KJ, Smidt U, et al. Beneficial effects of adding spironolactone to recommended antihypertensive treatment in diabetic nephropathy. Diabetes Care. 2005; 28:2106-2112.

[72] van den Meiracker AH, Baggen RG, Pauli S, et al. Spironolactone in type 2 diabetic nephropathy: effects on proteinuria, blood pressure and renal function. J Hypertens. 2006; 24:2285-2292.

[73] Sato A, Hyashi K, Sruta T. Antiproteinuric effects of mineralocorticoid receptor blockade in patients with chronic renal disease. Am J Hypertens. 2005; 18:44-49.

[74] Mehdi UF, Adams-Huet B, Raskin P, Vega GL and toto RD. Addition of Angiotensin receptor Blocade or Mineralocorticoid Antagonism to Maximal Angiotensin-Converting Enzyme Inhibition in Diabetic nephropathy. J Am soc Nephrol 2009; 20:2641-50.

[75] Chrysostomou A, Pedagogos E, MacGregor L, et al. Double-blind, placebo-controlled study on the effects of the aldosterone receptor antagonist spironolactone in patients who have persistent proteinuria and are on longterm angiotensin-converting enzyme inhibitory therapy, with or without an angiotensin II receptor blocker. Clin JAm Soc Nephrol. 2006; 1:256-262.

[76] Bianchi S, Bigazzi R, Campese VM. Long-term effects of spironolactone on proteinuria and kidney function in patients with chronic kidney disease. Kidney Int. 2006; 70:2116-2123.

[77] Epstein M, Buckalew V, Martinez F, et al. Antiproteinuric efficacy of eplerenone, enalapril, and eplerenone/enalapril combination in diabetic hypertensives with microalbuminuria [abstract]. Am J Hypertens. 2002; 15:24A.

[78] Epstein M, Williams GH, Weinberger M, et al. Selective aldosterone blockade with eplerenone reduces albuminuria in patients with type 2 diabetes. Clin J Am Soc Nephrol. 2006; 1:940-951.

[79] Rachmani R, Slavachevsky I, Amit M, et al. The effect of spironolactone, cilazapril and their combination on albuminuria in patients with hypertension and diabetic nephropathy is independent of blood pressure reduction: a randomized controlled study. Diabet Med. 2004; 21:471-475.

[80] Furumatsu Y, NagasawaY, Tomida K, et al. Effect of rennin-angiotensin-aldosterone system triple blockade on non-diabetic renal disease: addition of an aldosterone blocker,

spironolactone, to combination treatment with an angiotensin-converting enzyme inhibitor and angiotensin II receptor blocker. Hypertension Res 2008; 31: 59-67

[81] Swaminathan K, Davies J, George J, Rajendra N, Morris A, Struthers A. Spironolactone for poorly controlled hypertension in type 2 diabetes: conflicting effects on blood pressure, endothelial function, glycaemic control and hormonal profiles. Diabetologia 2008; 51: 762-768

[82] Saklayen MG, Gyebi L, Tasosa J , Yap J. Effects of Additive Therapy With Spironolactone on Proteinuria in Diabetic Patients Already on ACE Inhibitor or ARB Therapy: Results of a Randomized, Placebo-Controlled, Double-Blind, Crossover Trial. J Invest Med. 2008; 56:714-719.

[83] Yoneda T, Yoshiyu T, Usukura M, Oda N, Takata H, Yamamoto Y, Karashima S, Yamagishi M: Aldosterone Breakthrough During angiotensin II receptor blockade in hypertensive patients with diabetes mellitus. Am J Hypertension 2007; 20: 1329-1333

[84] Ogawa S, Takeuchi K, Mori T, Nako K, Ito S. Spironolactone Further Reduces Urinary Albumin Excretion and Plasma B-Type Natriuretic Peptide Levels in Hypertensive Type II diabetes treated with angiotensin-converting enzyme inhibitor. CLin Exp Pharmacol Physiol 2006; 33: 477-479.

[85] Chrysostomou A, Becker G. Spironolactone in addition to ACE inhibition to reduce proteinuria in patients with chronic renal disease. N Engl J Med. 2001;345:925-926.

[86] Bianchi S, Bigazzi R, Campese VM. Antagonists of aldosterone and proteinuria in patients with CKD: an uncontrolled pilot study. Am J Kidney Dis. 2005; 46:45-51.

[87] Schjoedt KJ, Rossing K, Juhl TR, et al. Beneficial impact of spironolactone on nephrotic range albuminuria in diabetic nephropathy. Kidney Int. 2006; 70:536-542.

[88] Mann JF, Schmieder RE, McQueen M, Dyal L, Schumacher H, Pogue J, Wang X, Maggioni A, Budaj A, Chaithiraphan S, Dickstein K, Keltai M, Metsärinne K, Oto A, Parkhomenko A, Piegas LS, Svendsen TL, Teo KK, Yusuf S, ONTARGET investigatorsRenal outcomes with telmisartan, ramipril, or both, in people at high vascular risk (the ONTARGET study): a multicentre, randomised, double-blind, controlled trial.Lancet. 2008;372(9638):547.

[89] McMurray JJ, Ostergren J, Swedberg K, Granger CB, Held P, Michelson EL, Olofsson B, Yusuf S, Pfeffer MA, CHARM Investigators and Committees. Effects of candesartan in patients with chronic heart failure and reduced left-ventricular systolic function taking angiotensin-converting-enzyme inhibitors: the CHARM-Added trial. Lancet. 2003; 362:767-771

[90] Zannad F, McMurray JJ, Krum H, van Veldhuisen DJ, Swedberg K, Shi H, Vincent J, Pocock SJ, Pitt B, EMPHASIS-HF Study Group. Eplerenone in patients with systolic heart failure and mild symptoms. N Engl J Med. 2011; 364:11-21

[91] Juurlink DN, Mamdani MM, Lee DS, Kopp A, Et al. Rates of hyperkalemia after publication of the Randomized Aldactone Evaluation study. N Eng J Med 2004; 351:543-51

[92] Parthasarathy HK, Menard J, White W et al. A double- blind, randomized study comparing the antihypertensive effect of epleronone and spironolactone in patients with hypertension and evidence of primary hyperaldosteronism. J Hypertension 2011;29:980-999.:

[93] Grossman C, Gekle M. New aspects of rapid aldosterone signaling. Molecular and Cellular Endocrinology. 2009; 308:53-62

4

Drug and Diabetic Nephropathy

Rozina Rani
Chattgram Maa-O-Shishu Hospital Medical College, Agrabad, Chittagong Bangladesh

1. Introduction

Diabetes mellitus is a group of metabolic disorders characterized by chronic hyperglycemia with disturbances of carbohydrate, fat and protein metabolism resulting from defect in insulin secretion, insulin action, or both. It is the leading cause of heart disease, adult blindness, and amputation of the lower extremities[1]. Diabetic patient suffer from a number of complications. Of these - hypertension, retinopathy, neuropathy, peripheral vascular disease - are most frequent ones and are responsible for considerable morbidity and mortality. Diabetic nephropathy (DN) is a chronic progressive kidney disease with high morbidity and mortality. There is a gradual loss of renal function ultimately leading to end stage renal disease (ESRD) where life is not sustainable without renal replacement therapy[2]. The course of DN is characterized by early elevation of arterial blood pressure, increasing albuminuria with gradual decline in glomerular filtration rate (GFR) of 10-12 ml.min-1.year-1[3,4,5]. The degree of albuminuria is closely related to the progression of DN[6]. Diabetic patients with nephrotic range proteinuria have the fastest decline in GFR[7] and the shortest survival time[8].

Proteinuria has been considered an indicator of glomerular disease severity[9]. The proposed effects of proteinuria on the kidney include increased severity of glomerulosclerosis, tubulointerstitial inflammation, and subsequent fibrosis, thereby contributing to progressive renal function loss. These facts have permitted the establishment of a "proteinuria hypothesis" that consists of three postulates: higher levels of proteinuria predict adverse clinical outcomes; reduction of proteinuria correlates with slowing of renal progression; and proteinuria is a surrogate end point and target of clinical interventions[10].

Key to the development of DN is the hyperglycemic state, which has been postulated to mediate its effect in several different ways. First, glucose in sustained high concentrations may be directly toxic to cells, altering cell growth and gene and protein expression and increasing extracellular matrix and growth factor production[11]. Second, glucose may induce its effects indirectly through the formation of metabolic derivatives such as oxidants and glycation products[12,13]. Formation of advanced glycation end-products (AGES) may damage cells because of modifications to extracellular matrix proteins and to cellular proteins[14].

The renin-angiotensin-aldosterone system (RAAS) is a coordinate cascade of proteins and peptide hormones, the principal effector of which is angiotensin II. In kidney it is regulated via a self-contained renin angiotensin system in a paracrine fashion[15]. Renin is an enzyme produced by the kidney in response to a number of factors including adrenergic activity (β_1-

receptor) and sodium depletion. Renin converts circulating glycoprotein, angiotensinogen, into the biologically a high potent vasoconstrictor angiotensin II[16].

Angiotensin II acts on the heart and the kidneys by binding to the G protein-coupled receptors type 1 and type 2. The angiotensin receptor type 1 mediates the more deleterious effects of angiotensin II – that is, vasoconstriction and cardiac and vessel hypertrophy[17].

In diabetes mellitus, local activation of the renin angiotensin system or increased intrarenal sensitivity to angiotensin II, especially angiotensin II receptor 1 occurs. Several studies have demonstrated that, in spite of normal or suppressed plasma renin activity, the intrarenal content of renin in increased. This increase can contribute to the progression of diabetic nephropathy via several hemodynamic, tubular and growth promoting actions[18].

Activation of the local renin angiotensin system also constricts the efferent more than the afferent arteriole. This glomerular hemodynamic change increases single nephron glomerular filtration rate in an attempt to maintain global glomerular filtration rate despite progressive loss of functioning nephrons in chronic kidney disease. However, if this change is sustained, it will likely result in glomerular injury and an accelerated loss of kidney function over time[19].

Angiotensin II is the main effector of the RAAS and exerts its vasoconstrictor effect predominantly on the postglomerular arterioles, thereby increasing the glomerular hydraulic pressure and the ultrafiltration of plasma proteins, effects that may contribute to the onset and progression of chronic renal damage. Angiotensin II may also directly contribute to accelerate renal damage by sustaining cell growth, inflammation, and fibrosis. Interventions that inhibit the activity of the RAAS are renoprotective and may slow or even halt the progression of chronic nepropathies[17].

A large number of studies established that progressive deterioration of renal function is the result of compensatory glomerular hemodynamic changes in response to nephron loss. In the widely used experimental model of renal mass reduction, the remaining nephrons undergo hypertrophy, reduced arterial resistance, and increased glomerular blood flow[20].

After nephron loss, the remaining nephrons develop glomerular capillary hypertension, and the single-nephron glomerular filtration rate (GFR) increase (hyperfiltration). These changes are thought to be adaptive in that they help to initially maintain the overall GFR. However, they have negative long-term effects and ultimately lead to renal insufficiency and ESRD.

Podocytes are glomerular epithelia cells for glomerular structure and function, surrounding glomerular capillaries and forming foot processes contributing to the filtration barrier and providing structural stabilization. The diabetic kidney abnormally regulates intraglomerular pressure with imbalance between afferent and efferent arteriolar vasodilatation leading to a 20 mmHg increase in glomerular pressure and allowing hypertension to be transmitted to the glomerulus[21].

Besides these glomerular hemodynamic effects, other studies have revealed several nonhemodynamic effects of angiotensin II that may also be important in renal disease progression. These findings have suggested that angiotensin II may alter permselective properties of the glomerular capillary barrier by mediating contraction of the foot processes, ultimately changing slit-diaphragm architecture and allowing proteins to escape more easily into the urinary space[22].

Nonhemodynamic effects of angiotensin II include increased production of reactive oxygen species; upregulation of cytokines, cell adhesion molecules, and profibrotic growth factors; induction of transforming growth factor-β (TGF-β) expression, increased synthesis of extracellular matrix proteins; stimulation of plasminogen activator inhibitor-1 production by endothelial and vascular smooth muscle cells; and macrophage activations and infiltrations[23].

There is increasing evidence that TGF-β is a major pro sclerotic mediator. Its production is stimulated by angiotensin II and by glucose directly. Preclinical studies have shown that TGF-β blockade prevents and also ameliorates DN[24,25].

In addition, to amplify some of the effects of angiotensin II, aldosterone may also directly contribute to endothelial dysfunction, aldosterone may also remodel human endothelium in vitro by increasing the size and stiffness of endothelial cells, which favors leakage through intracellular gaps[26].

In animal models, high intraglomerular capillary pressure impairs the size-selective function of the glomerular permeability barrier and causes protein ultrafiltration[27, 28]. The secondary process of reabsorption of filtered proteins can contribute to renal interstitial injury by activating intracellular events. Local recruitment of macrophages by tubular cells that are loaded with ultrafiltered plasma proteins may contribute to interstitial fibrosis by engaging matrix-producing interstitial myofibroblasts. Macrophages also regulate matrix accumulation via release of growth factors, such as TGF-β and platelet derived growth factor (PDGF). TGF-β stimulates the transformation of interstitial cells into myofibroblasts. In addition proximal tubular epithelial cells communicate with interstitial fibroblasts to promote fibrogenesis via paracrine release of TGF-β. In rats with remnant kidneys at day 14, after the onset of proteinuria, TGF-β mRNA was upregulated in proximal tubular cells in parallel with early accumulation of the peritubular interstitium, suggesting that interstitiall fibroblasts are the initial target of profibrogenic signals elicited by protein overreabsorption[29]. Treatment of these rats with an angiotensin converting enzyme inhibitor (ACEI) at the same time limited excess protein overload and interstitial inflammatory cell infiltration and abrogated the abnormal TGF-β 1 gene expression in tubular cells that in all likelihood was responsible of myofibroblasts in surrounding areas. ACEI exerts beneficial effects in the glomerulus primarily by preserving the permselective barrier to proteins[30], thereby limiting proteinuria and filtered protein-dependent inflammatory and fibrogenic signals. The ACEI also may act locally by preventing nonhemodynamic effects of angiotensin II via apical angiotensin receptors on tubular cells, including renal cell proliferation and TGF-β 1 expression[31].

In addition to albumin, transferring, and Immunoglobulin, glomerular proteinuria results in ultrafiltration of high molecular weight precursor forms or complexes of growth factor proteins such as insulin like growth factor 1, hepatocyte growth factor and TGF-β 1. Inflammatory and vasoactive substances formed in excessive amounts by proximal tubuli are secreted toward the basolateral compartment of the cell and give rise to a inflammatory reaction in the interstitium that consistently precedes renal scarring. These processes can be accelerated by cytokines released by tubular epithelial cells and by inflammatory cells that accumulate in the interstitium when proteinuria is present[32-36].

Both interstitial inflammation and progression of disease can be controlled by such drugs as ACEI, which strengthen the glomerular permeability barrier to proteins and thereby limit proteinuria and filtered protein-dependent inflammatory signals[37].

Lastly, the increased glomerular permeability may result in excess ultrafiltration of some complement protein fractions that may be directly toxic to proximal tubules and incite injury. In a subtotal nephrectomy model of renal insufficiency, C3 staining was associated with the appearance of interstitial infiltrated. Treatment with ACEI, which lowered proteinuria, also decreased C3 staining[38].

Recent studies utilizing transgenic rats with overexpression of the angiotensin II type 1 receptor in podocytes revealed that increased angiotensin receptor type 1 signaling in podocytes leads to structural podocyte damage and protein leakage[39]. To support this finding from a therapeutic point of view, recent studies showed that ACEI and angiotensin receptor blocker (ARB) induce redistribution of the molecules in the slit diaphragm, which determine leakage of protein through glomerular filtration barrier[40-42].

There are some data showing that some of the beneficial effects of the RAAS blockade may be related to anti-inflammatory properties of ACEI and ARB[43]. In a clinical study, Stevinkel et al found low plasma levels of tumor necrosis factor-α and C-reactive protein (CRP) in ESRD patients treated with ACEI[44]. The benefit seen with these drugs is beyond that which would be expected from their antihypertensive effects.

The disassociation between doses needed to inhibit local tissue actions of angiotensin II and circulatory concentrations directly involved in blood pressure regulation may be due to reduced tissue penetration or higher tissue concentration of angiotensin II or its receptor[45]. Increased RAAS activity and augmented angiotensin II receptor density in the diseased renal tissue together with reduced penetration of the drug may explain that higher doses are needed for complete RAAS blockade in the tissue responsible for antiproteinuric effects as compared to circulatory levels regulating systemic blood pressure[46].

Several underlying mechanisms may explain the blood pressure independent antiproteinuric effects of agents blocking the RAAS[47-50]. These include reduced intraglomerular hydraulic pressure independent of systemic blood pressure by vasodilatation preferentially of the post glomerular arterioles[51] and improved permselective properties of the glomerular membrane[52]. In addition, ARBs may prevent the occurrence of proteinuria by reducing the loss of glomerular nephrin[53] and by reducing renal levels of prosclerotic cytokines such as TGF-β and CTGF[54].

Doses of ACEI that exceed their maximal antihypertensive dose have not been examined adequately, because, ultrahigh doses of ACEI (doses above those approved for antihypertensive treatment according to the FDA and the European agency for the evaluation of medicinal products) was thought to be associated with serious side effects[55-57]. In contrast, ARB has tested over a wide range of doses, without showing an increase of side effects with ultrahigh doses. Various clinical studies support the notion that the dose of ARB is inversely related to proteinuria, independent of blood-pressure control[58-61].

2. Rationale for higher dose

ACEI and ARB have been shown to reduce proteinuria, blood pressure and thereby retarded deteriorating kidney function in diabetic subjects. Doses of ACEI and ARB currently employed in clinical practice and even in experimental protocols are based essentially on the observation of the maximal effects of these drugs on blood pressure.

"Conventional" doses of these drugs may be insufficient to completely neutralize the anomalous activation of the RAAS, thus helping to explain their failure to achieve complete renal protection[62].

So far reno protective therapy has been administered in doses extrapolated from the treatment of essential hypertension, with doses that may be suboptimal for reno protection. Studies of dose-related efficacy of ACEI or ARBs with dose titration based upon achieving the maximum antiproteinuric effect for reno protection have not been adequately performed[63].

The full reno- and cardiovascular protective potential of agents blocking the RAAS may not be reached in patients with diabetic renal disease when recommended doses of these agents are extrapolated from their blood pressure-lowering properties, which is currently the case for all ACEI and ARBs used for renoprotection. By exceeding currently recommended maximal dose, it has been demonstrated that within the recommended dose interval higher doses provide greater antiproteinuric effects than lower doses[64].

Recent trials investigating the ability of these agents to protect patients against target organ damage have now repeatedly shown that the higher doses were most effective, thus recommending more aggressive treatment in future[65].

The study of the Irbesartan in Patients with Type 2 Diabetes and Microalbuminuria Study (IRMA-2) investigated the reversibility of kidney function changes after withdrawal of 2 years' antihypertensive treatment. They included 133 hypertensive type 2 diabetic patients with persistent microalbuminuria, randomized to double-masked treatment with either placebo, irbesartan 150 mg, or irbesartan 300 mg once daily for 2 years. Arterial blood pressure, overnight urinary albumin excretion rate, and glomerular filtration rate (GFR) were determined repeatedly. In IRMA-2 trial the benefit of protein reduction was maintained only in the group that was treated with the higher dose of Irbesartan 300mg/day[66].

A double-masked randomized crossover trial included 52 (41 males) hypertensive type 2 diabetic patients with microalbuminuria on ongoing antihypertensive medication. Following 2 months wash-out (baseline), patients were treated randomly with irbesartan 300, 600, and 900 mg once daily, each dose for 2 months. This study by Rossing et al., revealed that ultrahigh dosing of irbesartan [900mg O.D (3 times higher maximal recommended dose)] was generally safe and offers additional nephroprotection independent of changes in systemic blood pressure and glomerular filtration rate in comparison to the currently recommended dose of 300mg[46]. In another study conducted by Andrei Forclaz et al., assessed the blockade of the rennin-angiotensin system (RAS) achieved with 2 angiotensin antagonists given either alone at different doses or with an ACE inhibitor. First, 20 normotensive subjects were randomly assigned to 100 mg Losartan once daily or 80 mg Telmisartan once daily for 1 week; during another week, the same dose of losartan and telmisartan were combined with 20 mg Lisinopril once daily. Then, 10 subjects were randomly assigned to 200 mg losartan once daily and 160 mg of Telmisartan once daily for 1 week and 100 mg losartan twice daily and 80 mg telmisartan twice daily during the second week. This study stated that the blockade of the renin angiotensin system (RAS) being only partial with 100mg Losartan and 80mg Telmisartan[67]. Previous studies with ACEI and angiotensin II receptor antagonists have shown that increasing the dose once daily has little effect on the peak inhibition but tends to prolong the duration of the inhibition. In accordance with this observation increasing the dose of Losartan to 200mg (2 times higher than maximal recommended dose) once daily and that of Telmisartan to 160mg once daily significantly improved the trough blockade[68,69,70]. Another study with a total of 23 hypertensive patients with type 2 diabetes and nephropathy was carried out with four treatment periods, each lasting 2 months. This study stated that, albuminuria was reduced significantly more by Candesartan 16 and 32mg (recommended maximal dose) as compared with 8mg daily, without differences between the two highest doses[45]. Study with 64mg (2 times maximal recommended dose) was more effective in reducing proteinuria in patients with chronic kidney disease than 16 and 32mg/day Candesartan[71]. Data from another study of 10 older patients with heavy proteinuria (>1.5 g/day) of different eitiology have suggested that additional reduction in proteinuria can be obtained by increasing the dose of Candesartan from 32 to 96mg (3 times maximal recommended dose) daily[72]. A recent short-term safety study of 12 patients with various forms of chronic renal diseases with severe proteinuria also demonstrated good tolerability of the ARB Candesartan in doses 5 times higher than currently approved maximum dose[58].

Vogt et al., conducted study with Lisinopril 10, 20, 30 and 40mg/day (2 times higher the usual dose) in 12 (8 of whom were finally selected for the study) nondiabetic proteinuric patients. The eligible patients entered the run-in phase in which previous medication was replaced for the highest recommended daily dose irbesartan 300 mg combined with the diuretic hydrochlorothiazide 12.5 mg once daily. Then, patients with proteinuria >1 g/d and serum potassium concentration <5.5 mmol/L entered the phase of dose titration. In this phase, lisinopril was added in increasing daily doses to a maximum of 40 mg. All periods of treatment (run-in and up-titration) lasted at least 6 weeks. Their study concluded that, dose titration induced further reduction of residual proteinuria[73]. Fujihara et al., concluded that the renal protection afforded by ARB in renal ablation was dose dependent and maximal protection may require doses several fold higher than those currently employed. In rat model, treatment with Losartan at a dose 10 fold higher than dose 50mg/kg/day and 50 fold higher than those usually employed in experimental studies, arrested the progression of both glomerulosclerosis and interstitial expansion. This dose dependence of Losartan is likely to be observed in human as well, since clinical studies showed that the human responses can be predicted with reasonable accuracy from animal experiments[62]. The effects of different dosage of ramipril, from a minimum of 5mg/day to a maximum of 20 mg/day (4 times the recommended maximum dosage) were evaluated on the level of proteinuria. Although the higher dosage had no additional effect on blood pressure, urinary protein excretion rates were further reduced[37].

In a study by Ruggenenti P, uptitration of lisinopril from 10 to 40 mg was done in 28 patients with nondiabetic chronic nephropathies. These patients entered 4-week lisinopril uptitration periods (from 10, to 20, 30, and 40 mg/d), followed by a 6-week backtitration period to lisinopril 10 mg/d and 4-week recovery period (lisinopril withdrawal). Maximum lisinopril doses significantly and safely reduced proteinuria, serum total, LDL cholesterol, and triglycerides without substantially affecting serum HDL and renal hemodynamics[74]. More recently in a preliminary report, Schjoedt et al.[75] studied 56 patients with type 1 diabetes and nephropathy, who in a double masked crossover trial received 20, 40 or 60 mg/day of lisinopril. The 40 mg/day dose provided a great antiproteinuric effect than 20 mg/day but 60 mg/day did not afford further renoprotection.

Tang et al., in their study on 75 patients with chronic heart failure with low Enalapril (5 mg) dose and high dose (40 mg) over six months and found that there was not any significant reduction in systolic and diastolic blood pressure between the two dose groups. They also measured serum aldosterone and angiotensin II levels in their study and they observed that these renin system hormones weren't adequately suppressed even with the higher dose[76].

Most studies that showed effective reduction of blood pressure and proteinuria included mostly normotensive and/ or microalbuminuric group of patients. In the study conducted by Adrienne et al.,[77] the antiproteinuric effects of losartan in 147 normotensive patients with type 2 diabetes and microalbuminuria was assessed. The losartan dose was 50 mg during the first 5 weeks and 100 mg during the subsequent 5 weeks. A significant 25% relative reduction in the albumin excretion rate occurred after 5 weeks of the 50 mg losartan dose, with further improvement over the subsequent 5 weeks with the 100 mg dose. Losartan was safe and well tolerated in these normotensive patients.

Lacouriciere et al.,[78] in their studies after using Losartan and Enalapril found significantly decreased blood pressure in hypetensive type 2 diabetics with early nephropathy. The study was a one-year prospective, double blind trial with losartan and enalapril administered alone or in combination with hydrochlorothiazide and other antihypertensive agents. Arterial Blood Pressure and renal and biochemical parameters were measured at baseline and after 12, 28, and 52 weeks of active treatment. 92 hypertensive type 2 diabetics with early nephropathy completed the study.

It may be possible that advanced renal failure patients with proteinuria may not respond to increasing doses of Enalapril. Similar findings were also seen by Jensen et al.,[79]. They conducted study with normal to high Enalapril dose (5 to 40 mg) including macroproteinuric patients with advanced renal insufficiency of variable etiologies. They found that at study end blood pressure and proteinuria didn't change significantly in both dose groups.

Anderson et al.,[63] in their study with 50 consecutive hypertensive type 1 diabetic patients with diabetic nephropathy received increasing doses of losartan 50, 100, and 150 mg once daily in three periods each lasting 2 months. Using Losartan from 50 to 150 mg among macroproteinuric patients with normal renal function found that maximum antiproteinuric effect was at 100 mg dose without any adverse effect at 150 mg. No significant benefit of increasing dose from 100 to 150 mg was observed in their study groups.

Huo et al.,[80] undertook a study with Losartan starting with 50 mg and then increasing to 200 mg in a total 360 proteinuric nephropathy patients for a period of 3 years and found significant reduction in blood pressure and proteinuria. But in their study, to control blood pressure, concomitant antihypertensive drugs were used in their patients. It may be possible that antihypertensive drugs in Hou's study reduced blood pressure significantly which influenced the proteinuria reduction to a significant level unlike ours.

Woo et al.,[81] carried out a study in nondiabetic proteinuric subjects with renal dysfunction using 10 mg Enalapril and 100 mg Losartan. 41 patients with biopsy-proven IgAN entered a control trial, with 21 in the treatment group and 20 in the control group. Patients in the treatment group received ACEI/ATRA or both with 3 monthly increases in dosage. They found that blood pressure or proteinuria was reduced only in 30% to 50 % patients. The non responder patients were those who had heavy proteinuria (>2 g/day) and more advanced renal dysfunction (serum creatinine > 2.5 mg/dl). Study results indicate that combination of heavy proteinuria with advanced renal impairment may be less or non responsive to angiotensin converting enzyme inhibitors or angiotensin receptor blocker even at higher doses.

Rocca et al.,[82] in 45 chronic heart failure patients showed increasing dose of Enalapril from 5 to 40 mg reduced blood pressure more and cough was more common on highest than lowest dose. The dosage was changed three times to treat all patients with lower, higher, and finally, the initial dosage for 4 weeks each. Within patient comparison revealed that serum potassium and creatinine were higher on the highest than the lowest dose. The patient's included in that trial were suffering from chronic heart failure and were primarily non diabetic and non proteinuric patients. It is possible that these patients are more susceptible to adverse effect with increasing doses of angiotensin converting enzyme inhibitor.

Brenner et al.,[83] conducted a study with a total 1513 patients having hypertension, type 2 DM and nephropathy (S. cr 1.3-3 mg/dl) for a mean of 3.4 years. A total of 327 patients in the losartan group reached the primary end point, as compared with 359 in the placebo group. Their study established that losartan, along with conventional antihypertensive treatment as needed, conferred strong renal protection in these patients. The risk of the primary end point a composite of doubling of the S. creatinine concentration, ESRD was reduced by 25% & 28% respectively with losartan but had no effect on the rate of death. The level of proteinuria declined by 35% with losartan.

3. Safety monitoring

Enalapril was well tolerated even at 40mg (maximal recommended dose) once daily dose, as compared with 5mg once daily dose. In fact, there were more reported adverse events and death (requiring withdrawal from the trial) in the low-dose group than in the high-dose group. As seen in previous studies, a large proportion of patients with advanced chronic heart failure could receive up to very high doses of Lisinopril (medium-dose 12.5 or 15.0 mg once daily for 2 to 4 weeks and then randomized to high 35.0 or 32.5 mg once daily or low-dose 5.0 or 2.5 mg once daily) and Enalapril without significantly more adverse effects[84,85]. Losartan could be administered at an extremely high dose without any perceptible toxic effect. In rat model, treated with 500mg/kg/day, had no hypotension and plasma K^+ concentration was not higher[63]. In the trial with lisinopril (where a total of 3164 patients were assigned randomly with either low dose of 2.5 to 5.0 mg daily lisinopril in 1596 patients or high doses of 32.5 to 35 mg daily lisinopril to 1568 patients for 39 to 58 months), increase in serum creatinine in the high-dose group (35mg/day) was slightly greater than in the low-dose group (5mg/day), but the number of patients with major increase in serum creatinine (>1mg/dl) was not different[86]. There was a therapy with Candesartan 8, 16, 32mg (maximal recommended dose) in a total of 23 hypertensive patients with type 2 diabetes and nephropathy with four treatment periods, each lasting for 2 months. The therapy was well tolerated without associated adverse events. A slight increase in serum K^+ was found, but no incidence of hyperkalamia and hypotension was observed in these patients[45]. No serious adverse event was reported in relation to the ultrahigh dose (64mg i.e.2 times maximal recommended dose) of candesartan. This confirmed previous studies observing no dose-response curves of serious adverse effect of increasing dose of ARB[70].

In a pilot study, 12 patients (10 males; age = 57± 14 years) with a history of diabetic or non-diabetic chronic kidney disease received candesartan in an 8-week open-label trial in which drug was titrated to a targeted dosage of 160 mg/day (5 times above the currently approved maximum dose) and remained at that dosage for the subsequent 4 weeks. Candesartan was well tolerated with no serious drug-related adverse events reported. Serum creatinine concentrations throughout the study were not different from baseline levels. Plasma potassium concentrations at 160 mg/day candesartan were similar to those at baseline. The results of this pilot study suggest that supramaximal doses of ARBs are safe and well tolerated in patients with chronic kidney disease, while reducing both blood pressure and proteinuria[58].

In Irbesartan Diabetic Nephropathy Trial (IDNT), Irbesartan (titrated to 300mg/day i.e. maximal recommended dose) slowed the deterioration of renal function by decreasing risk of doubling of serum creatinine, development of end stage renal disease, or death by 20%. Fewer patients receiving Irbesartan had a doubling of their serum creatinine concentration than placebo[87].

Treatment with Irbesartan was carried out in 52 (41 males) hypertensive type 2 diabetic patients with microalbuminuria. Following 2 months of wash-out (baseline), patients were treated randomly with irbesartan 300, 600, and 900mg/day (3 times higher maximal recommended dose), each dose for 2 months. The therapy induced an increase in plasma K^+ and these changes were only marginally greater when exceeding the currently recommended dose of Irbesartan. None of the patients developed hyperkalemia[46].

In RENAAL (Reduction of Endpoints in NIDDM with the AngiotensinII II Antagonist Losartan) study, 50 consecutive hypertensive type 1 diabetic patients with diabetic nephropathy received increasing dose of losartan, 50, 100, and 150 mg once daily in three periods each lasting 2 months. Losartan 50mg to 100mg reduced the primary end point (doubling of baseline serum creatinine, end stage renal disease, or death). Potassium, sodium, and cholesterol, including HDL-cholesterol, remained unchanged at 50, 100 and 150mg/day with Losartan. Levels of uric acid in serum did not exceed the upper normal range in this study[63].

Serum K^+ and serum creatinine were slightly, higher at high [40mg/day (4 times the recommended dose)] than at low (10mg/day) enalapril levels. Most patients show an only mild increase in serum creatinine, and ACEI therapy did not have to be discontinued in these patients. An increase in enalapril dose did not lead to hyperkalemia. Serious adverse events (i.e. worsening of chronic heart failure, anuria and serious arrhythmia) tended to be more common after downward than after upward titration of enalapril[82]. In the ValHeft (Valsartan in Heart Failure) trial, patients received 160mg valsartan twice daily without any serious adverse effect[88]. In a study by Hou et al. , the incidence of cough was significantly higher in the benazepril arm as compared to losartan arm, but it did not seem to be dosage related. Hyperkalemia occurred in eight (4.4%) patients in the benazepril arm and eight (4.4%) patients in the losartan arm. Of these 16 patients, six were successfully treated with dietary modification, concomitant diuretic therapy, and optimized acid-base balance. The remaining 10 patients withdrew from the study[80]. In the study with ultrahigh dose of Irbesartan (900 mg) total 58 patients having hypertension, type 2 diabetes mellitus with microalbuminuria (persistent Urinary Albumin Excretion between 30 & 300 mg/24hours) on ongoing antihypertensive (wash out done) were included. 4 patients were excluded due to adverse clinical events, which were not considered related to the study medication. 1 patient discontinued the study after 2 weeks on Irbesartan 900 mg before any clinical examination was performed due to complaints of dizziness & general discomfort. Among 52 patients completing the study, 7 patients complained of mild & transient dizziness, 1 patient during 300 mg, 3 patients during 600 mg & 3 during 900 mg. There was a significant increase in plasma K^+ of 0.3 mmol/L during treatment with irbesartan 300 & 600 mg & by 0.4 mmol/L during treatment with 900 mg. However, none of the patients included in the study developed hyperkalemia (plasma $K^+ > 5.5$ mmol/L). Plasma hemoglobin decreased significantly from 8.7 mmo/L at baseline to 8.2 mmol/L during treatment with 300 & 600 mg & to 8.1 mmol/L during irbesartan 900 mg[46].

4. Dual blockage of RAAS with ACEIs and ARBs

An insufficient response to ACE inhibition might be explained by the incomplete blockade of the RAS obtained with ACE inhibitors, which are unable to block completely the formation of angiotensin II (Ang II), because some generation of Ang II is produced via other non-ACE pathways[89]. Furthermore, Ang II levels return to normal values after chronic therapy with ACE inhibition, the so-called "ACE escape phenomenon"[90].

The demonstration of local angiotensin II (Ang II) synthesis in numerous tissues and organs has led to the concept of local or tissue-based RAASs that are independent of but can interact with the traditional circulating RAAS[91]. These local RAASs appear to act in a paracrine/autocrine manner to regulate organ function and are involved in pathologic events associated with end-organ damage. The kidney contains all the elements of the RAAS, and intrarenal formation of Ang II independent of the circulating RAAS was first demonstrated more than 30 years ago[92].

Local AngII in the kidney has multiple roles contributing in hypertension and kidney damage. It enhances capillary filtration pressure, directly by efferent arterial vasoconstriction and indirectly through TGF-β1 (transforming growth factor beta1) mediated impaired afferent arteriole autoregulation[93]. AngII decreases the synthesis of negatively charged proteoglycans and suppresses nephrin transcription[94, 95], which results in podocyte apoptosis. Through VEGF (vascular endothelial growth factor) and TGF-β1, induces synthesis of the α3 chain of collagen type IV, the principal ingredient of the glomerular basement membrane[96], stimulates upregulation of adhesion molecules such as vascular cellular adhesion molecule-1 (VCAM-1), intracellular adhesion molecule-1 (ICAM-1), and integrins, allowing circulating immune cells to adhere on capillaries. Ang II induces nuclear factor Kβ (NF-κB) -mediated transcription of chemokines, including monocyte chemoattractant protein-1 (MCP-1), RANTES, and others, resulting in renal tissue infiltration with leukocytes and also induces plasminogen activator inhibitor-1 (PAI-1) and tissue inhibitor of matrix metalloproteinases-1 (TIMP-1) which inhibits metalloproteinases resulting in accumulation of extracellular matrix. Through all these mechanisms, AngII induces proteinuria, inflammation, growth effects, apoptosis and fibrosis[97].

Chymase-dependent Ang II formation may be at least partly responsible for 'ACE escape'. This term refers to the observation that, in a high proportion of patients chronically treated with ACE inhibitors, Ang II levels gradually return to baseline after an initial decline. This increase in Ang II formation in the presence of ACE inhibitors is likely due to a compensatory increase in plasma renin activity (PRA) caused by disruption of the feedback loop by which

AngII normally inhibits renin release[98]. Under these circumstances, Ang II can be formed from Ang I by alternative, ACE-independent pathways, such as chymase, which has been shown to be upregulated in diabetic and hypertension-related nephropathies[99].

ACE-I inhibits the angiotensin-converting enzyme (ACE), thereby reducing the synthesis of Ag II. In addition, it inhibits the degradation of bradykinin, a vasodilator that stimulates nitric oxide, prostaglandin E2, prostacyclin and cyclic guanosine monophosphate production. This might confer additional renal protection, beyond that achieved by the inhibition of Ag II. However, with prolonged ACE-I therapy, the Ag II level can increase through an escape mechanism via peripheral chymase action[89,99]. ARB, on the other hand, acts directly on the Ag II type 1 receptor (AT 1) and thus blocks all the known actions of Ag II. In addition, by blocking AT 1, it provides unopposed stimulation of the Ag II type 2 receptor (AT 2) in the kidney. Stimulation of the AT 2 receptor has been associated with increased nitric oxide production, increased natriuresis as well as growth inhibitory effects[100]. In order to take advantage of the distinct properties of both these medications, a number of studies have explored the possibility of dual blockade of the RAAS with ACE-I and ARB.

In the search of new alternatives that could improve the antiproteinuric and nephroprotective effects of RAS blockers, we believe that the association of ACE inhibitors and ARB might prove useful. ARB produces a complete blockade of the RAS and stimulates the vasodilating and non-proliferative actions of Ang II via the AT2 receptor[101]. Furthermore, ACE inhibitors, but not ARB, inhibit the metabolism of kinins, which increases the levels of bradykinin, also a potent vasodilator[102].

Recently, some authors have reported a superior effect of the combination of ACE inhibition and ARB on microalbuminuria and on clinical proteinuria in patients with primary nephropathies[103-105], and in type 1 and type 2 diabetic patients[106, 107].

The rationale for combined therapy with ACE inhibitors and ARB is based on the different mechanism of these two drugs in the RAS blockade. Both drugs inhibit the action of Ang II. It is known that Ang II plays a pivotal role in the pathophysiological course of renal disease progression. ACE inhibition could not completely inhibit the generation of Ang II, which may be produced via other non-ACE pathways[89]. In contrast, ARB completely abolishes the action of Ang II through blockading theAT1 receptor, producing an accumulation of Ang II that stimulates the vasodilatory and antiproliferative actions of Ang II mediated through the AT2 receptor[101]. On the other hand, ACE inhibitors but not ARB, decreases degradation of bradykinin, which is a potent vasodilator[102].

A recent meta-analysis by Jennings et al reported a greater reduction in proteinuria with combination therapy when compared with ACE-I alone[108]. The response to treatment with ACE-I and ARB may differ among different races[109].

Mogensen et al studied 197 hypertensive patients with type 2 DM and microproteinuria, and found that combination therapy with once daily candesartan 16 mg and lisinopril 20 mg was more effective in reducing BP and albuminuria than monotherapy with either drug alone[106].

Cetinkaya et al found that a combination of enalapril 10 mg daily and losartan 50 mg daily decreased both the proteinuria and MAP by a greater extent when compared with the administration of either drug alone[110].

In two separate randomised double-blind crossover studies, Rossing et al found a further reduction in albuminuria when candesartan 16 mg was added to the pre-existing ACE-I therapy in hypertensive type 2 diabetic patients. In the first study involving 18 type 2 diabetic patients who were taking the recommended doses of ACE-I, corresponding to 20 mg of enalapril/lisinopril once daily or 100 mg of captopril daily, the administration of candesartan 16 mg daily for two months induced a 25% reduction in albuminuria, together with a 10 mmHg reduction in 24-hour systolic BP[111]. In the second study involving 20 type 2 diabetic patients on a maximal recommended dose of ACE-I (enalapril/lisinopril 40 mg daily or captopril 150 mg daily), there was a further 28% significant reduction in albuminuria, and a modest but non-significant reduction in BP after two months of being administered candesartan at 16 mg daily[112]. On the other hand, the addition of Losartan 50 mg daily for one month did not improve proteinuria in 16 obese, hypertensive patients (12 with diabetic nephropathy) with moderately advanced renal failure and heavy proteinuria (mean urinary protein 3.8 g/day)[113]. A Korean group also reported no beneficial effect on proteinuria when candesartan was added to ramipril therapy in type 2 diabetic patients with nephropathy despite the positive anti-proteinuric effect seen in patients with IgA nephropathy following the same regimen[114, 115].

Dual blockade of RAAS at different steps with ACEI and ARB would be an attractive alternative.

In meta-analysis, Doulton et al demonstrated that combination therapy provided a further 30%- 39% drop in proteinuria compared to monotherapy[116] and in MacKinnon et al resulted in a significant decline in proteinuria both in diabetic and nondiabetic patients with a slight but significant increase in potassium, and an insignificant drop in GFR[117].

The IMPROVE (Irbesartan in the Management of Proteinuric Patients at High Risk for Vascular Events) study has shown no further benefit on albuminuria reduction in patients treated with combination therapy despite the fact that BP reduction was slightly better in the combination group. Subgroup analyses showed the largest reduction in albuminuria occurred in patients with overt nephropathy but it did not reach statistical significance[118].

In contrast to these studies, the VALERIA (Valsartan in Combination With Lisinopril Versus the Respective High Dose Monotherapies in Hypertensive Patients With Microalbuminuria) trial demonstrated that combination therapy was more effective in reducing microalbuminuria despite the fact that patients received the maximal recommended doses of lisinopril or valsartan as monotherapy[119].

5. Direct renin inhibition

Aliskiren is the first orally active Direct Renin Inhibitor (DRI) to receive regulatory approval for hypertension. By inhibiting the enzymatic conversion by renin of Angiotensinogen to Angiotensin I, DRIs inhibit the initial and rate-limiting step in the RAAS cascade, thus reducing the product ion of al l downstream products derived from Angiotensin[120, 121]. Furthermore, in both clinical studies[122] and in experimental animals[123], aliskiren reduces plasma and/or urinary excretion of aldosterone. The role of aldosterone in endothelial dysfunction, inflammation, proteinuria and fibrosis is well known[97].

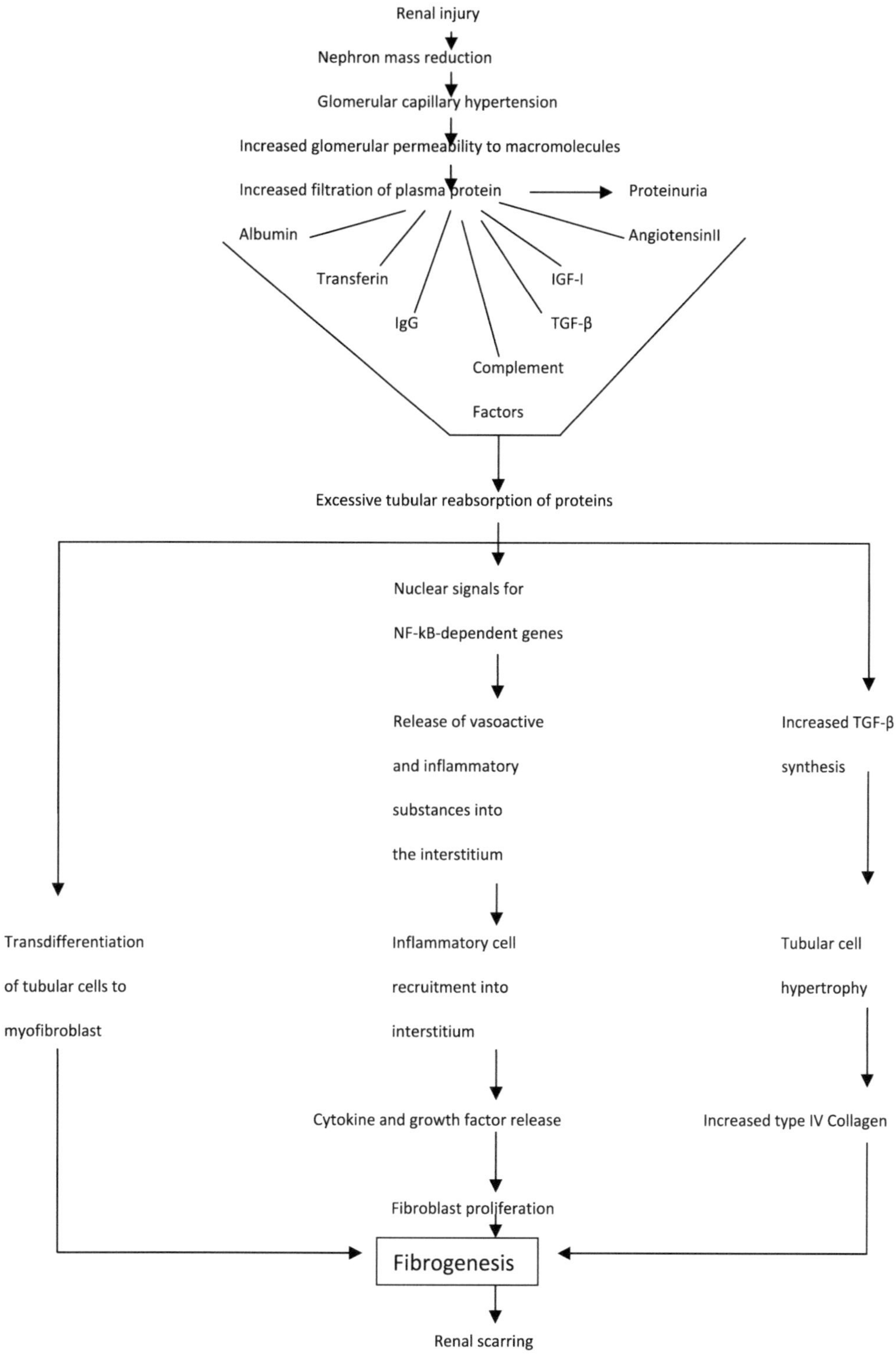

Fig. 1. Effect of increased glomerular permeability to proteins on progressive renal injury

The mechanisms by which aliskiren may impart renoprotection are still under investigation. However, a number of possible mechanisms can be envisioned. First, aliskiren not only inhibits renin but also inhibits the activity of prorenin[124] following its non-proteolytic activation upon binding to the (pro)renin receptor[125]. This may be of particular importance in diabetes in which prorenin levels are elevated and may contribute to local Ang II formation[126]. Second, aliskiren blocks the circulating RAAS and lowers blood pressure[127]. Hypertension is one of the most common comorbidities in CKD and its control is essential in reducing further renal damage and cardiovascular risk in CKD patients[128]. Third, aliskiren blocks the intrarenal RAAS and lowers renal Ang I and Ang II levels[129], thus reducing the deleterious renal effects of Ang II[97] (fig. 1). Finally, aliskiren has been shown to reduce the renal expression of the (pro)renin receptor in an animal model of diabetes[124]. If the (pro)renin receptor plays a role in CKD, downregulation of this receptor may reduce the Ang II-independent effects of (pro)renin receptor activation on renal fibrotic pathways[130] (Fig. 3).

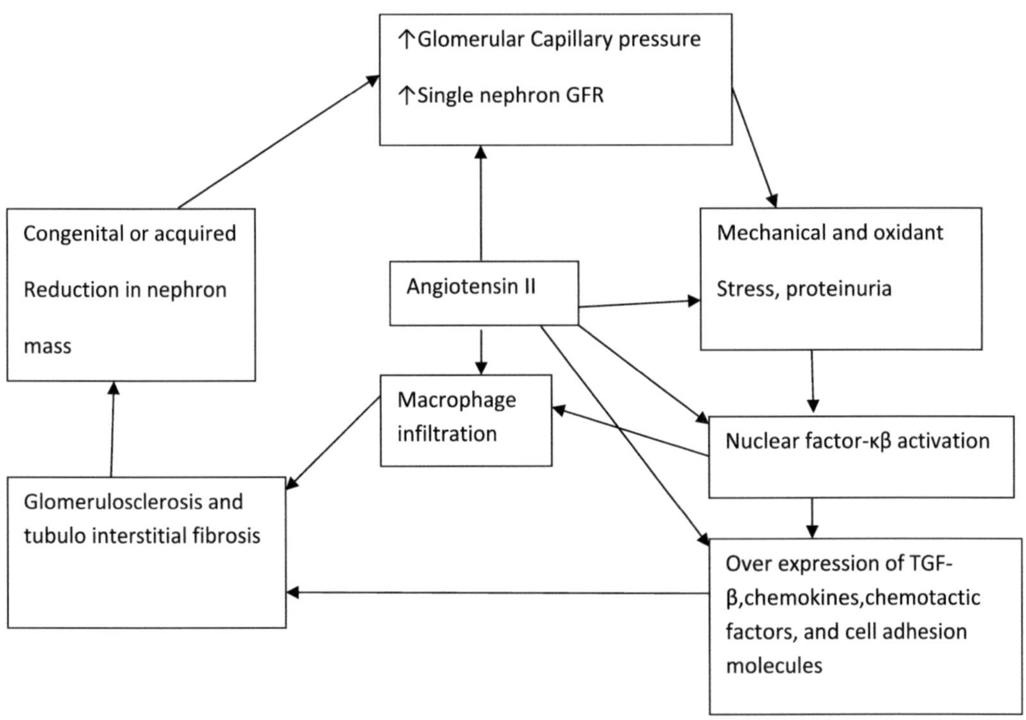

Fig. 2. Final common pathway for progression of chronic renal disease

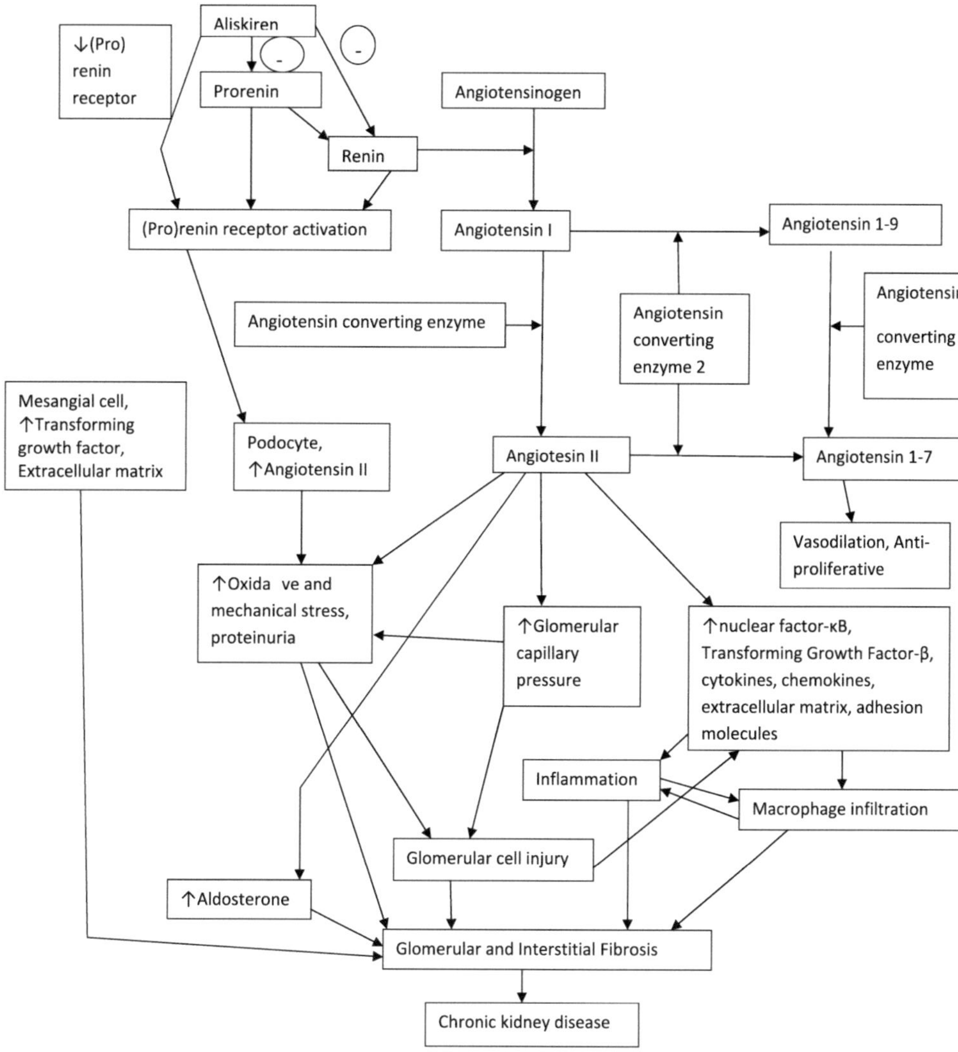

Fig. 3. Multiple role of the Renin angiotensin aldosterone system in the pathogenesis of chronic kidney disease

In patients who have vascular disease or high risk diabetes without heart failure, angiotensin-converting-enzyme inhibitors reduce mortality and morbidity from cardiovascular causes, but the role of angiotensin-receptor blockers in such patients is unknown. The Ongoing Telmisartan Alone and in Combination with Ramipril Global Endpoint Trial (ONTARGET) was carried out for the comparative study between ramipril, telmisartan and the combination of both in patients with vascular disease or high risk diabetes. After a 3 week, single-blind run-in period, patients underwent double-blind randomization, with 8576 assigned to receive 10 mg of ramipri per day, 8542 assigned to receive 80 mg telmisartan per day, and 8502 assigned to receive both drugs (combination therapy). Telmisartan was equivalent to ramipril in patients with vascular disease or high risk diabetes and was associated with less angioedema. The combination of the two drugs was associated with more adverse events without an increase in benefit[131].

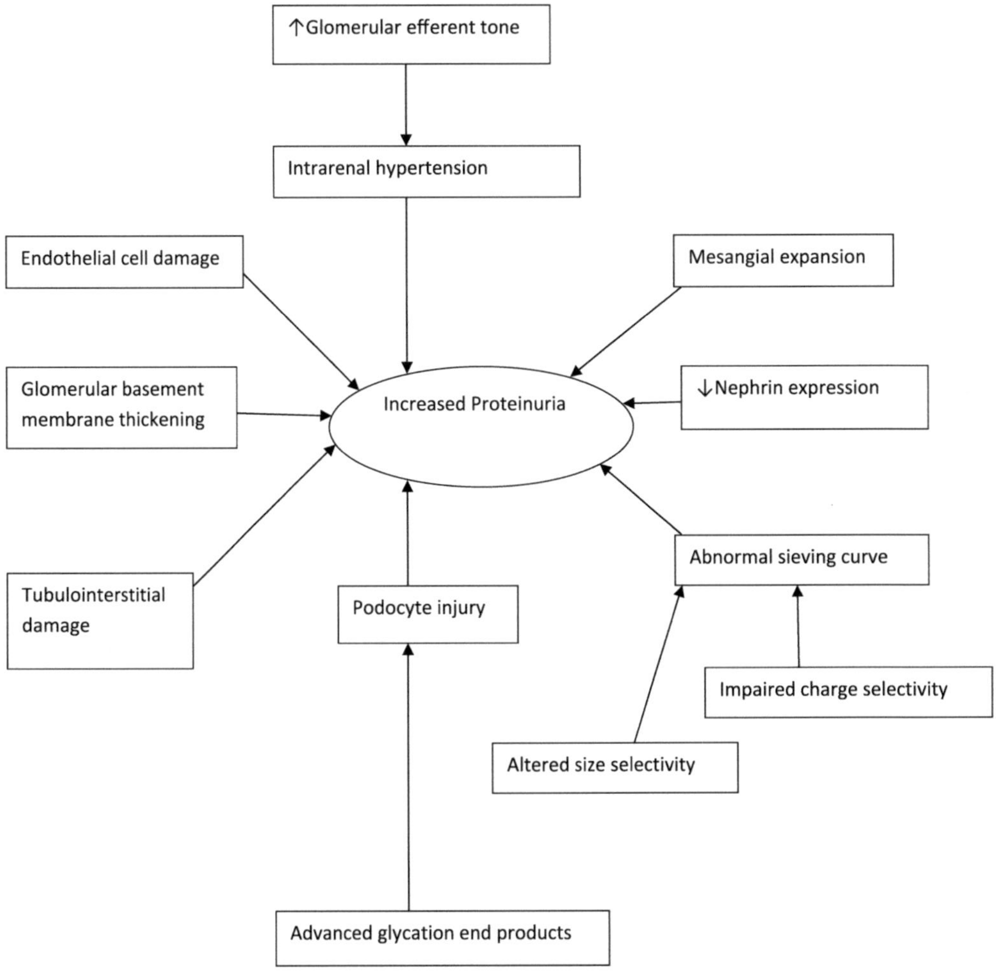

Fig. 4. Mechanism of proteinuria in diabetic nephropathy

Stage	Glomerular Filtration Rate	Urinary albumin excretion (mg/d)	Blood pressure	Years after diagnosis
i. Hyperfiltration	Supernormal	<30	Normal	0
ii. Microalbuminuria	High normal To normal	30-300	Rising	5-15
iii. Proteinuria	Normal To decreasing	>300	Elevated	10-20
iv. Progressive nephropathy	Decreasing	Increasing	Elevated	15-20
v. End stage renal disease	<15ml/min	Nephrotic	Elevated	20-30

Table 1. Stages of Diabetic Nephropathy

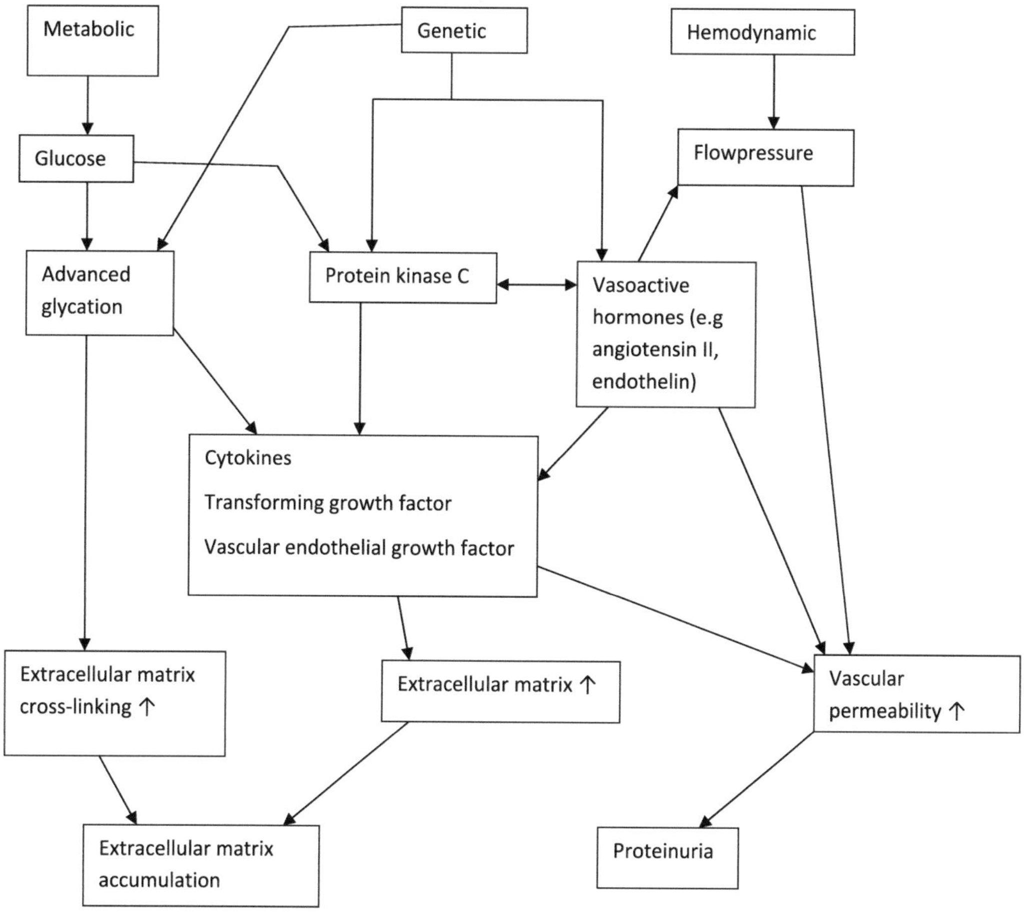

Fig. 5. Pathogenesis of Diabetic nephropathy

6. Conclusion

ACE inhibitors and ARBs, as monotherapy or in combination, have evolved as accepted first-line agents for delaying the progression of diabetic nephropathy. Currently, recommendations favor ACE inhibitors for type 1 and ARBs or ACE inhibitors for type 2 diabetes as a result of large, controlled clinical trials. Therapeutic goals should be addressed not only for BP reduction, but in diminishing albuminuria as well. In subjects with microalbuminuria, the dose of ARBs or ACE inhibitors should be titrated by the clinician until normoalbuminuria is induced, even if supramaximal doses or a combination of ARBs and ACE inhibitors are necessary. There is evidence that achieving reduction in both microalbuminuria and in heavy proteinuria at greater doses than those used to control BP may be required using monotherapy or a combination of these RAS blockers[132].

Different studies showed that higher doses of angiotensin converting enzyme inhibitors and angiotensin receptor blocker are safer and beneficial. Rationale to use higher doses of angiotensin converting enzyme inhibitors or angiotensin receptor blocker is not only to reduce proteinuria and or to control blood pressure. Additional beneficial effects are observed at higher doses other than renal systems. Losartan showed cardio protection by cardiac remodeling, vascular remodeling, atherosclerosis, endothelial function, inhibition of thrombus formation and platelet aggregation, reduction of risk factor for stroke in addition to renal effects[133].

Higher drug doses can reduce nephrotoxic components like TGF β[134], connective tissue growth factor[135], inflammatory mediators like cytokines[63] etc. It is evident that, these drugs, even when do not reduce proteinuria or blood pressure significantly, may provide the additional renoprotection with higher doses.

Dual blockade of the RAS provides superior short-term renoprotection independent of systemic blood pressure changes in comparison with maximally recommended doses of ACEI in patients with type 2 diabetes as well as nephropathy.

The ability of these two therapeutic agents to synergistically antagonize the RAAS can also be explained by their complimentary mechanisms of action. For example, ACE inhibition leads to a prolonged half-life of bradykinin, a potent vasodilator believed to be renoprotective. ARBs do not increase the half-life of bradykinin. They can further ablate the damaging effects resulting from the production of angiotensin II by non-ACE pathways, which is not completely blocked by an ACEI. Thus, it seems plausible that combining these two agents could more effectively oppose the RAAS than either agent alone[136].

7. References

[1] Anderson RN. Deaths: Leading causes for 1999. Natl Vital Stat Rep. 2001; 49: 1-87.

[2] Turnar R, Holman R, Stratton I, Cull C, Frighi V, Manley S, Matthews D, Neil A, McElroy H, Kohner E, Fox C, Hadden D, Wright D. Tight blood pressure control and risk of macrovascular and microvasular complications type 2 diabetes. BMJ. 1998; 317: 703-13.

[3] Rahman M, Roy AC, Chowdhury D, Hossain M. Clinicopathological spectrum of renal diseases in IPGMR. An analysis of 2000 cases in 11 years. Journal of BCPS 1985; 11: 3-11.

[4] Mogensen CE. Progression of nephropathy in long-term diabetics with proteinuria and effect of initial antihypertensive treatment. Scand J Clin Lab Invest 1976; 36: 383-88.

[5] Parving HH, Andersen AR, Smidt UM, Svendsen PA. Early aggressive antihypertensive treatment reduces rate of decline in kidney function in Diabetic Nephropathy. Lancet 1 1983: 1175-79.

[6] Wilmer WA, Hebert LA, Lewis EJ, Rohd RD, Whittier F, Cattran D, Levey AS, Lewis JB, Spitalewitz S, Blumenthal S, Bain RP. Remission of nephritic syndrome in type 1 diabetes: long term follow of patients in the captopril study. Am J Kidney Dis. 1999; 34: 308-14

[7] Lewis E, Hunsicker L, Bain R, Rhode R. The effect of angiotensin converting enzyme inhibition on Diabetic nephropathy. N Engle J Med. 1993; 329: 1456-62.

[8] Björck S, Mulec H, Johnsen SA, Norden G, Aurell M. Renal protective effect of enalapril in diabetic nephropathy. BMJ 1992; 304: 339-43.

[9] Campese Vm, Bianchi S, Bigazzi R. Is microalbuminuria a predictor of cardiovascular and renal disease in patients with essential hypertension? Curr Opin Nephron Hypertens. 2000; 9: 143-47.

[10] Williams ME. Diabetic nephropathy: The proteinuria hypothesis. Am J Nephrol. 2005; 25: 77-94.
[11] Raptis AE, Viberti G. Pathogenesis of diabetic nephropathy. Exp Clin Endocrinol Diabetes. 2001; 109 (Suppl 2): S424-S437.
[12] Sheetz MJ, King GL. Molecular understanding of hyperglycemia's adverse effects for diabetic complications. JAMA. 2002; 288 (20): 2579-88.
[13] Brownlee M. Biochemistry and molecular cell biology of diabetic complications. Nature. 2001; 414: 813-20.
[14] Vlassara H, Palace MR. Diabetes and advanced glycation end products. J Intern Med. 2002; 251 (2): 87-101.
[15] Carey RM and Siragy HM. The intrarenal renin angiotensin system and diabetic nephropathy. TRENDS in Endocrin and Met. 2003; 14: 274-81.
[16] Bennett PN and Brown MJ. Arterial hypertension, angina pectoris, myocardial infarction. In: Clinical Pharmacology; Ninth edition. New York: Churchill Livingstone; 2003: pp 467.
[17] Remuzzi G, Perico N, Macia M, Ruggenenti P. The role of renin-angiotensin-aldosterone system in the progression of chronic kidney disease. Kidney Int. 2005; 68, Supplement 99: S57-S65.
[18] Andersen S, Jung FF, Ingelfinger JR. Renal renin-angiotensin system in diabetes. Functional, immunohisochemical and molecular biological correlations. AM J Physiol. 1993; 265: F477-F86.
[19] Brenner BM, Lawler EV, Mackenzie HS. The hyperfiltration theory: a paradigm shift in nephrology. Kidney Int. 1996; 49: 1774-77.
[20] Anderson S, Rennke HG, Brenner BM. Therapeutic advantage of converting enzyme inhibitors in arresting progressive renal disease associated with systemic hypertension in the rat. J Clin Invest. 1986; 77 (6): 1993-2000.
[21] Zachary T, Bloomgarden MD. Diabetic nephropathy. Diabetes care. 2005;28:745-75.
[22] Shake JG, Brandt RC, Daniels BS. Angiotensin II induces actin polymerization within the glomerular filtration barrier: Possible role in the local regulation of ultrafiltration. J Am Soc Nephrol. 1992; 3: 568A.
[23] Ruiz-Ortega M, Lorenzo O, Suzuki Y, Rupérez M, Egido J. Pro-inflammatory actions of angiotensins. Curr Opin Nephrol Hypertens. 2001; 10" 321-29.
[24] Choles HR, Kasinath BS, Gorin Y, Abboud He. Angiotensin II and growth factors in the pathogenesis of diabetic nephropathy. Kidney Int Suppl. 2002; 82: 8-11.
[25] Brenner BM. Remission of renal disease: Recounting the challenge, acquiring the goal. J Clin Invest. 2002; 110: 1753-58.
[26] Oberleithner H. Aldosterone makes human endothelium stiff and vulnerable. Kidney Int. 2005; 67: 1680-82.
[27] Yoshioka T, Mitarai T, Kon V, Deen WM, Rennke HG, Ichikawa I. Role for angiotensin II in an overt functional proteinuria. Kidney Int. 1986; 30: 538-45.
[28] Yoshioka T, Rennke HG, Salant DJ, Deen WM, Ichikawa I. Role of abnormally high transmural pressure in the permselectivity defect of glomerular capillary wall: a study in early passive Heymann nepritis. Circ Res. 1987; 61: 531-38.
[29] Abbate M, Zoja C, Rottoli D, Corna D, Tomasoni S, Remuzzi G. Proximal tubular cells promote fibrogenesis by TGF β1 mediated induction of peritubular myofibroblasts. Kidney Int. 2002; 61: 2066-77.

[30] Abbate M, Zoja C, Morigi M, Rottoli D, Angioletti S, Tomasoni S, Zanchi C, Longeretti L, Donadelli R, Remuzzi G. Transforming growth factor beta 1 is upregulated by podocytes in response to excess intraglomerular passage of proteins. Am J PAthol. 2002; 161: 2179-93.
[31] Cao Z, Cooper ME. Role of angiotensin II in tubule interstitial injury. Semin Nephrol. 2001; 21: 554-62.
[32] Eddy AA. Molecular insights into renal interstitial fibrosis [Editorial]. J AM Soc Nephrol. 1996; 7: 2495-508.
[33] Border WA, Nobble NA. Transforming growth factor beta in tissue fibrosis. N Engl J Med. 1994; 331: 1286-92.
[34] Postlethwaite AE, Holness MA, Katali H, Raghow R. Human fibroblasts synthesize elevated levels of extracellular matrix proteins in response to interleukin 4. J Clin Invest. 1992; 90: 1479-85.
[35] Jarma K, Ziyadeh FN. The transforming growth factor-beta system and the kidney. Semin Nephrol. 1993; 13: 116-28.
[36] AC, Jowett TP, Firth JD, Burton S, Kitamura M, Fine LG. A new paracrine loop implicated in human tubulo-interstitial fibrosis: tubular derived endothelins modulate renal interstitial fibroblast function [Abstract]. J Am Soc Nephrol. 1993, 4: 473.
[37] Remuzzi G MD, Ruggenenti P. Chronic renal disease: Renoprotective benefits of renin angiotensin system inhibition. Ann Intern Med. 2002; 136: 604-15.
[38] Abbate M, Zoja C, Rottoli D, Corna D, Perico N, Bertani T, Remuzzi G. Antiproteinuric therapy while preventing the abnormal protein tubule abrogates protein and complement dependent interstitial inflammation in experimental renal disease. J Am Soc Nephrol. 1999; 10: 804-13
[39] Hoffmann S, Podlich D, Hahnel B,Kriz W, Gretz N. Angiotensin II type 1 receptor overexpression in podocytes induces glomerulosclerosis in transgenic rats. J Am Soc Nephrol. 2004; 15: 1475-87.
[40] Macconi D, Ghilarrdi M, Bonassi ME, Mohamed EI, Abbate M, Colombi F, Remuzzi G, Remuzzi A. Effect of Angiotensin-Converting Enzyme Inhibition on Glomerular Basement Membrane Permeability and Distribution of Zonula Occludens-1 in MWF Rats. J Am Soc Nephrol. 2000; 11: 477-89.
[41] Benigni A, Tomasoni S Gagliardini E, Zoja C, James A, Grunkemeyer, Kalluri R, Remuzzi G. Blocking angiotensin II synthesis/activity preserves glomerular nephrin in rats with severe nephrosis. J Am Soc Nephrol. 2001; 12: 941-48.
[42] Bonnet F, Cooper ME, Kawachi H, Allen TJ, Boner G, Cao Z. Irbesartan normalizes the defficiency in glomerular nephrin expression in a model of diabetes and hypertension. Diabetologia. 2001; 44: 874-77.
[43] Stevinkel P, Ketteles M, Johnson R, Lindholm B, Pecotis-Filho R, Riella M, HeimbÜrger O, Cederholm T, Girndt M. IL-10, IL-6, and TNF-alpha: central factors in the altered cytokine network of uremia- The good, the bad, and the ugly. Kidney Int. 2005;67: 1216-33.
[44] Stevinkel P, Anderson A, Wang T, Lindholm B, Bergstrom J, Palmblad J, , HeimbÜrger O, Cederholm T. Do ACE-inhibitors suppress tumor necrosis factor alpha production in advanced chronic renal failure? J Int Med. 1999; 246 (5): 503-7.
[45] Rossing K, Christensen PK, Hansen BV, Carstensen B, Parving HH. Optimal dose of candesartan for renoprotection in type 2 diabetic patients with nephropathy. Diabetes care. 2003; 26: 150-55.

[46] Rossing K, Schjoedt KJ, Jensen BR, Boomsma F, Parving HH. Enhanced renoprotective effects of ultrahigh doses of irbesartan in patients with type 2 diabetes and microalbuminuria. Kidney Int. 2005. 68: 1190-98.
[47] Parving HH, Lehnert H, Jens B, Mortensen C, Gomis R, Andersen S, Arner P. The effect of irbesartan on the development of diabetic nephropathy in patients with type 2 diabetes. N Engl J Med. 2001; 345: 870-78.
[48] Brenner BM, Cooper ME, de Zeeuw D, Keane WF, Mitch WE, Parving HH, Remuzzi G, Snapinn V, Zhang Z, Shahnaz. Effects of losartan on renal and cardiovascular outcomes in patients with type 2 diabetes mellitus and nephropathy. N Engl J Med. 2001; 345: 861-69.
[49] Lewis EJ, Hunsicker LG, Clarke WR, Berl T, Pohl MA, Lewis JB, Ritz E, Atkins RC, Rohde R, Itamar Raz. Reno protective effects of the angiotensin receptor antagonists irbesartan in patients with nephropathy due to type 2 diabetes. N Engl J Med. 2001; 345: 851-60.
[50] Viberti G and Wheeldon NM. Microalbuminuria reduction with valsartan in patients with type 2 diabetes mellitus- A blood pressure independent effect. Circulation. 2002; 106: 672-78.
[51] Imanishi M, Yoshika K, Konish Y. Glomerular hypertension as one of albuminuria in type 2 diabetic patients. Diabetologia. 1999; 42: 999-1005.
[52] Andersen S, Blouch K, Bialek J, Deckert M, Parving HH, Myers BD. Glomerular permselectivity in early stages of overt diabetic nephropathy. Kidney Int. 2000. 58: 2129-37.
[53] Bennet P, Cooper ME, Kawachi H, Allen TJ, Boner G, Cao Z. Irbesartan normalizes the deficiency in glomerular nephrin expression in a model of diabetes and hypertension. Diabetologia. 2001; 44: 874-77.
[54] Maciasaac RJ, Jerums G, Cooper ME. New insights into the significance of microalbuminuria. Curr Opin Nephrol Hypertens. 2004; 13: 83-91.
[55] Sturgill BC and Shearlock KT. Membranous glomerulopathy and nephrotic syndrome after captopril therapy. JAMA. 1983; 250: 2343-45.
[56] Textor SC, Gephardt GN, Bravo EL, Tarazi RC, Fouad FM, Tubbs R, McMahon JT. Membranous glomerulopathy associated with captopril therapy. Am J Med. 1983; 74: 705-12.
[57] Hoorntje SJ, Kallenberg CG, Weening JJ, Donkar AJ, The TH, Hoedemaeker PJ. Immune-complex glomerulopathy in patients treated with captopril. Lancet. 1980; 1: 1212-15.
[58] Weinberg AJ, Zappe DH, Ashton M, Weinberg MS. Safety and tolerability of high dose angiotensin blocker therapy in patients with chronic kidney disease: A pilot study. Am J Nephrol. 2004; 24: 340-45.
[59] Schmieder RE. Talmesartan/hydrochlorothiazide combination therapy in the treatment of essential hypertension. Expert Opin Pharmacother. 2004; 5: 2303-10.
[60] Benigni A and Remuzzi G. How renal cytokines and growth factors contribute to renal disease progression. Am J Kidney Dis. 2001; 37[Suppl 2]: S21-S24.
[61] Donadelli R, Zanchi C, Morigi M, Buelli S, Batani C, Tomasoni S, Corna D, Rottoli D, Benigni A, Abbate M, Remuzzi G, Zoja C. Protein overload induces fractalkine upregulation in proximal tubular cells through nuclear factor kappaB- and p38 mitogen activated protein kinase dependent pathways. J Am Soc Nephrol. 2003; 14: 2436-46.

[62] Fujihara C K, Velho M, Malheiros DMAC, Zatz R. An extremely high dose of losartan affords superior renoprotection in the remnant model. Kidney Int. 2005; 67: 1913-1924.

[63] Anderson S, Rossing P, Juhl TR, Deinum J, Parving HH. Optimal dose of losartan for renoprotection in diabetic nephropathy. Nephrol Dial Transplant 2002; 17: 1413-18.

[64] Laverman GD, Navis G, Henning RH, De Jong PE, de Zeeuw D. Dual renin-angiotensin system blockade at optimal doses for proteinuria. Kidney Int 2002; 62: 1020-25.

[65] Dahlof B, Devereux RB, Kjeldsen SE, Julius S, Beevers G, Faire U, Fyhrquist F, Ibsen H, Kristiansson K, Lederballe-Pedersen O, Lindholm LH, Nieminen MS, Omvik P, Oparil S, Wedel H. Cardiovascular morbidity and mortality in the Losartan Intervention For Endpoint reduction in hypertension study (LIFE): a randomized trial against atenolol. Lancet. 2002; 359: 995–1003.

[66] Andersen S, Brochuer - Mortensen J, Parving HH. For the Irbesartan in patients with type 2 Diabetes & Microalbuminuria. Study Group: Kidney function during & after withdrawal of long-term irbesartan treatment in patients with type 2 diabetes and microalbuminuria. Diabetes Care. 2003; 26: 3296-3302.

[67] Forclaz A, Maillard M, Nussberger J, Brunner H R, Burnier M. Angiotensin II Receptor Blockade. Is There a Benefit of Adding an ACE Inhibitor? Hypertension. 2003; 41: 31-36.

[68] Maillard MP, Wurzner G, Nussberger J, Centeno C, Burnier M, Brunner HR. Comparative angiotensin II Receptor blockade in healthy volunteers: the importance of dosing. Clinical Pharmacol Ther. 2002; 71: 68-76.

[69] Maillard MP, Mazzolai L, Daven V, Centeno C, Nussberger J, Brunner HR, Burnier M. Assessment of angiotensin II receptor blockade in humans using a standardized angiotensin II receptor-binding assay. Am J Hypertens. 1999; 12:1201–1208.

[70] Ferguson RK, Turini GA, Brunner HR, Gavras H, McKinstry DN. A specific orally active inhibitor of angiotensin-converting enzyme in man. Lancet. 1977; 309:775–778.

[71] Schmieder RE, Klingbeil AU, Fleiscgmann EH, Veelken R, Delles C. Additional antiproteinuric effect of ultra high dose candesartan: A double-blind, randomized, prospective study. J Am Soc Nephrol 2005; 16: 3038-45.

[72] Weinberg MS, Weinberg AJ, Cor R, Zapper DH. The effect of high-dose angiotensin II receptor blockade beyond maximal recommended doses in reducing urinary protein excretion. J Renin Angiotensin Aldosterone Syst. 2001; 2: S 196 –S 198.

[73] Vogt L, Navis G, de Zeeuw D. Individual titration for maximal blockade of renin-angiotensin system in proteinuric patients: A feasible strategy? J Am Soc Nephrol 2005; 16: S53-S57.

[74] Ruggenenti P, Mise N, Pisoni R, Arnoldi F, Pezzotta A, Perna A, Catteneo D, Remuzzi G. Diverse effects of increasing lisinopril doses on lipid abnormalities in chronic nephropathies. Circulation 2003; 107: 586 - 592.

[75] Schjoedt KJ, Astrup A, Persson F et al. Optimal dose of lisinopril for renoprotection in type 1 diabetic patients with diabetic nephropathy. Proceeding from the European Association for the Study of Diabetes (EASD), 2007.

[76] Tang WHW, Vagelos RH, Yee YG, Benedict CR, Willson KRN, Liss CL, LaBella P, Fowler MB, Neurohormonal and clinical response to high versus low-dose Enalapril therapy in chronic heart failure. J Am Coll Cardiolo. 2002; 39: 70-78.

[77] Adrienne AM, Zandbergen, Marinus GA, Baggen, Lamberts SWJ, Bootsma A H, de Zeeuw D, Ouwendjik RJT. Effect of Losartan on Microalbuminuria in Normotensive Patients with Type 2 Diabetes Mellitus. Ann intern Med. 2003; 139: 90-96.

[78] Lacourciere Y, Belanger A, Godin C, Halle JP, Ross S, Wright N, Marion J. Long-term comparison of losartan and enalapril on the kidney function in hypertensive type 2 diabetics with early nephropathy. Kidney Int. 2000; 58: 762-769.
[79] Jensen TE, Heusterberg J, Sonne J, Strndgaard S, Kamper AL. Enalapril dosage in progressive chronic nephropathy: a randomised, controlled trial. Eur J Clin Pharmacol. 2005; 61: 87-96.
[80] Hou FF, Xie D, Zhang X, Chen PY, Zhang WR, Liang M, Guo ZJ, Jiang JP. Renoprotection of optimal antiproteinuric dose (ROAD) study: A randomized controlled study of Benajepril and Losartan in chronic renal insufficiency. J Am Soc Nephrol. 2007; 18: 1889-98.
[81] Woo KT, Lau YK, Wong KSGSC. ACEI/ATRA therapy decreases proteinuria by improving glomerular permselectivity in IgA nephritis. Kidney Int. 2000; 58: 2485-91.
[82] Rocca HPBLA, Weilenmann D, Kiowski W, Friedrich E, Maly, Follath F. Plasma level of Enalaprilat in chronic therapy of heart failure: Relationship to adverse events. J Pharmacol and Exp Ther. 1999; 289: 565-571.
[83] Brenner BM, Cooper ME, de Zeeuw D, Keane WF, Mitch WE, Parving HH, Remuzzi G, Snapinn V, Zhang Z, Shahnaz. Effects of losartan on renal and cardiovascular outcomes in patients with type 2 diabetes mellitus and nephropathy. N. Engl. J. Med. 2001; 345: 861–869.
[84] Massie BM, Armstrong PW, Cleland JGF. Toleration of high doses of angiotensin-converting enzyme inhibitors in patients with chronic heart failure. Arch Intern Med. 2001; 161:165-71.
[85] Kostis JB, Shelton BJ, Yusuf S. Tolerability of enalapril initiation by patients with left ventricular dysfunction: results of the medication of challenge phase of the Studies of Left Ventricular Dysfunction. Am Heart J. 1994; 128: 358-64.
[86] Packer M, Wilson P A P, Armstrong P W, Cleland JGE, Horowitz JD, Massie BM, Ryden L, Thygesen K, Uretsky BF. Comparative Effects of Low and High Doses of the Angiotensin-Converting Enzyme Inhibitor, Lisinopril, on Morbidity and Mortality in Chronic Heart Failure. Circulation 1999; 100: 2312-2318.
[87] Lewis EJ, Hunsicker LG, Clarke WR, Berl T, Pohl MA, Lewis JB, Ritz E, Atkins R C, Rohde R, Itamar Raz. Reno protective effect of the angiotensin receptor antagonist irbesartan in patients with nephropathy due to type 2 diabetes. N. Engl. J. Med.2001; 345: 851–860.
[88] Cohn JN, Tognoni G. A randomized trial of the angiotensin-receptor blocker valsartan in chronic heart failure. N Eng J Med 2001; 345: 1667-75.
[89] Hollenberg NK, Fisher NDL, Price DA: Pathways for angiotensin II generation in intact human tissue-evidence fromcomparative pharmacological interruption of the renin system. Hypertension 1998; 32:387–392.
[90] Nussberger J, Brunner DB, Waeber B, Brunner HR: Plasma angiotensins under sustained converting enzyme inhibition with enalapril in normal humans. J Hypertens 1985; 3(Suppl 3):S269–S270.
[91] Kobori H, Nangaku M, Navar LG, Nishiyama A: The intrarenal renin-angiotensin system: from physiology to the pathobiology of hypertension and kidney disease. Pharmacol Rev 2007; 59: 251–87.
[92] Kimbrough HM Jr, Vaughan ED Jr, Carey RM, Ayers CR: Effect of intrarenal angiotensin II blockade on renal function in conscious dogs. Circ Res 1977; 40: 174–78.

[93] Sharma K, Cook A, Smith M, Valancius C, Inscho EW: TGF-beta impairs renal autoregulation via generation of ROS. Am J Physiol Renal Physiol 2005; 288: F1069-F1077.
[94] Wolf G, Butzmann U, Wenzel UO: The renin-angiotensin system and progression or renal disease: From hemodynamics to cell biology. Nephron Physiol 2003; 93: 3 –13.
[95] Chen S, Lee JS, Iglesias-de la Cruz MC, Kasama Y, Izquier-do-Lahuerta A, Wolf G, Ziyadeh FN: Angiotensin II stimulates alpha3(IV) collagen production in mouse podocytes via TGF-beta and VEGF signaling: Implications for diabetic nephropathy. Nephrol Dial Transplant 2005; 20: 1320–28.
[96] Sarnak MJ, Levey AS, Schoolwerth AC, Coresh J, Culleton B, Hamm LL, et al. Kidney disease as a risk factor for development of cardiovascular disease: a statement from the American Heart Association Councils on Kidney in Cardiovascular Disease, High Blood Pressure Research, Clinical Cardiology and Epidimiology and Prevention. Circulation 2003; 108: 2154-2169.
[97] Ruster C, Wolf G. Renin-Angiotensin-Aldosterone System and Progression of Renal Disease.J Am Soc Nephrol 2006; 17:2985-91.
[98] Atlas SA: The renin-angiotensin aldosterone system: pathophysiological role and pharmacologic inhibition. J Manag Care Pharm 2007; 13: 9–20.
[99] Huang XR, Chen WY, Truong LD, Lan HY: Chymase is upregulated in diabetic nephropathy: implications for an alternative pathway of angiotensin II-mediated diabetic renal and vascular disease. J Am Soc Nephrol 2003; 14: 1738–47.
[100] Burns KD. Angiotensin II and its receptors in the diabetic kidney. Am J Kidney Dis 2000; 36:449-67.
[101] Siragy HM: The role of the AT2 receptor in hypertension. Am J Hypertens 2000; 3 Suppl(5 Pt 2):62S–67S.
[102] Allen TJ, Cao Z, Youssef S, et al: The role of angiotensin II and bradykinin in experimental diabetic nephropathy: Functional and structural studies. Diabetes 1997; 46:1612–1618.
[103] Russo D, Pisano A, Balletta MM, et al: Additive antiproteinuric effects of converting enzyme inhibitor and losartan in normotensive patients with IgA nephropathy. Am J Kidney Dis 1999; 33:851–856.
[104] Ruilope LM,Aldigier JC, Ponticelli C, et al: Safety of the combination of valsartan and benazepril in patients with chronic renal disease. European Group for the Investigation of Valsartan in Chronic Renal Disease. J Hypertens 2000; 18:89–95.
[105] Ferrari P,MartiHP, PfisterM, Frey JF:Additive antiproteinuric effect of combined ACE inhibition and angiotensin II receptor blockade. J Hypertens 2002; 20:125–130.
[106] Mogensen CE, Neldam S, Tikkanen I, et al: Randomised controlled trial of dual blockade of renin-angiotensin systemin patients with hypertension, microalbuminuria, and non-insulin dependent diabetes: The candesartan and lisinopril microalbuminuria (CALM) study. BMJ 2000; 321:1440–1444.
[107] Jacobsen P, Andersen S, Rossing K, et al: Dual blockade of the renin angiotensin system in type 1 patients with diabetic nephropathy. Nephrol Dial Transplant 2002; 17:1019–1024.
[108] Jennings DL, Kalus JS, Coleman CI, Manierski C, Yee J. Combination therapy with an ACE inhibitor and an angiotensin receptor blocker for diabetic nephropathy: a meta-analysis. Diabet Med. 2007; 24:486-93.

[109] Hostetter TH. Prevention of end-stage renal disease due to type 2 diabetes. N Engl J Med 2001; 345:910-2.
[110] Cetinkaya R, Odabas AR, Selcuk Y. Anti-proteinuric effects of combination therapy with enalapril and losartan in patients with nephropathy due to type 2 diabetes. Int J Clin Pract 2004; 58:432-5.
[111] Rossing K, Christensen PK, Jensen BR, Parving HH. Dual blockade of the renin-angiotensin system in diabetic nephropathy: a randomized double-blind crossover study. Diabetes Care 2002; 25:95-100.
[112] Rossing K, Jacobsen P, Pietraszek L, Parving HH. Renoprotective effects of adding angiotensin II receptor blocker to maximal recommended doses of ACE inhibitor in diabetic nephropathy: a randomized double-blind crossover trial. Diabetes Care 2003; 26:2268-74.
[113] Agarwal R. Add-on angiotensin receptor blockade with maximized ACE inhibition. Kidney Int 2001; 59:2282-9.
[114] Song JH, Lee SW, Suh JH, et al. The effects of dual blockade of the renin-angiotensin system on urinary protein and transforming growth factor-beta excretion in 2 groups of patients with IgA and diabetic nephropathy. Clin Nephrol 2003; 60:318-26.
[115] Kim MJ, Song JH, Suh JH, Lee SW, Kim GA. Additive antiproteinuric effect of combination therapy with ACE inhibitor and angiotensin II receptor antagonist: differential short-term response between IgA nephropathy and diabetic nephropathy. Yonsei Med J 2003; 44:463-72.
[116] Doulton TW, He FJ, MacGregor GA. Systematic review of combined angiotensin-converting enzyme inhibition and angiotensin receptor blockade in hypertension. Hypertension 2005; 45: 880-86.
[117] MacKinnon M, Shurraw S, Akbari A, Knoll GA, Jaffey J, Clark HD: Combination therapy with an angiotensin receptor blocker and an ACE inhibitor in proteinuric renal disease: a systematic review of the efficacy and safety data. Am J Kidney Dis 2006; 48: 8-20.
[118] Bakris GL, Ruilope L, Locatelli F, et al: Treatment of microalbuminuria in hypertensive subjects with elevated cardiovascular risk: results of the IMPROVE trial. Kidney Int 2007; 72: 879-85.
[119] Menne J, Farsang C, Deak L, Klebs S, Meier M, Handrock R, et al: Valsartan in combination with lisinopril versus the respective high dose monotherapies in hypertensive patients with microalbuminuria: the VALERIA trial. J Hypertens 2008; 26: 1860-67.
[120] Persson F, Rossing P, Schjoedt KJ, Juhl T, Tarnow L, Stehouwer CD, Schalkwijk C, Boomsma F, Frandsen E, Parving HH: Time course of the antiproteinuric and antihypertensive effects of direct renin inhibition in type 2 diabetes. Kidney Int 2008; 73: 1419–25.
[121] Persson F, Rossing P, Reinhard H, Juhl T, Stehouwer CD, Schalkwijk C, Danser AH, Boomsma F, Frandsen E, Parving HH: Renal effects of aliskiren compared with and in combination with irbesartan in patients with type 2 diabetes, hypertension, and albuminuria. Diabetes Care 2009; 32: 1873–79.
[122] Yarows SA: Aliskiren/valsartan combination for the treatment of cardiovascular and renal diseases. Expert Rev Cardiovasc Ther 2010; 8: 19–33.
[123] Feldman DL: New insights into the renoprotective actions of the renin inhibitor aliskiren in experimental renal disease. Hypertens Res 2010; 33: 279–287.

[124] Feldman DL, Jin L, Xuan H, Contrepas A, Zhou Y, Webb RL, Mueller DN, Feldt S, Cumin F, Maniara W, Persohn E, Schuetz H, Jan Danser AH, Nguyen G: Effects of aliskiren on blood pressure, albuminuria, and (pro)renin receptor expression in diabetic TG(mRen-2)27 rats. Hypertension 2008; 52: 130–136.

[125] Danser AH: The increase in renin during renin inhibition: does it result in harmful effects by the (pro)renin receptor? Hypertens Res 2010; 33:4–10.

[126] Feldman DL: New insights into the renoprotective actions of the renin inhibitor aliskiren in experimental renal disease. Hypertens Res 2010; 33: 279–287.

[127] Pimenta E, Oparil S: Role of aliskiren in cardiorenal protection and use in hypertensives with multiple risk factors. Ther Clin Risk Manag 2009; 5: 459–464.

[128] KDOQI Clinical Practice Guidelines and Clinical Practice Recommendations for Diabetes and Chronic Kidney Disease. Am J Kidney Dis 2007; 49:S12–S154.

[129] Pilz B, Shagdarsuren E, Wellner M, Fiebeler A, Dechend R, Gratze P, Meiners S, Feldman DL, Webb RL, Garrelds IM, Jan Danser AH, Luft FC, Muller DN: Aliskiren, a human renin inhibitor, ameliorates cardiac and renal damage in double-transgenic rats. Hypertension 2005; 46: 569–576.

[130] Huang Y, Wongamorntham S, Kasting J, Mc-Quillan D, Owens RT, Yu L, Noble NA, Border W: Renin increases mesangial cell transforming growth factor- β_1 and matrix proteins through receptor-mediated, angiotensin II-independent mechanisms. Kidney Int 2006; 69: 105–113.

[131] Yusuf S, Teo KK, Pogue J, Dyal L, Copland I, Hamilton ON, Schumacher H, Ingelheim B, Dagenais G, Sleight P, Anderson C. Telmisartan, Ramipril, or Both in patients at high risk for vascular events. N Engl J Med 2008; 358: 1547-59.

[132] Marc S. Weinberg, MD, Nicholas Kaperonis, MD, and George L. Bakris, MD. How High Should an ACE Inhibitor or Angiotensin Receptor Blocker Be Dosed in Patients with Diabetic Nephropathy? Current Hypertension Reports 2003; 5:418–425.

[133] Dahlof B, Devereux R, de Faire U. The Losartan Intervention For Endpoint reduction (LIFE) in Hypertension study: rationale, design, and methods. The LIFE Study Group. Am J Hypertens. 1997; 10: 705-713.

[134] Anderson S, Rossing P, Juhl TR, Deinum J, Parving HH. Optimal dose of losartan for renoprotection in diabetic nephropathy. Nephrol Dial Transplant 2002; 17: 1413-18.

[135] Andersen S, Frans A, Nieuwenhoven V, Tarnow L, Rossing P, Rossing K, Wieten L, Goldschmeding R, Parving HH. Reduction of urinary connective tissue growth factor by Losartan in type 1 patients with diabetic nephropathy. Kidney Int. 2005; 67: 2325-29.

[136] Imig JD. ACE inhibition and bradykinin-mediated renal vascular responses. Hypertension 2004; 43: 533.

Section 2

Novel Therapeutic Molecules in Diabetic Nephropathy

5

Kidney ADP-Ribosyl Cyclase Inhibitors as a Therapeutic Tool for Diabetic Nephropathy

Uh-Hyun Kim
Department of Biochemistry and the Institute of Cardiovascular Research, Chonbuk National University Medical School, Jeonju Republic of Korea

1. Introduction

ADP-ribosyl cyclases (ADPR-cyclases)/CD38 have emerged as effecter molecules for generating novel Ca^{2+} signaling messengers, cyclic ADP-ribose (cADPR) and nicotinic acid adenine dinucleotide phosphate (NAADP) (1, 2) (see Figure 1). Mounting evidence has indicated that G protein-coupled receptors, including the angiotensin II (Ang II) receptor, mediate activation of ADPR-cyclase to generate Ca^{2+} signaling messengers (3-5). We have studied Ang II receptor-mediated activation of ADPR-cyclase, resulting in Ca^{2+} dysfunction

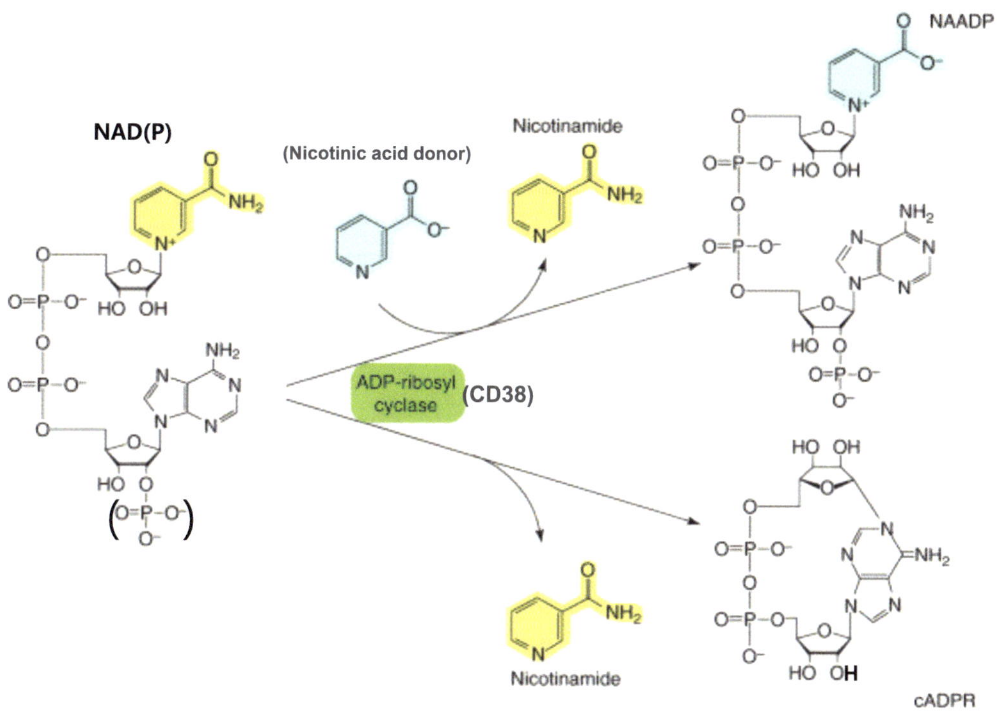

Fig. 1. CD38/ADPR-cyclase-catalyzed reactions for the production of two Ca^{2+} mobilizing second messengers, NAADP and cADPR.

which plays an important role in the pathogenesis of renal failure using an in vitro and an in vivo model (4, 6). In this review article, I would like to give an overview on the current worldwide status of diabetic nephropathy (DN) as a leading cause of end-stage renal disease (ESDR), the causative role of renin-angiotensin-aldosterone system (RAAS) for DN, the role of ADPR-cyclase in pathogenesis of DN and a potential therapeutic tool for DN by the intervention of Ang II receptor-mediated Ca^{2+} signaling with a kidney-specific ADPR-cyclase inhibitor.

2. Diabetic nephropathy and the renin-angiotensin-aldosterone system

Chronic kidney disease (CKD) is a major worldwide public-health problem affecting about 10% of the population (7). CKD has an increased annual incidence rate of about 5–8% (8). A leading cause of CKD is diabetic nephropathy (DN) throughout much of the world. This disease is characterized by the thickening of the glomerular basement membrane and mesangial matrix expansion (9). The early stage of DN is associated with glomerular hyperfiltration and glomerular hypertrophy, but not the collapse of the glomerular capillaries. DN results from an interaction between metabolic and hemodynamic factors. Glucose-dependent pathways are activated within the diabetic kidney, such as increasing oxidative stress, polyol formation, and advanced glycation end product accumulation (10).

In addition to elevated blood glucose, hypertension and inappropriate activation of the RAAS have been identified as contributing to the development and progression of diabetic renal disease (11). Clinical studies have demonstrated an important role for blood glucose control in reducing the development and progression of DN (12, 13) and they also have shown the importance of blood pressure reduction (14, 15) and the blockade of the RAAS (16–18) in slowing the progression of renal dysfunction in diabetes.

The pharmacological inhibition of the RAAS with angiotensin converting enzyme inhibitors (ACEIs) or angiotensin II receptor antagonists (ARBs) are the first-line treatments for CKD patients. Despite several advantages of these agents, a number of side-effects do occur (19-21). Moreover, the incidence of end-stage renal disease as a result of diabetes continues to rise in the world.

RAAS is a major regulatory system of cardiovascular and renal function. The final step of the RAAS cascade is the activation of Ang II receptors by Ang II. In the kidney, Ang II plays critical roles in the regulation of the glomerular filtration rate (GFR) and renal blood flow, and salt water retention (22-24). Effects of Ang II are mediated by at least two structurally and pharmacologically distinct Ang II type 1 and 2 receptors (AT1R and AT2R, respectively) (23, 24). The physiological and pathophysiological effects of Ang II are mainly exerted by AT1R activation (24-26) via complex interacting signaling pathways involving the primary stimulation of phospholipase C (PLC) and Ca^{2+} mobilization and the secondary activation of protein tyrosine kinase (PTK), extracellular signal-regulated kinases-1 and -2, and phosphatidylinositol 3-kinase (PI3K)-dependent kinase Akt (23-26). We extended these signaling pathways mainly focusing on the molecular basis of Ca^{2+} signaling by ADPR-cyclase activation in Ang II signaling in murine mesangial cells (MMCs) and other cells (see below).

3. ADP-ribosyl cyclase (ADPR-cyclase)/CD38

CD38, a type II transmembrane glycoprotein, represents a mammalian ADPR-cyclase and is involved in T cell activation (27) and oxytocin secretion, which is closely associated with social behavior (28). CD38 acts mainly as an NAD glycohydrolase therewith regulating intracellular NAD levels (29, 30). CD38 was initially identified as a cell surface marker on thymocytes and T lymphocytes, showing discrete expression during lymphocyte differentiation (31). Further studies revealed that CD38 expression is ubiquitous in the immune system as well as in various organs, including prostate epithelial cells, pancreatic islet cells, and brain cells (32-35). From a study on new intracellular messengers in the sea mollusk *Aplysia*, a surprising finding of the striking similarity between human CD38 and the ADPR-cyclase enzyme purified from *Aplysia* was made (36). ADPR-cyclase generates two important Ca^{2+}-mobilizing second messengers, cADPR and NAADP, from NAD^+ and $NADP^+$, respectively (37-39). The second messenger, cADPR, increases intracellular Ca^{2+} concentration ($[Ca^{2+}]i$) through the release of Ca^{2+} from intracellular endoplasmic reticulum (ER) stores via ryanodine receptors and/or Ca^{2+} influx through plasma membrane Ca^{2+} channels (5, 39,40, 41). The other second messenger, NAADP, increases intracellular Ca^{2+} concentration ($[Ca^{2+}]i$) through the release of Ca^{2+} from a discrete intracellular store, called acidic organelles, via Two-pore channels (TPCs) (42). Production of NAADP by ADPR-cyclases including CD38 is stimulated by various G protein-coupled receptors (GPCRs), including, AT1R (43, 44).

Mounting evidence has indicated that ADPR-cyclase(s) other than CD38 may exist in the kidney, brain, and the heart (40, 45), including various cells (30, 45-47). The first clues to the existence of novel ADPR-cyclase(s) emerged from experiments of the comparison of tissue cADPR levels in CD38 wild type and knockout mice (40). Levels of cADPR in spleen, bone marrow and lungs of CD38 knockout mice were significantly decreased, compared to those of CD38 wild type mice, whereas levels of cADPR in brain, heart and kidneys of CD38 knockout mice were comparable to those of CD38 wild type mice (40). These results suggest that ADPR-cyclase(s) other than CD38 may exist in the kidney, brain, and the heart. We recently demonstrated that Ang II-stimulated Ca^{2+} signals were not significantly different between CD38 wild type and CD38 knockout cardiomyocytes (48). However a cADPR antagonistic analog, 8-bromo-cADPR (8-Br-cADPR) completely inhibited the Ang II-induced sustained Ca^{2+} increase. These findings indicate that cADPR is generated by a novel unidentified ADPR-cyclase other than CD38. In addition, a bisphenyl compound 4,4'-dihydroxyazobenzene (4-DAB) has been shown to inhibit kidney ADPR-cyclase, but not CD38, with a high potency (47). The kidney ADPR-cyclase inhibitor inhibits kidney ADPR-cyclase activity with a 10,000-fold more potency than it does with heart ADPR-cyclase activity. However, an analog of 4-DAB, 2,2'-dihydroxyazobenzene (2-DAB), inhibits kidney and heart ADPR-cyclase activity with similar effects (see below). These results suggest that ADPR-cyclases in the kidney and the heart are different. Therefore, the signaling pathways of Ang II-induced ADPR-cyclase activation in rat cardiomyocytes (48) and mesangial cells (4) are different due to different ADPR-cyclases (see below).

4. The role of ADPR-cyclase/CD38 in GPCR-mediated Ca^{2+} signaling

Evidence from our and other laboratories has indicated that various G protein-coupled receptors (GPCRs) mediate the activation of ADP-ribosyl cyclase (ADPR-cyclase) (3-6). ADPR-cyclase-involved GPCRs include the β-adrenergic receptor, muscarinic receptor, interleukin 8 receptor (IL8R) and AT1R. The mechanism by which GPCR activates ADPR-cyclase was discovered from the functional loop involving IL-8 and CD38 in lymphokine-activated killer (LAK) cells (5). Stimulation of IL8R results in protein kinase G-dependent phosphorylation of nonmuscle myosin heavy chain IIA (MHCIIA) and the association of phosphorylated MHCIIA with CD38 through Lck, which are essential for CD38 internalization for cADPR formation (49). Ensuing cADPR-mediated Ca^{2+} release from ER stores induces NAADP production by Rap1 activation via cAMP/Epac/PKA, resulting in the release of Ca^{2+} from lysosome-related acidic organelles (44). Although the result of IL8-mediated CD38 activation mechanism in LAK cells shows us one representative model, whether a similar mechanism by which other GPCRs use to activate ADPR-cyclase in other cells as that in IL8R-LAK cells remains to be clarified.

Initially we assumed that ADPR-cyclase plays a role in Ang II receptor-mediated Ca^{2+} signaling in the kidney. Therefore, we chose mouse mesangial cells (MMCs) as a model system to study Ang II signaling because MMCs are believed to be the center for the pathogenesis of CKD (4). Treatment of MMCs with Ang II induced an increase in intracellular Ca^{2+} concentrations through a transient Ca^{2+} release via an inositol 1,4,5-trisphosphate receptor (IP_3R) and a sustained Ca^{2+} influx via L-type Ca^{2+} channels. The sustained Ca^{2+} signal, but not the transient Ca^{2+} signal, was blocked by 8-Br-cADPR, and an ADPR cyclase inhibitor, 4-DAB. In support of the results, 4-DAB inhibited Ang II-induced cADPR production. Application of pharmacological inhibitors revealed that the activation of ADPR-cyclase by Ang II involved AT1R, PI3K, PTK, and PLC-γ1 (Figure 2).

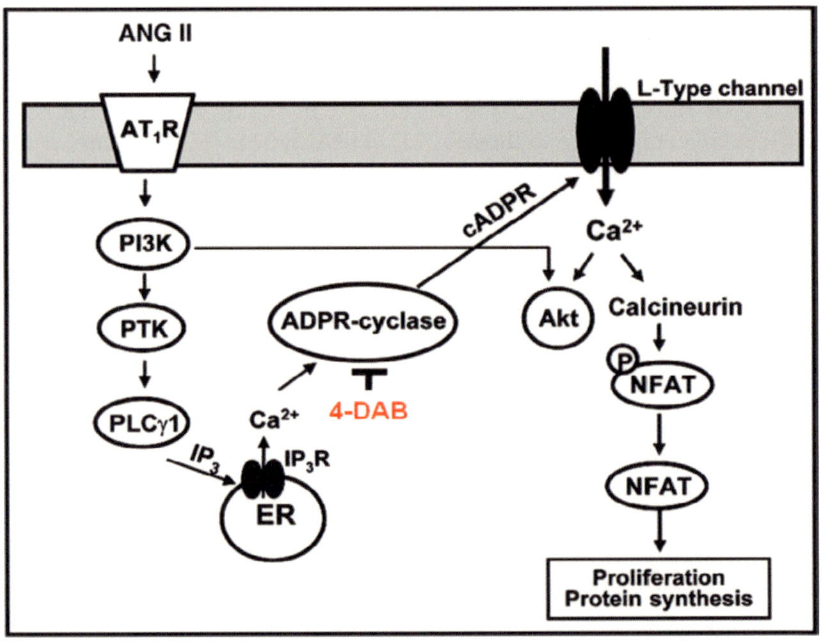

Fig. 2. Schematic model of ADPR-cyclase activation in Ang II signaling pathway (adopted from [4]). Stimulation of AT1R by Ang II leads to sequential activation of PI3K, PTK, and PLCγ1, in turn causing a Ca^{2+} release by IP_3R from ER, resulting in activation of ADPR-cyclase. Activation of ADPR-cyclase induces Ca^{2+} influx via L-type calcium channels, Akt phosphorylation, NFAT nuclear translocation, cell proliferation, and protein synthesis. 4-DAB abrogates the sustained Ca^{2+} signal, thereby blocking downstream events.

Moreover, 4-DAB as well as 8-Br-cADPR abrogated Ang II-mediated Akt phosphorylation, nuclear translocation of nuclear factor of activated T cell (NFAT), and the uptake of

[^{3}H]thymidine and [^{3}H]leucine in MMCs. These results demonstrate that ADPR-cyclase in MMCs plays a pivotal role in Ang II signaling for cell proliferation and protein synthesis. The Ang II-induced ADPR-cyclase activation has also been observed in rat cardiomyocytes (48) and MMCs (4), and hepatic stellate cells (50), although the signaling pathways in those cells are different from each other (see below, Figure 3).

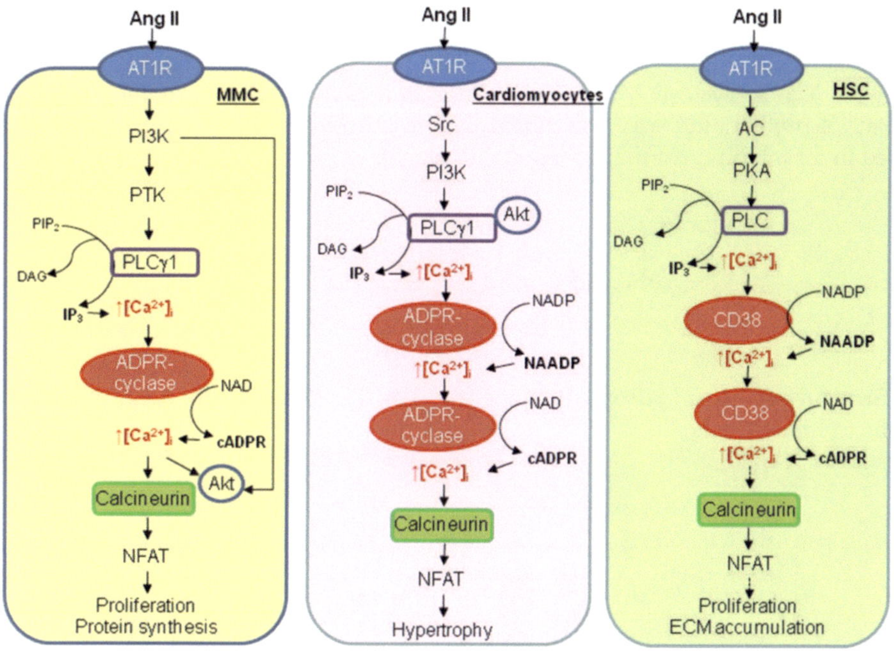

Fig. 3. Variation on the theme of angiotensin II-induced Ca^{2+} signaling. AT1R, angiotensin II type 1 receptor; MMC, mouse mesangial cell; HSC, hepatic stellate cell.

5. The discovery of a small-molecule inhibitor for kidney ADPR-cyclase and its application to diabetic nephropathy

In order to get small-molecule inhibitors of kidney ADPR-cyclase, which make it possible to elucidate the involvement of ADPR-cyclase/cADPR in Ang II signaling in the kidney (4, 6), we screened a chemical library of approximately 10,000 compounds using a partially purified ADPR-cyclase from rat kidneys (47). This screen resulted in the selection of 4-DAB as a small molecule inhibitor (Figure 4). The compound was able to inhibit the generation of cGDPR and ε-ADPR from NGD^+ and ε-NAD^+, respectively, by the kidney ADPR-cyclase in a concentration-dependent manner. These data suggest that the compound may bind to the active site of the enzyme. Half maximal inhibition (IC_{50}) of the enzyme activity was approximately 100 μM. CD38 and ADPR-cyclases partially purified from rat brain, heart, and spleen tissues were insensitive to 4-DAB at 200 μM.

Although a number of GPCRs have been shown to utilize ADPR-cyclase in the regulation of $[Ca^{2+}]$i, we chose the extracellular calcium ion ($[Ca^{2+}]_o$)-sensing receptor (CaSR) to test 4-DAB as a possible candidate inhibitor of ADPR-cyclase in MMCs. Stimulation of CaSR with $[Ca^{2+}]_o$ resulted in a significant increase of [cADPR]i and a generation of long-lasting increase of $[Ca^{2+}]$i, involving an initial peak rise followed by a sustained increase that was gradually decreased. The sustained Ca^{2+} signal, but not the initial peak, was blocked by pre-treatment with 8-Br-cADPR. On the basis of these results that show the stimulation of CaSR activates ADPR-cyclase in MMC, we next evaluated 4-DAB as a possible candidate inhibitor of ADPR-cyclase. This compound was able to inhibit $[Ca^{2+}]_o$-mediated later sustained elevation of $[Ca^{2+}]i$ but not the initial rise of $[Ca^{2+}]i$ in a dose-dependent manner. Further, $[Ca^{2+}]_o$ -induced production of cADPR was also blocked by pre-treatment of 4-DAB in a concentration-dependent manner. IC_{50} was approximately 2.5 nM. In addition, since it has been reported that CaSR-mediated Ca^{2+} signals is involved in MMC proliferation, we examined whether 4-DAB inhibits the $[Ca^{2+}]_o$-induced MMC proliferation and demonstrated that the $[Ca^{2+}]_o$-induced increment of proliferation was also inhibited by 4-DAB in a similar range of concentrations observed in the inhibition of the sustained Ca^{2+} signal.

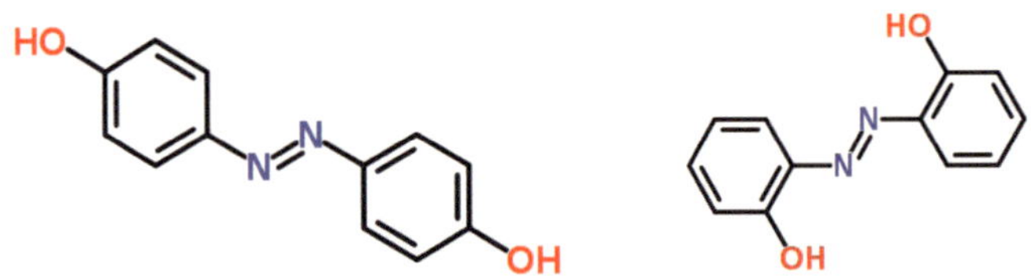

Fig. 4. Structure of 4,4'-dihydroazobenzene (4-DAB), left, and 2,2'-dihydroazobenzene (2-DAB), right.

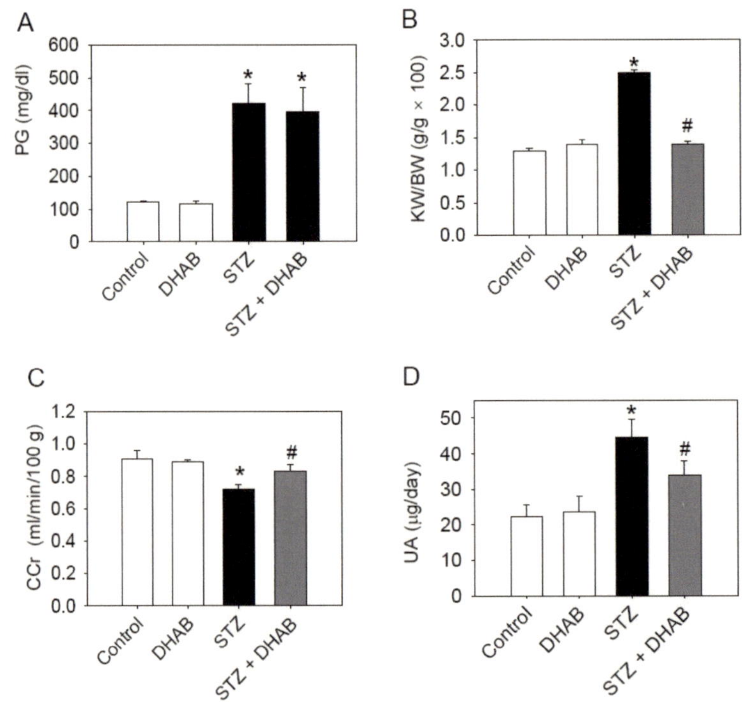

Fig. 5. Effect of 4,4'-dihydroazobenzene (DHAB) on streptozotocin (STZ)-treated mice. (adopted from [6]). A: Plasma glucose level (PG), B: Ratio of kidney weight per body weight (KW/BW), C: Creatinine clearance (CCr) level, and D: Urinary albuminuria (UA) of 6 wk diabetic and control mice after DHAB treatment. Data are means ± SE. $*P < 0.05$ vs. control, $\#P < 0.05$ vs. STZ group.

We utilized the specific inhibitor for kidney ADPR-cyclase to corroborate the evidence that there are ADPR-cyclases different from CD38. We utilized a human T cell-derived cell line, Jurkat T cell, which exclusively expresses CD38 that is regulated by CD3/TCR (51). Treatment of Jurkat T cells with OKT3, which is a ligand for CD3/TCR, showed a typical biphasic increase of $[Ca^{2+}]i$, involving an initial peak rise followed by a sustained increase. Pre-treatment with 8-Br-cADPR inhibited only the sustained Ca^{2+} rise. In contrast, 4-DAB did not show any effects on OKT3-mediated Ca^{2+} rise even at 10 μM.

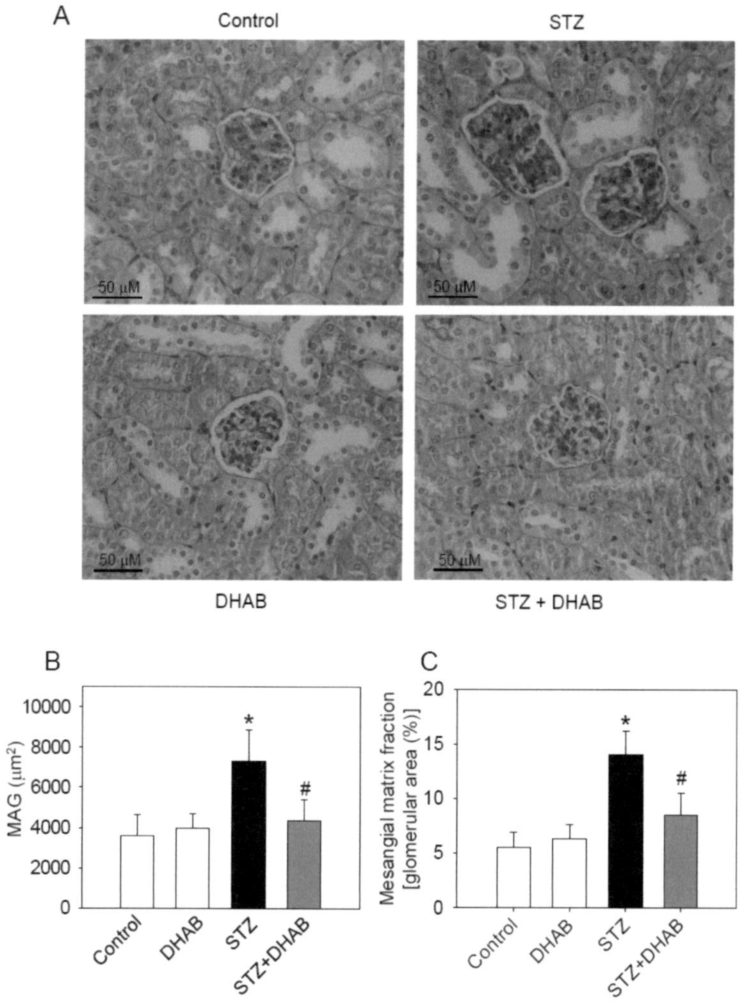

Fig. 6. Light microscopic appearance of glomeruli. (adopted from [6]). A: Representative photomicrographs of the kidney sections stained with periodic acid-Schiff (PAS). Scale bars; 50 μm. B: Quantification of glomerular size from A. Glomerular cross-sectional areas were determined by using a computer-assisted color image analyzer. MAG; mean area of glomeruli. C: Quantification of extracellular mesangial matrix expansion is expressed as PAS-positive mesangial material per total glomerular tuft cross-sectional area (mesangial area/total glomerular tuft area X 100). Values are means ± SE from 25 individual glomeruli in kidney sections from 6 mice in each group. *$P < 0.05$ vs. control; #$P < 0.05$ vs. STZ.

Based on our earlier observation that 4-DAB was a potent inhibitor of kidney ADPR-cyclase and could protect Ang II-mediated mesangial cell growth (4, 47), we further investigated the effects of 4-DAB on a mouse model of DN (6). Male mice were randomly assigned to normal control and diabetic groups of comparable age. The diabetic group received 45 μg/kg of 4-DAB for 6 wk via daily intraperitoneal injections. Alterations of mesangial cell proliferation and extracellular matrix (ECM) production are believed to play predominant roles in the pathogenesis of progressive glomerulosclerosis which leads to ESRD (52, 53). In the process of tissue development and wound healing, TGF-β1 plays a crucial role in controlling ECM deposition and remodeling: TGF- β1 stimulates the synthesis of major components of ECM proteins, such as collagen and fibronectin (54-56). In diabetic kidneys, the overexpression of TGF- β1 is believed to be the major mediator responsible for early pathological changes of DN, including glomerular basement membrane thickening and mesangial matrix expansion (52, 55).

4-DAB treatment significantly ameliorated albuminuria and downregulated the expression of fibrogenic factor TGF-β1, subsequently reducing mesangial matrix protein production in diabetic mice kidney, without, however, changing serum glucose levels (Figures 5 and 6, Ref. 6). ADPR-cyclase was significantly activated, and cADPR levels were also increased in diabetic kidneys, which were prevented by 4-DAB treatment. On the other hand, plasma and kidney Ang II levels were elevated in both the diabetic and 4-DAB -treated diabetic mice group. This result suggests that 4-DAB affects only ADPR-cyclase activation, but not plasma and kidney Ang II levels in the diabetic experimental model. Furthermore, 4-DAB inhibited the phosphorylation of Akt and the NFAT3 nuclear translocation in the kidneys of the diabetic group. These findings indicate a crucial role of ADPR-cyclase signaling in the renal pathogenesis of diabetes and provide a therapeutic tool for the treatment of renal diseases.

6. Perspectives

A potent small-molecule inhibitor 4-DAB, that inhibits specifically the kidney ADPR-cyclase, has been discovered. The discovery of the specific inhibitor for the enzyme enables us to provide further evidence that there are ADPR-cyclases different from CD38. Benefits of the kidney ADPR-cyclase specific inhibitor are several folds: the use of 4-DAB may facilitate in the understanding of kidney functions involving the regulation of Ca^{2+} homeostasis; the inhibitor may help to understand the pathogenesis of the kidney; this compound can be the basis for the development of tissue specific inhibitors of ADPR-cyclases; and finally, the compound may be applied for therapeutic purposes for the prevention and management of human CKD. Furthermore, a similar strategy can be applied for the development of tissue specific inhibitors of ADPR-cyclases with the intent to intervene in other diseases, such as hypertension. For instance, the identification of an inhibitor for ADPR-cyclase of arterial smooth muscle cells can be a potential anti-hypertensive drug.

7. Acknowledgments

This work was supported by the Korea Science and Engineering Foundation (National Research Laboratory Grant R0A-2007-000-20121-0). The author thanks Dr. Gabor Raffai and John Kang for critically reading the manuscript.

8. References

[1] Malavasi, F., Deaglio, S., Funaro, A., Ferrero, E., Horenstein, A. L., Ortolan, E., Vaisitti, T., and Aydin, S. (2008) Evolution and function of the ADP ribosyl cyclase/CD38 gene family in physiology and pathology. Physiol. Rev. 88:841 - 886

[2] Lee, HC (1997) Mechanisms of calcium signaling by cyclic ADP-ribose and NAADP. Physiol. Rev. 77:1133 - 1164

[3] Higashida H, Zhang JS, Hashi M, Shintaku M, Higashida C, and Takeda Y. (2000) Angiotensin II stimulates cyclic ADP-ribose formation in neonatal rat cardiac myocytes. Biochem J 352:197–202

[4] Kim SY, Gul R, Rah SY, Kim SH, Park SK, Im MJ, Kwon HJ, and Kim UH. (2008) Molecular mechanism of ADP-ribosyl cyclase activation in angiotensin II signaling in murine mesangial cells. Am J Physiol Renal Physiol 294: F982–F989

[5] Rah SY, Park KH, Han MK, Im MJ, and Kim UH. (2005) Activation of CD38 by interleukin-8 signaling regulates intracellular Ca^{2+} level and motility of lymphokine-activated killer cells. J Biol Chem 280: 2888–2895

[6] Kim SY, Park KH, Gul R, Jang KY, and Kim UH. (2009) Role of kidney ADP-ribosyl cyclase in diabetic nephropathy. Am J Physiol Renal Physiol 296: F291–F297

[7] USRD 2006 ADR/reference tables. Available at: http://www.usrds.org/reference_2006.htm 2008

[8] El-Nahas M (2005) The global challenge of chronic kidney disease. Kidney Int 68:2918–2929

[9] Vestra MD, Saller A, Mauer M, and Fioretto P. (2001) Role of mesangial expansion in the pathogenesis of diabetic nephropathy. J Nephrol 14: S51–S57

[10] Cooper ME. Interaction of metabolic and haemodynamic factors in mediating experimental diabetic nephropathy. (2001) Diabetologia 44: 1957–1972

[11] Coresh J, Astor BC, Greene T, Eknoyan G, and Levey AS (2003) Prevalence of chronic kidney disease and decreased kidney function in the adult US population: Third National Health and Nutrition Examination Survey. Am J Kidney Dis 41:1–12

[12] Harris RC. (2004) Diabetes and the kidney. In Cecil Textbook of Medicine, 22nd Ed. 750-753

[13] Diabetes Control and Complications Trial Research Group: The effect of intensive treatment of diabetes on the development and progression of long-term complications in insulin-dependent diabetes mellitus. (1993) N Engl J Med 329:977–986

[14] Parving H-H, Andersen ER, Smidt U, Hommel E, and Mathiesen E (1987) Antihypertensive treatment postpones endstage renal failure in diabetic nephropathy. Br Med J 294:1443–1447

[15] Bakris GL, Williams M, Dworkin L, Elliott WJ, Epstein M, Toto R, Tuttle K, Douglas J, Hsueh W, and Sowers J (2000) Preserving renal function in adults with hypertension and diabetes: a consensus approach. National Kidney Foundation Hypertension and Diabetes Executive Committees Working Group. Am J Kidney Dis 36:646–661

[16] Lewis EJ, Hunsicker LG, and Bain RP. (1993) The effect of angiotensin-converting-enzyme inhibition on diabetic nephropathy. The Collaborative Study Group. N Engl J Med 329: 1456–1462

[17] Barnett AH, Bain SC, Bouter P, Karlberg B, Madsbad S, Jervell J, and Mustonen J. (2004) Angiotensin-receptor blockade versus converting-enzyme inhibition in type 2 diabetes and nephropathy. N Engl J Med 351: 1952–1961

[18] Brenner BM, Cooper ME, de Zeeuw D, Keane WF, Mitch WE, Parving HH, Remuzzi G, Snapinn SM, Zhang Z, and Shahinfar S (2001) Effects of losartan on renal and cardiovascular outcomes in patients with type 2 diabetes and nephropathy. N Engl J Med 345:861–869

[19] Kostis JB, Shelton B, Gosselin G, Goulet C, Hood WB Jr, Kohn RM, Kubo SH, Schron E, Weiss MB, Willis PW 3rd, Young JB, and Probstfield J (1996) Adverse effects of enalapril in the Studies of Left Ventricular Dysfunction (SOLVD). SOLVD Investigators. Am Heart J 131:350–355

[20] Oparil S, Yarows SA, Patel S, Fang H, Zhang J, and Satlin A (2007) Efficacy and safety of combined use of aliskiren and valsartan in patients with hypertension: a randomised, double-blind trial. Lancet 370:221–229

[21] Nakao N, Yoshimura A, Morita H, Takada M, Kayano T, and Ideura T (2003) Combination treatment of angiotensin-II receptor blocker and angiotensin-converting-enzyme inhibitor in non-diabetic renal disease (COOPERATE): a randomised controlled trial. Lancet 361:117–124

[22] Anderson PW, Do YS, and Hsueh WA. (1993) Angiotensin II causes mesangial cell hypertrophy. Hypertension 21: 29–35

[23] Feng Z, Wei C, Chen X, Wang J, Cheng H, Zhang X, Hong Q, Shi S, Fu B, and Wei R. (2006) Essential role of Ca^{2+} release channels in angiotensin II-induced Ca^{2+} oscillations and mesangial cell contraction. Kidney Int 70:130–138

[24] Kim S, and Iwao H. (2000) Molecular and cellular mechanisms of angiotensin II-mediated cardiovascular and renal diseases. Pharmacol Rev 52: 11–34

[25] Guo DF, Sun YL, Hamet P, and Inagami T. (2001) The angiotensin II type 1 receptor and receptor-associated proteins. Cell Res 11: 165–180

[26] Seta K, Nanamori M, Modrall G, Neubig RR, and Sadoshima J. (2002) AT1 receptor mutant lacking heretotrimeric G protein coupling activates the Src-Ras-ERK pathway without nuclear translocation of ERKs. J Biol Chem 277: 9268–9277

[27] Howard M, Grimaldi JC, Bazan JF, Lund FE, Santos-Argumedo L, Parkhouse RME, Walseth TF, and Lee HC. (1993) Formation and hydrolysis of cyclic ADP-ribose catalyzed by lymphocyte antigen CD38. Science 262:1056–1059

[28] Jin D, Liu HX, Hirai H, Torashima T, Nagai T, Lopatina O, Shnayder NA, Yamada K, Noda M, Seike T, Fujita K, Takasawa S, Yokoyama S, Koizumi K, Shiraishi Y, Tanaka S, Hashii M, Yoshihara T, Higashida K, Islam MS, Yamada N, Hayashi K, Noguchi N, Kato I, Okamoto H, Matsushima A, Salmina A, Munesue T, Shimizu N, Mochida S, Asano M, and Higashida H. (2007) CD38 is critical for social behavior by regulating oxytocin secretion. Nature 446: 41–45

[29] Barbosa MT, Soares SM, Novak CM, Sinclair D, Levine JA, Aksoy P, and Chini EN. (2007) The enzyme CD38 (a NAD glycohydrolase, EC 3.2.2.5) is necessary for the development of diet-induced obesity. FASEB J 21:3629–3639

[30] Young GS, Choleris E, Lund FE, and Kirkland JB. Decreased cADPR and increased NAD^+ in the $Cd38^{-/-}$ mouse. Biochem Biophys Res Commun 346: 188–192, 2006.

[31] Reinherz EL, Kung PC, Goldstein G, Levey RH, and Schlossman SF. (1980) Discrete stages of human intrathymic differentiation: analysis of normal thymocytes and leukemic lymphoblasts of T-cell lineage. Proc Natl Acad Sci U S A 77: 1588-1592
[32] Koguma T, Takasawa S, Tohgo A, Karasawa T, Furuya Y, Yonekura H, and Okamoto H. (1994) Cloning and characterization of cDNA encoding rat ADP-ribosyl cyclase/cyclic ADP-ribose hydrolase (homologue to human CD38) from islets of Langerhans. Biochim Biophys Acta 1223: 160-162
[33] Kramer G, Steiner G, Fodinger D, Fiebiger E, Rappersberger C, Binder S, Hofbauer J, and Marberger M. (1995) High expression of a CD38-like molecule in normal prostatic epithelium and its differential loss in benign and malignant disease. J Urol 154: 1636-1641
[34] Mizuguchi M, Otsuka N, Sato M, Ishii Y, Kon S, Yamada M, Nishina H, Katada T, and Ikeda K. (1995) Neuronal localization of CD38 antigen in the human brain. Brain Res 697: 235-240
[35] Verderio C, Bruzzone S, Zocchi E, Fedele E, Schenk U, De Flora A, and Matteoli M. (2001) Evidence of a role for cyclic ADP-ribose in calcium signalling and neurotransmitter release in cultured astrocytes. J Neurochem 78: 646-657
[36] States DJ, Walseth TF, and Lee HC. (1992) Similarities in amino acid sequences of Aplysia ADP-ribosyl cyclase and human lymphocyte antigen CD38. Trends Biochem Sci 17: 495
[37] Galione A, and Churchill GC. (2000) Cyclic ADP-ribose as a calcium-mobilizing messenger. Sci STKE 41: pe1
[38] Guse AH, Silva CP, Berg I, Skapenko AL, Weber K, Heyer P, Hohenegger M, Pitter BV, and Mayr GW. (1999) Regulation of calcium signaling in T lymphocytes by the second messenger cyclic ADP-ribose. Nature 398: 70–73
[39] Lee HC. (2001) Physiological functions of cyclic ADP-ribose and NAADP as calcium messengers. Annu Rev Pharmacol Toxicol 41: 317–345
[40] Partida-Sanchez S, Cockayne DA, Monard S, Jacobson EL, Oppenheimer N, Garvy B, Kusser K, Goodrich S, Howard M, Harmsen A, Randall TD, and Lund FE. (2001) Cyclic ADP-ribose production by CD38 regulates intracellular calcium release, extracellular calcium influx and chemotaxis in neutrophils and is required for bacterial clearance in vivo. Nat Med 7:1209–1216
[41] Higashida H, Salmina AB, Olovyannikova RY, Hashii M, Yokoyama S, Koizumi K, Jin D, Liu HX, Lopatina O, Amina S, Islam MS, Huang JJ, and Noda M. (2007) Cyclic ADP-ribose as a universal calcium signal molecule in the nervous system. Neurochem Int 51: 192–199
[42] Calcraft, PJ, Ruas, M., Pan, Z., Cheng, X., Arredouani, A., Hao, X., Tang, J., Rietdorf, K., Teboul, L., Chuang, KT, Lin, P., Xiao, R., Wang, C., Zhu, Y., Lin, Y., Wyatt, CN, Parrington, J., Ma, J., Evans, AM, Galione, A., and Zhu, MX (2009) NAADP mobilizes calcium from acidic organelles through two-pore channels. Nature 459, 596 - 600
[43] Kim B.-J., Park K., Yim C., Takasawa S., Okamoto H., Im M. , and Kim UH. (2008) Generation of nicotinic acid adenine dinucleotide phosphate and cyclic ADP-ribose by glucagon-like peptide-1 evokes Ca^{2+} signal that is essential for insulin secretion in mouse pancreatic islets. Diabetes 57, 868–878

[44] Rah SY, Mushtaq M, Nam TS, Kim SH, and Kim UH. (2010) Generation of Cyclic ADP-ribose and Nicotinic Acid Adenine Dinucleotide Phosphate by CD38 for Ca^{2+} Signaling in Interleukin-8-treated Lymphokine-activated Killer Cells. J Biol Chem 285: 21877–21887

[45] Ceni C, Muller-Steffner H, Lund F, Pochon N, Schweitzer A, De Waard M, Schuber F, Villaz M, and Moutin MJ. (2003) Evidence for an intracellular ADP-ribosyl cyclase/NAD^{+}-glycohydrolase in brain from CD38- deficient mice. J Biol Chem 278: 40670–40678

[46] de Toledo FG, Cheng J, Liang M, Chini EN, and Dousa TP. (2000) ADP-ribosyl cyclase in rat vascular smooth muscle cells: properties and regulation. Circ Res 86: 1153–1159

[47] Nam TS, Choi SH, Rah SY, Kim SY, Jang W, Im MJ, Kwon HJ, and Kim UH. (2006) Discovery of a small-molecule inhibitor for kidney ADP-ribosyl cyclase: implication for intracellular calcium signal mediated by cyclic ADP-ribose. Exp Mol Med 38: 718–726

[48] Gul R, Kim SY, Park KH, Kim BJ, Kim SJ, Im MJ, and Kim UH. (2008) A novel signaling pathway of ADP-ribosyl cyclase activation by angiotensin II in adult rat cardiomyocytes. Am J Physiol Heart Circ Physiol 295:H77–H88

[49] Rah SY, Park KH, Nam TS, Kim SJ, Kim H, Im MJ, and Kim UH. (2007) Association of CD38 with nonmuscle myosin heavy chain IIA and Lck is essential for the internalization and activation of CD38. J Biol Chem 282: 5653-5660

[50] Kim SY, Cho BH, and Kim UH. (2010) CD38-mediated Ca^{2+} Signaling Contributes to Angiotensin II-induced Activation of Hepatic Stellate Cells. J Biol Chem 285: 576-582

[51] Zubiaur M, Izquierdo M, Terhorst C, Malavasi F, and Sancho J. (1997) CD38 ligation results in activation of the Raf-1/mitogen-activated protein kinase and the CD3-zeta/zeta-associated protein-70 signaling pathways in Jurkat T lymphocytes. J Immunol 159: 193-205

[52] Liu Y. (2006) Renal fibrosis: new insights into the pathogenesis and therapeutics. Kidndy Int 69: 213–217

[53] Ruiz-Torres MP, Lopez-Ongil S, Griera M, Diez-Marques ML, Rodriguez-Puyol M, and Rodriguez-Puyol D. (2005) The accumulation of extracellular matrix in the kidney: consequences on cellular function. J Nephrol 18:334–340.

[54] Chen S, Hong SW, Iglesias-de la Cruz MC, Isono M, Casaretto A, and Ziyadeh FN. (2001) The key role of the transforming growth factor-beta system in the pathogenesis of diabetic nephropathy. Renal Fail 23: 471–481

[55] Mezzano SA, Ortega MR, and Egido J. (2001) Angiotensin II and renal fibrosis. Hypertension 38: 635–638

[56] Ziyadeh FN, Sharma K, Ericksen M, and Wolf G. (1994) Stimulation of collagen gene expression and protein synthesis in murine mesangial cells by high glucose is mediated by autocrine activation of transforming growth factor beta. J Clin Invest 93: 536–542

6

Significance of Advanced Glycation End-Products (AGE) and the Receptor for AGE (RAGE) in Diabetic Nephropathy

Tarek Kamal[1,2], Yasuhiko Yamamoto[1,*] and Hiroshi Yamamoto[1]
[1]*Department of Biochemistry and Molecular Vascular Biology*
Kanazawa University Graduate School of Medical Science, Kanazawa
[2]*On leave from Kafr EL-Sheikh University*
[1]*Japan*
[2]*Egypt*

1. Introduction

Diabetic nephropathy is a life-threatening complication of *diabetes mellitus* and the leading cause of end-stage renal disease (ESRD) in developed countries. Diabetes is responsible for over 40% of all new cases with ESRD in the United States and Japan, eventually undergoing renal dialysis or transplantation. Diabetic nephropathy is characterized by glomerular hyperfiltration and thickening of glomerular basement membranes, followed by expansion of extracellular matrix in mesangial area. There are many factors and pathways that are involved in the pathogenesis of diabetic nephropathy. In this chapter, we will focus on advanced glycation end-products (AGE) and the receptor for AGE (RAGE) in the development and prevention of diabetic nephropathy.

2. Possible molecular mechanisms for the development of diabetic nephropathy

Diabetic nephropathy occurs in 20-40% of patients with diabetes and accounts for disabilities and the high mortality rate in patients with diabetes (1). In proportion to the rapid increase of diabetic population, diabetic nephropathy is now the major cause of ESRD in developed countries. There are many factors influencing the development of diabetic nephropathy, this including genetic, hemodynamic, environmental, and metabolic factors. The epidemiological studies have revealed that hyperglycemia *per se* is the most important factor in the onset and progression of diabetic vascular complications (2). Potential mechanisms underlying diabetic nephropathy include activations of polyol and hexosamine pathways, oxidative and nitrosative stress, ER stress, protein kinase C activation, poly(ADP-ribose) polymerase activation, and inflammation (3). Extensive intracellular and extracellular formation of AGE can also become a pathogenic factor in sustained hyperglycemia-induced kidney injuries. Both receptor-dependent and -independent mechanisms are involved in AGE-induced cellular dysfunction and tissue damage.

---

* Corresponding Author

3. AGE

Reducing sugars like glucose can react nonenzymatically with amino groups of proteins, and a series of further complex molecular rearrangements of dehydration, condensation and crosslinking yield irreversible and heterogeneous derivatives termed AGE (4). AGE are also generated by the reaction of aldehydes and metabolites from glycolysis pathway such as dicarbonyls of methylglyoxal (MG), glyoxal and 3-deoxyglucosone (3DG) with amino acids, lipids and nucleic acids, and through lipid peroxidation (5,6). Although this process takes place continuously within the body during aging, it is extremely accelerated in diabetes (7). There are a large portion of these agents can be exogenous. Tobacco smoke has already been recognized as an important exogenous source of AGE (8). The diet, especially the modern western diet, also provides a relatively large portion of formed AGE and AGE-precursors; *e.g.* $^{\varepsilon}$N -carboxymethyl-lysine (CML) and MG (9). However, the exact nature of various diet-derived AGE derivatives has not yet been fully elucidated.

In vitro, AGE stimulate the generation of reactive oxygen species (ROS), insulin-like growth factor-1 (IGF-1), platelet-derived growth factor (PDGF), and transforming growth factor-β (TGF- β) in mesangial cells (10, 11), the features characteristic of glomerulosclerosis. AGE also induce TGF- β production in tubular cells, which links to the pathogenesis of tubulointerstitial fibrosis (12). Podocytes undergo apoptosis when exposed to AGE (13), this being implicated in podocyte injuries in diabetes (Fig. 1).

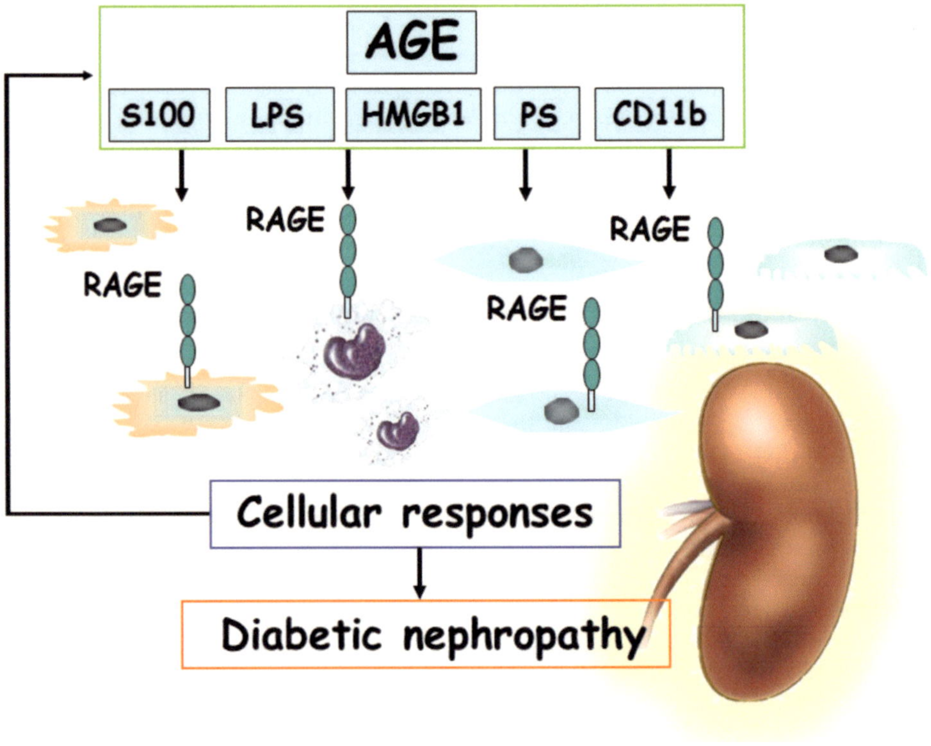

Fig. 1. AGE-RAGE axis and the interaction of other ligands with RAGE contribute to cellular responses and development of diabetic nephropathy. LPS, lipopolysaccharides; PS, phosphatidylserine.

There are three lines of evidence for the role of AGE in diabetic nephropathy. The first line concerns the association between the accumulation of AGE-modified proteins and severity of diabetic nephropathy in both diabetic animals and man (14-17). The second comes from the fact that kidney injuries develop following injection of AGE-modified proteins in non-diabetic animals (18). The third kind of evidence is that the development and progression of diabetic nephropathy is attenuated by the treatment with inhibitors of AGE formation and AGE breakers such as aminoguanidine, pyridoxamine and ALT-711 (19-22).

4. AGE receptors

Accumulating evidence indicates that the interaction of AGE with their receptor can play an important role in the pathogenesis of diabetic nephropathy (23). The best characterized AGE receptor is RAGE. Many other AGE receptors and soluble binding proteins interacting with AGE may also participate in the AGE homeostasis: scavenger receptors class A (MSR-A), class B (MSR-B) (CD36 and LOX1), AGE-R1 (OST48 oligosaccharyltransferase), AGE-R2 (80K-H protein kinase C substrate), AGE-R3 (galectin-3), and toll-like receptor (TLR) 4 (24-28). There are also other molecules like lysozyme and lactoferrin-like polypeptide that play a role in cellular uptake and degradation of AGE (29).

RAGE is a member of the immunoglobulin superfamily, having a total of 394 amino acid residues in the case with human ortholog with a single hydrophobic transmembrane domain (19 amino acids) and a highly charged C-terminal cytosolic tail (43 amino acids) that mediates intracellular signaling pathways (30). Extracellularly, RAGE has an N-terminal immunoglobulin (Ig) V-type ligand binding domain and two Ig C-type domains (V-C-C') (Fig. 2).

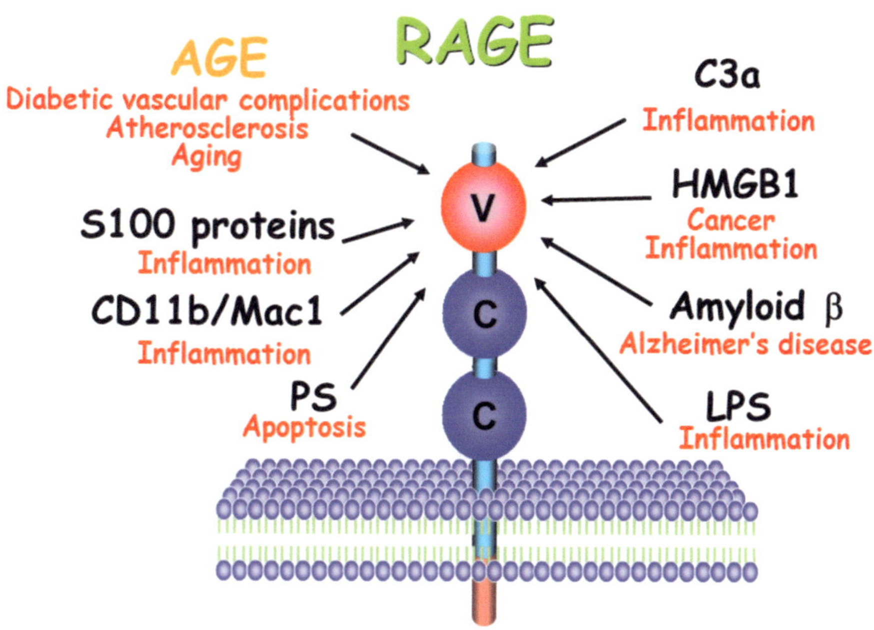

Fig. 2. RAGE belongs to an immunoglobulin superfamily and functions as a member of PRRs. LPS, lipopolysaccharides; PS, phosphatidylserine.

AGE-RAGE interaction can induce expressions of genes for vascular endothelial growth factor (VEGF) and for vascular cell adhesion molecule-1 (VCAM-1) in endothelial cells (EC) (31, 32), leading to enhancement of vascular permeability and local inflammation. Secretion of various cytokines such as tumor necrosis factor α (TNFα), interleukin 1β (IL1β), IL6, and monocyte chemotactic protein-1 (MCP-1) were induced by the AGE-RAGE system in monocytes and macrophages (33) (Fig. 1). Mammalian homologue of Drosophila gene Diaphanous 1 (mDia1) has been identified as a directly binding molecule with an intracellular domain of RAGE and subsequently proven to act as a part of the machinery of RAGE intracellular signaling (34). It is very recently reported that AGE-RAGE interaction can cause phosphorylation of cytoplasmic domain at Ser391 of RAGE by PKCζ (35) (Fig. 3).

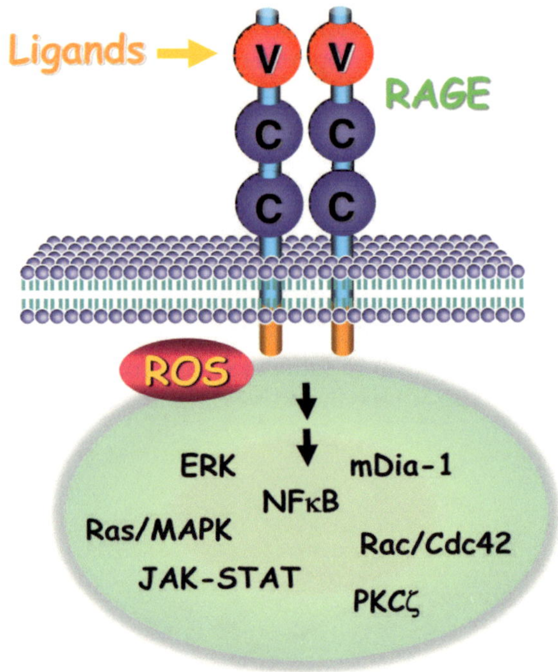

Fig. 3. RAGE intracellular signaling pathways. ERK, extracellular signal-regulated kinase; mDia-1, mammalian Diaphanous-related formin-1; NFκB, nuclear factor κB; PKCζ, protein kinase C ζ; JAK-STAT, The Janus kinase-signal transducers and activators of transcription; Ras/MAPK, Ras/mitogen-activated protein kinase; Rac/Cdc42, Rac/Cell division control protein 42 homolog.

RAGE ligands other than AGE have been identified, including high-mobility group box protein 1 (HMGB1), calcium-binding S100 protein group, β2-integrin Mac/CD11b, amyloid β peptide, β-sheet fibrils, advanced oxidation protein products (AOPP), complement C3a, lipopolysaccharides (LPS), and phosphatidylserine on the surface of apoptotic cells (36-41) (Fig. 2). RAGE is thus considered a member of pattern-recognition receptors like TLRs, actively participating not only in diabetic vascular complications but in the interface of innate and adaptive immunity and in inflammation.

Ligand engagement of RAGE activates the nuclear factor-κB (NF-κB) and other signaling pathways through stimulation of ERK (extracellular signal-regulated kinase)1/2, p38 MAPK (mitogen-activated protein kinase)-JNK (c-Jun N-terminal kinases), JAK (Janus kinase)-STAT (signal transducer and activator of transcription), and Rac-Cdc42 (42) (Fig. 3). Expression of RAGE is basically low in vascular cells but apparently constitutively induced during diabetes and inflammation. This is explained by the fact that the gene for RAGE *per se* is under the control of NF-κB, which thus constitutes a positive loop of regulation (43), thereby resulting in the superdrive of the AGE-RAGE system during prolonged hyperglycemic exposure.

5. RAGE and diabetic nephropathy in mice

Development of diabetic nephropathy is characterized by glomerular hyperfiltration and thickening of glomerular basement membranes, followed by an expansion of extracellular matrix in mesangial areas and increased albuminuria. Diabetic nephropathy ultimately proceeds to glomerular sclerosis associated with renal dysfunction.

Because diabetic nephropathy is the major cause of ESRD, the development of effective remedies to retard the progression of diabetic nephropathy has become a pharmaceutical goal. However, it has been hampered by the lack of adequate experimental models to test them (44). We created transgenic (Tg) mice that overexpressed human RAGE in vascular cells by introducing fertilized ovum a transgene carrying human RAGE gene under the control of the murine *flk-1* promoter which works in EC (45). The Tg mice were made

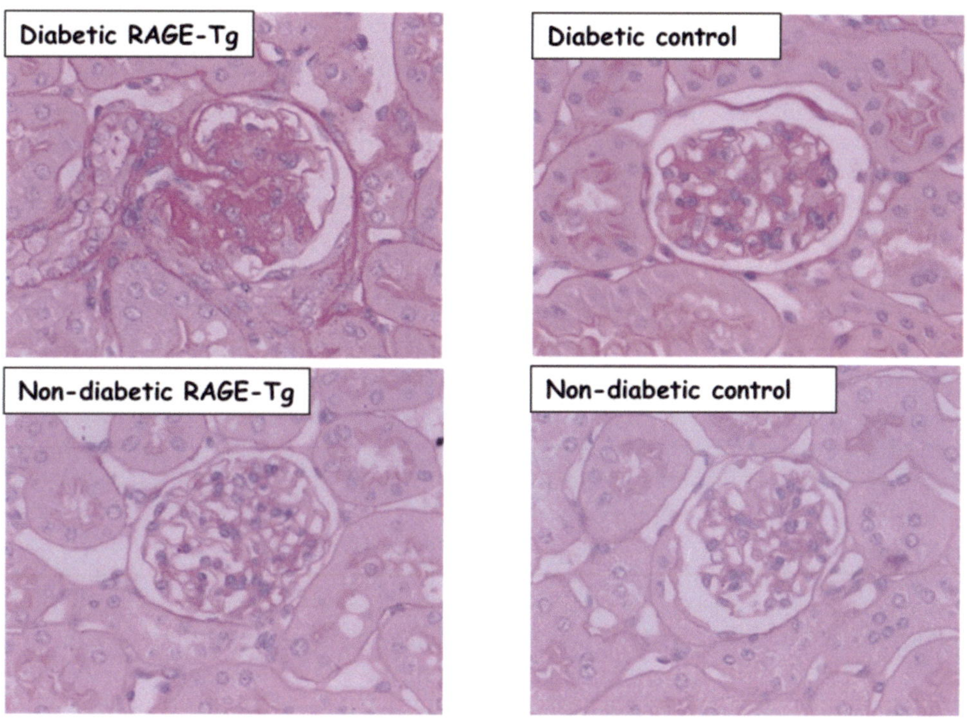

Fig. 4. Periodic acid-Schiff (PAS) stain of the mouse kidneys at 16 weeks of age (ref. 45). Diabetic RAGE-Tg, diabetes-induced RAGE-overexpressing transgenic mice; Diabetic control, diabetes-induced non-transgenic mice; Non-diabetic RAGE-Tg, non-diabetic RAGE-overexpressing transgenic mice; Non-diabetic control, non-diabetic non-transgenic mice.

diabetic by crossbreeding with another Tg line carrying inducible nitric oxide synthase (iNOS) cDNA under the control of insulin promoter (46). The resultant double Tg mice showed significant increases in kidney weight, albuminuria, glomerulosclerosis, and serum creatinine compared with the diabetic iNOS Tg controls (45) (Fig. 4). The sole iNOS Tg mice also showed progression of diabetic nephropathy accompanied by expression of TGF-β in glomeruli (47). Inagi and our group introduced megsin (mesangial cell-specific gene with homology to serine protease inhibitor) as the third transgene into RAGE-iNOS double Tg mice, this resulting in further acceleration of the development of nephropathy signs such as mesangial expansion, nodule-like lesion, and tubulointerstitial damage with an increase in local oxidative stress (48). Our group also generated homozygous RAGE knockout (KO) mice and found that the RAGE KO mice displayed suppression of all of the following features of advanced glomerular disease: kidney enlargement, increase in glomerular cell number, mesangial expansion, advanced glomerulosclerosis, albuminuria and the increase in serum creatinine (49). The endothelial-mesenchymal-transition (EndoMT) was also attenuated by the deletion of RAGE (50). That RAGE axis is a crucial cause of diabetic nephropathy has thus clearly emerged from experiments with RAGE-gene manipulated animals. Another model is the OVE26 mouse, in which diabetes is induced by transgene-mediated introduction of calmodulin in pancreatic β-cells (51). RAGE deletion was also beneficial to diabetic nephropathy in the OVE26 diabetic mice (52).

6. Inhibition of AGE and RAGE for the treatment of diabetic nephropathy

A key aim of therapy in diabetic patients is to reduce hyperglycemia by modification of the diet. However, dietary compliance is often difficult, and the alternative is to use pharmacological compounds that can reduce AGE and inhibit RAGE action. There are several endogenous molecular devices that can serve to protect the body from glycation and AGE such as α-ketogluteraldehyde dehydrogenase, glyoxalase and scavengers (53, 54). Hyperglycemia and RAGE activation are suggested to down-regulate glyoxalase I production and the enzyme activity (55). It is, therefore, rational to take pharmacologic strategies against the down-regulation of those endogenous detoxication enzymes.

Applications of inhibitors for AGE and RAGE may be promising therapeutic approaches for diabetic nephropathy (Table 1). Antioxidants may protect against free radicals derived from autoxidative glycation and AGE. Benfotiamine is a synthetic S-acyl derivative of thiamine and has anti-oxidant and anti-AGE formation (56). Amadoriases may be used to deglycate Amadori products or to inactivate intermediates such as 3DG. AGE-crosslink breakers such as ALT-711 (algebrium) and *N*-phenylthiazolium bromide (PTB) offer the potential of reversing diabetic nephropathy, although their precise mechanism of action is still unclear (57, 58). TTP488 is an antagonist against RAGE, which is under clinical studies, and neutralizing anti-RAGE antibody may also be useful (59). Low-molecular weight heparin (LMWH) can bind RAGE and act as an antagonist to RAGE [31]. LMWH treatment of the mouse model of diabetic nephropathy showed both the preventive and therapeutic effects on albuminuria and glomerulosclerosis in a dose-dependent manner (49). Thiazolidinediones, calcium channel blockers, angiotensin-converting enzyme inhibitors (ACEI), angiotensin II receptor blockers (ARB), and statins are reported to suppress RAGE expression (60, 61). There are numerous compounds that have been investigated for the anti-glycation activity but their use in humans is still debatable (62). Decoy type receptors of

RAGE, namely soluble RAGE (sRAGE), is also applicable for the treatment of diabetic nephropathy. sRAGE corresponds to the extracellular domain of RAGE lacking the transmembrane and cytosolic domains. As the N-terminal V-type domain is included, sRAGE has the same ligand-binding ability as membrane RAGE and thus is able to act as a decoy by preventing the ligands to reach the membrane-bound counterpart. In *db/db* mice, treatment with murine sRAGE (50 mg/day for 19 weeks) decreased albuminuria, glomeruloslerosis and GBM thickening (63); the sRAGE employed in that study was the truncated form of RAGE artificially produced by recombinant gene technology. Endogenous sRAGE exists in the circulation of humans. To generate sRAGE endogenously, two mechanisms are considered: (1) the alternative splicing to remove the transmembrane region and (2) the proteolytic cleavage from the cell surface. We identified and reported a splice variant form of soluble RAGE and named it endogenous secretory RAGE (esRAGE) (64, 65). Reinforcing sRAGE genesis by ectodomain shedding will decrease an amount of signal-transducing RAGE and will in turn reciprocally increase an amount of decoy receptor sRAGE; this can control ligand-RAGE signaling and subsequent cellular derangement in the kidney. Treatment with statins and ACEI is reported to stimulate circulating sRAGE production in human studies (66, 67). Further investigations are needed for better understanding of the regulation of sRAGE production and for developing drugs that can simultaneously upregulate sRAGE and downregulate mRAGE.

AGE inhibitors	Pyridoxamine Benfotiamine GLY-230
AGE-crosslink brakers	PTB ALT-711 (Algebrium) C36 TRC4186
RAGE inhibitors	LMWH TTP488/PF04494700
sRAGE	TTP3000, TTP4000 ACEI ARB TZD

PTB, N-phenacylthiazolium bromide; LMWH, low-molecular weight heparin; ACEI, angiotensin converting enzyme inhibitor; ARB, angiotensin receptor blockers; TZD, thiazolidinedione; sRAGE, soluble RAGE.

Table 1. Inhibitors of AGE and RAGE

7. Conclusions

Accumulating evidence has supported the concept that AGE and RAGE play an active role in the development and progression of diabetic nephropathy. Prophylactic and therapeutic strategies focusing on RAGE and its ligand axis will be of great importance in conquering diabetic kidney injuries.

8. References

[1] Gross JL, de Azevedo MJ, Silveiro SP, Canani LH, Caramori ML, Zelmanovitz T. Diabetic nephropathy: diagnosis, prevention, and treatment. *Diabetes Care* 2005; 28:164-176.

[2] The Diabetes Control and Complications Trial Research Group. The effect of intensive treatment of diabetes on the development and progression of long-term complications in insulin-dependent diabetes mellitus. *N Engl J Med* 1993; 329: 977-986.

[3] Pacher P, Szabó C. Role of poly(ADP-ribose) polymerase-1 activation in the pathogenesis of diabetic complications: endothelial dysfunction, as a common underlying theme. *Antioxid Redox Signal* 2005; 7(11-12): 1568-1580.

[4] Brownlee M, Cerami A, Vlassara H. Advanced glycosylation end products in tissue and the biochemical basis of diabetic complications. *N Eng J Med* 1988; 318(20): 1315-1321.

[5] Nagai R, Mori T, Yamamoto Y, Kaji Y, Yonei Y. Significance of advanced glycation endproducts (AGEs) in aging-related disease. *Anti-Aging Med* 2010; 7(10): 112-119.

[6] Fu MX, Requena JR, Jenkins AJ, Lyons TJ, Baynes JW, Thorpe SR. The advanced glycation end products, Nepsilon-(carboxymethyl)lysine, is a product of both lipid peroxidation and glycoxidation reactions. *J Biol Chem* 1996; 271:9982-9986.

[7] Thorpe SR, Baynes JW. Role of the Millard reaction in diabetes mellitus and diseases of aging. *Drugs Aging* 1996; 9: 69-77.

[8] Cerami C, Founds H, Nicholl I, Mitsuhashi T, Giordano D, Vanpatten S, Lee A, Al-Abed Y, Vlassara H, Bucala R, Cerami A. Tobacco smoke is a source of toxic reactive glycation products. *Proc Natl Acad Sci USA* 1997; 94(25): 13915-13920.

[9] Vlassara H, Palace MR. Diabetes and advanced glycation endproducts. *J Intern Med* 2002; 251: 87-101.

[10] Yamagishi S, Inagaki Y, Okamoto T, et al. Advanced glycation end products inhibit de novo protein synthesis and induce TGF-beta overexpression in proximal tubular cells. *Kidney Int* 2003; 63: 464-473.

[11] Doi T, Vlassara H, Kirstein M, Yamada Y, Striker GE, Striker LJ. Receptor-specific increase in extracellular matrix production in mouse mesangial cells by advanced glycosylation end products is mediated via platelet-derived growth factor. *Proc Natl Acad Sci USA* 1992; 89(7): 2873-2877.

[12] Sharma K, Ziyadeh FN. Hyperglycemia and diabetic kidney disease. The case for transforming growth factor-beta as a key mediator. *Diabetes* 1995; 44: 1139-1146.

[13] Chuang PY, Yu Q, Fang W, Uribarri J, He JC. Advanced glycation endproducts induce podocyte apoptosis by activation of the FOXO4 transcription factor. *Kidney Int* 2007; 72(8): 965-976.

[14] Sugiyama S, Miyata T, Horie K, Lida Y, Tsuyuki M, Tanaka H, et al. Advanced glycation endproducts in diabetic nephropathy. Nephrol Dial Transplant 1996; 11: 91-94.

[15] Sell DR, Lapolla A, Odetti P, Fogarty J, Monnier VM. Pentosidine formation in skin correlates with severity of complications in individuals with long-standing IDDM. *Diabetes* 1992; 41; 1286-1292.

[16] McCance DR, Dyer DG, Dunn JA, Bailie KE, Thorpe SR, Baynes JW, Lyons TJ. Millard reaction products and their relation to complications in insulin-dependent diabetes mellitus. *J Clin Invest* 1993; 91: 2470-2478.

[17] Beisswenger PJ, Makita Z, Curphey TJ, Moore LL, Jean S, Brinck-Johnsen T, Bucala R, Vlassara H. Formation of immunochemical advanced glycation endproducts

preceds and correlates with early manifestations of renal and retinal disease in diabetes. *Diabetes* 1995; 44: 824-829.

[18] Vlassara H, Striker LJ, Teichberg S, Fuh H, Li YM, Steffes M. Advanced glycation endproducts induce glomerular Sclerosis and albuminuria in normal rats. *Proc Natl Acad Sci USA* 1994; 91: 11704-11708.

[19] Hammes HP, Strodter D, Weiss A, Bretzel RG, Federlin K, Brownlee M. Secondary intervention with aminoguanidine retards the progression of diabetic nephropathy in the rat model. *Diabetologia* 1995; 38: 656-660.

[20] Soulis T, Cooper ME, Satra S, Thallas V, Panagiotopoulos S, BJerrum OJ, Jerums G. Relative contributions of advanced glycation and nitric oxide synthase inhibition to aminoguandine-mediated renoprotection in diabetic rats. Diabetologia 1997; 40: 1141-1151.

[21] Degenhardt TP, Alderson NL, Arrington DD, Beattie RJ, Basgen JM, Steffes MW, Thorpe SR, Baynes JW. Pyridoxamine inhibits early renal disease and dyslipidemia in the streptozotocin-diabetic rat. *Kidneys Int* 2002; 61: 939-950.

[22] Thallas-Bonke V, Lindschau C, Rizkalla B, Bach LA, Boner G, Meier M, Haller H, Cooper ME, Forbes JM. Attenuation of extracellular matrix accumulation in diabetic nephropathy by the advanced glycation end product cross-link breaker ALT-711 via a protein kinase C-alpha-dependent pathway. *Diabetes* 2004; 53(11): 2921-2930.

[23] Yamamoto H, Watanabe T, Yamamoto Y, *et al.* RAGE in diabetic nephropathy. *Curr Mol Med* 2007; 7 (8): 752-757.

[24] Yang Z, Makita Z, Horii Y, *et al.* Two novel rat liver membrane proteins that bind advanced glycosylation endproducts: relationship to macrophage receptor for glucose-modified proteins. *J Exp Med* 1991; 174(3): 515-524.

[25] Vlassara H, Li YM, Imani Y, *et al.* Identification of galectin-3 as a high-affinity binding protein for advanced glycation end products (AGE): a new member of the AGE-receptor complex. *Mol Med* 1995; 1(6): 634-646.

[26] Zhu W, Sano H, Nagai R, Fukuhara K, Miyazaki A, Horiuchi S. The role of galectin-3 in endocytosis of advanced glycation end products and modified low density lipoproteins. *Biochem Biophys Res Commun* 2001; 280(4): 1183-1188.

[27] Suzuki H, Kurihara Y, Takeya M, *et al.* A role for macrophage scavenger receptors in atherosclerosis and susceptibility to infection. *Nature* 1997; 386(6633): 292-296.

[28] Hodgkinson CP, Laxton RC, Patel K, Ye S. Advanced glycation end-product of low density lipoprotein activates the toll-like 4 receptor pathway implications for diabetic atherosclerosis. *Arterioscler Thromb Vasc Biol* 2008; 28(12): 2275-2281.

[29] Mitsuhashi T, Li YM, Fishbane S, Vlassara H. Depletion of reactive advanced glycation endproducts from diabetic uremic sera using a lysozyme-linked matrix. *J Clin Invest* 1997; 100(4): 847-854.

[30] Bierhaus A, Humpert PM, Morcos M, et al. Understanding RAGE, the receptor for advanced glycation endproducts. *J Mol Med* 2005; 83: 876-886.

[31] Yamagishi S, Yonekura H, Yamamoto Y, *et al.* Advanced glycation end products-driven angiogenesis in vitro. Induction of the growth and tube formation of human microvascular endothelial cells through autocrine vascular endothelial growth factor. *J Biol Chem* 1997; 272(13):8723-8730.

[32] Yamamoto Y, Yonekura H, Watanabe T, *et al.* Short-chain aldehyde-derived ligands for RAGE and their actions on endothelial cells. *Diabetes Res Clin Pract* 2007; 77 (S1): 30-40.

[33] Hou FF, Miyata T, Boyce J, *et al.* beta(2)-Microglobulin modified with advanced glycation end products delays monocyte apoptosis. *Kidney Int* 2001; 59(3): 990-1002.

[34] Hudson BI, Kalea AZ, Arriero MDM, *et al.* Interaction of the RAGE cytoplasmic domain with diaphanous-1 is required for ligand-stimulated cellular migration through activation of Rac1 and Cdc42. *J Biol Chem* 2008; 283(49): 34457-34468.

[35] Sakaguchi M, Murata H, Yamamoto K, *et al.* TIRAP, an adaptor protein for TLR2/4, transduces a signal from RAGE phosphorylated upon ligand binding. *PLoS One* 2011; 6(8): e23132.

[36] Hori O, Brett J, Slattery T, *et al.* The receptor for advanced glycation end products (RAGE) is a cellular binding site for amphoterin. Mediation of neurite outgrowth and co-expression of rage and amphoterin in the developing nervous system. *J Biol Chem* 1995; 270(43): 25752-25761.

[37] Hofmann MA, Drury S, Fu C, *et al.* RAGE mediates a novel proinflammatory axis: a central cell surface receptor for S100/calgranulin polypeptides. *Cell* 1999; 97(7): 889-901.

[38] Yan SD, Chen X, Fu J, *et al.* RAGE and amyloid-beta peptide neurotoxicity in Alzheimer's disease. *Nature* 1996; 382(6593): 685-691.

[39] Chavakis T, Bierhaus A, Al-Fakhri N, *et al.* The pattern recognition receptor (RAGE) is a counter receptor for leukocyte integrins: a novel pathway for inflammatory cell recruitment. *J Exp Med* 2003; 198(10): 1507-1515.

[40] Yamamoto Y, Harashima A, Saito H, *et al.* Septic shock is associated with receptor for advanced glycation end products ligation of LPS. *J Immunol* 2011; 186(5): 3248-3257.

[41] He M, Kubo H, Morimoto K, *et al.* Receptor for advanced glycation end products binds to phosphatidylserine and assists in the clearance of apoptotic cells. *EMBO Rep* 2011; 12(4): 358-364.

[42] Barlovic DP, Soro-Paavonen A, Jandeleit-Dahm KA. RAGE biology, atherosclerosis and diabetes. *Clin Sci (Lond)* 2011; 121(2): 43-55.

[43] Tanaka N, Yonekura H, Yamagishi S, *et al.* The receptor for advanced glycation end products is induced by the glycation products themselves and tumor necrosis factor-alpha through nuclear factor-kappa B, and by 17beta-estradiol through Sp-1 in human vascular endothelial cells. *J Biol Chem* 2000; 275(33): 25781-25790.

[44] Inagi R, Nanagaku M, Miyata T. Synergistic contribution of carbonyl stress and megsin in diabetic nephropathy. Ann NY Acad Sci 2005; 1043: 605-608.

[45] Yamamoto Y, Kato I, Doi T, *et al.* Development and prevention of advanced diabetic nephropathy in RAGE-overexpressing mice. *J Clin Invest* 2001; 108(2): 261-268.

[46] Takamura T, Kato I, Kimura N, *et al.* Transgenic mice overexpressing type 2 nitric-oxide synthase in pancreatic beta cells develop insulin-dependent diabetes without insulitis. *J Biol Chem* 1998; 273(5): 2493-2496.

[47] Ohashi S, Abe H, Takahashi T, Yamamoto Y, Takeuchi M, Arai H, Nagata K, Kita T, Okamoto H, Yamamoto H, Doi T. Advanced glycation end products increase collagen-specific chaperone protein in mouse diabetic nephropathy. *J Biol Chem* 2004; 279: 19816-19823.

[48] Inagi R, Yamamoto Y, Nangaku M, *et al.* A severe diabetic nephropathy model with early development of nodule-like lesions induced by megsin overexpression in RAGE/iNOS transgenic mice. *Diabetes* 2006; 55(2): 356-366.

[49] Myint KM, Yamamoto Y, Doi T, *et al.* RAGE control of diabetic nephropathy in a mouse model: effects of RAGE gene disruption and administration of low-molecular weight heparin. *Diabetes* 2006; 55(9):2510-2522.

[50] Li L, Qu X, Yao J, *et al.* Blockade of endothelial-mesenchymal transition by a Smad 3 inhibitor delays the early development of streptozotocin-induced diabetic nephropathy. *Diabetes* 2010; 59(10): 2612-2624.

[51] Zheng S, Noonan WT, Metreveli NS, Coventry S, Kralik PM, Carlson EC, Epstein PN. Development of late-stage diabetic nephropathy in OVE26 diabetic mice. *Diabetes* 2004; 53(12): 3248-3257.

[52] Reinger N, Lau K, McCalla D, *et al.* Deletion of the receptor for advanced glycation end products reduces glomerulosclerosis and preserves renal function in the diabetic OVE26 mouse. *Diabetes* 2010; 59(8): 2043-2054.

[53] Hata F, Igaki N, Nakamichi T, Masuda S, Nishimoto S, Oimomi M, et al. Suppressive effect of α-Ketogluteraldehyde dehydrogenase on the advanced process of the Millard reaction. *Diabetes Res Clin Practice* 1988; 5: 5413.

[54] Thornalley PJ. The glyoxalase system: new developments towards functional characterization of a metabolic pathway fundamental to biological life. *Biochem J* 1990; 269(1): 1–11.

[55] Xue M, Rabbani N, Thornalley PJ. Glyoxalase in ageing. *Semin Cell Dev Biol* 2011; 22(3): 293-301.

[56] Stirban A, Negrean M, Stratmann B, *et al.* Benfotiamine prevents macro- and microvascular endothelial dysfunction and oxidative stress following a meal rich in advanced glycation end products in individuals with type 2 diabetes. *Diabetes Care* 2006; 29(9): 2064-2071.

[57] Schwedler SB, Verbeke P, Bakala H, *et al.* N-phenacylthiazolium bromide decreases renal and increases urinary advanced glycation end products excretion without ameliorating diabetic nephropathy in C57BL/6 mice. *Diabetes Obes Metab* 2001; 3(4): 230-239.

[58] Wolffenbuttel BH, Bouanger CM, Crijns FR, *et al.* Breakers of advanced glycation endproducts restore large artery properties in experimental diabetes. *Proc Natl Acad Sci USA* 1998; 95(8): 4630-4634.

[59] Jensen IJ, Denner I, Schrijers BF, Tilton RG, Rash R, Flyvgerg A. Renal effects of a neutralizing RAGE-antibody in long term streptozotocin-diabetic mice. *J Endocrinol* 2006; 188: 493-501.

[60] Marx N, Walcher D, Ivanova N, *et al.* Thiazolidinediones reduce endothelial expression of receptors for advanced glycation end products. *Diabetes* 2004; 53(10): 2662-2668.

[61] Yamagishi S, Takeuchi M. Nifedipine inhibits gene expression of receptor for advanced glycation end products (RAGE) in endothelial cells by suppressing reactive oxygen species generation. *Drugs Exp Clin Res* 2004; 30(4): 169–175.

[62] Ahmed N. Advanced glycation endproducts-role in pathology of diabetic complications. *Diabetes Res Clin Pract* 2005; 67: 3-21.

[63] Wendt T, Tanji N, Guo J, Kislinger TR, Qu W, Lu Y, et al. RAGE drives the development of glomeruloslerosis and implicates podocyte activation in the pathogenesis of diabetic nephropathy. *Am J Pathol* 2003; 162: 1123-1137.

[64] Yonekura H, Yamamoto Y, Sakurai S, *et al.* Novel splice variants of the receptor for advanced glycation end-products expressed in human vascular endothelial cells and pericytes, and their putative roles in diabetes-induced vascular injury. *Biochem J* 2003; 370(3): 1097-1109.

[65] Harashima A, Yamamoto Y, Cheng C, *et al.* Identification of mouse orthologue of endogenous secretory receptor for advanced glycation end-products: structure, function and expression. *Biochem J* 2006; 396(1): 109-115.

[66] Cuccurullo C, Lezzi A, Fazia ML, *et al.* Suppression of RAGE as a basis of simvastatin-dependent plaque stabilization in type 2 diabetes. *Arterioscler Thromb Vasc Biol* 2006; 26(12): 2716-2723.

[67] Santilli F, Bucciarelli L, Noto D, *et al.* Decreased plasma soluble RAGE in patients with hypercholesterolemia: effects of statins. *Free Radic Biol Med* 2007; 43(9): 1255-1262.

7

The Contribution of Fibronectin ED-A Expression to Myofibroblast Transdifferentiation in Diabetic Renal Fibrosis

Keisuke Ina, Hirokazu Kitamura,
Shuji Tatsukawa and Yoshihisa Fujikura
Oita University
Japan

1. Introduction

The number of cases in which hemodialysis therapy for diabetic nephropathy is required has been increasing. Currently, the goal of treatment for renal fibrosis is not only to prevent the development and progression of the disease, but also to promote its remission and regression.

It is well known that glomerulosclerosis and tubulointerstitial fibrosis occur during the early stages of diabetic nephropathy. It has been demonstrated that the development of tubulointerstitial lesions is more closely correlated with a progressive decline in renal function compared to glomerular lesions (Bohle et al., 1991). Tubulointerstitial fibrosis ultimately leads to renal failure as a result of renal atrophy. The myofibroblasts emerging in tubulointerstitial fibrosis tissue have been indicated to play a crucial role in the development and progression of fibrosis (Simonson, 2007). They overproduce extracellular matrix (ECM) molecules, including type I collagen and fibronectin, and repress ECM degradation through the production of tissue inhibitor of metalloproteinase-1 (TIMP-1) (Edwards et al., 1987) and plasminogen activator inhibitor-1 (PAI-1) in response to transforming growth factor-β_1 (TGF-β_1), which is increased in DN (Laiho et al., 1987), followed by ECM accumulation (i.e. fibrosis). Furthermore, the myofibroblasts may induce fibrosis tissue contraction via increased cell contraction promoted by α-smooth muscle actin (α-SMA) expression, leading to renal atrophy and failure. Myofibroblasts are considered to be derived from various kinds of cells, e.g. fibroblasts (Strutz and Zeisberg, 2006), epithelial cells (Iwano et al., 2002), endothelial cells (Zeisberg et al., 2008), pericytes (Humphreys et al., 2010), and bone marrow-originated cells (Keeley et al., 2010), via stimulation by TGF-β_1.

Although α-SMA expression, which is the most pronounced characteristic of myofibroblasts, has been considered to cause tissue contraction, the detailed mechanism has not yet been determined. Myofiboblasts were first described in wound-healing granulation tissue

(Gabbiani et al., 1971), where they were referred to as "modified fibroblasts" on the basis of their ultrastructural identification in transmission electron microscopic studies. These cells include a fibrillar system corresponding to stress fibers, nuclear indentation implying cell contraction, and cell-to-ECM and cell-to-cell junctions. Thus, modified fibroblasts (myofibroblasts) were described as an intermediate type of cell between fibroblasts and smooth muscle cells due to their ability to produce ECM and contract. Later investigators have noted that α-SMA expression in the stress fibers was the major characteristic of myofibroblasts.

At present, cells with α-SMA-positive stress fibers in the interstitium, except for vascular components, are recognized to be myofibroblasts. In vertebrate tissues, six actin isoforms have been identified. Four actin isoforms, including the α-skeletal, α-cardiac, α-vascular and γ-enteric isoforms, are tissue-restricted and involved in cell contraction. The other two actin isoforms, the β-cytoplasmic and γ-cytoplasmic isoforms, are ubiquitously expressed. These have been considered to constitute noncontractile cytoskeletons. The α-vascular actin is the SMA isoform, referred to as "α-SMA". During myofibroblast transdifferentiation, the actin isoform transitions, at least in part, from the cytosolic actin to α-SMA. It has been proposed that myofibroblasts have the ability to contract due to their expression of α-SMA.

Fibronectin, a 440 kDa dimeric glycoprotein, is one of the ECM molecules that exerts various functions, including adhesion, migration and differentiation. The fibronectin subunit is composed of three internally homologous repeats and contains binding sites for cell surface receptors and for other ECM components (Magnusson & Mosher, 1998; Peterson et al., 1983). Fibronectin polymorphisms arise from the alternative splicing of mRNA at three regions, ED-A, ED-B and IIICS (Norton & Hynes, 1987) (Fig. 1). The two former sequences are either omitted or included, while the latter one varies in length. Fibronectins are present in an insoluble form in the ECM, and in a soluble form in circulation, namely as cellular fibronectin and plasma fibronectin. Only cellular fibronectin contains ED-A and ED-B (Vartio et al., 1987). The fibronectin ED-A and fibronectin ED-B isoforms are predominantly expressed in embryonic tissue, and are seldom found in normal adult tissues. However, fibronectin ED-A has been demonstrated to be re-expressed in a variety of reactive and pathological processes, such as wound healing (Ffrench-Constant et al., 1989), arterial internal thickening (Glukhova et al., 1989) and liver fibrosis (Jamagin et al., 1994). *In vitro*, TGF-β_1 has been shown to increase fibronectin production, and it regulates the splicing pattern of fibronectin pre-messenger RNA, followed by expression of the ED-A domain (Balza et al., 1988; Borsi et al., 1990). Moreover, it has been suggested that the fibronectin ED-A isoform modulates various cells to generate myofibroblasts which express α-SMA (Bochaton-Piallat et al., 2000; Ffrench-Constant et al., 1989; Jamagin et al., 1994). Gabbiani and coworkers demonstrated that the fibronectin ED-A isoform plays a crucial role in TGF-β_1-induced myofibroblast transdifferentiation in an *in vitro* study using human subcutaneous fibroblasts (Serini et al., 1998).

In the present study, we examined whether TGF-β_1 induces the expression of the ED-A domain in fibronectin, and whether this, in turn, leads to α-SMA expression in renal fibroblasts by using an *in vitro* model of fibrosis due to diabetic nephropathy. Furthermore, whether the fibronectin ED-A isoform stimulates the contraction of the collagen gel through the expression of α-SMA and the accumulation of type I collagen was examined.

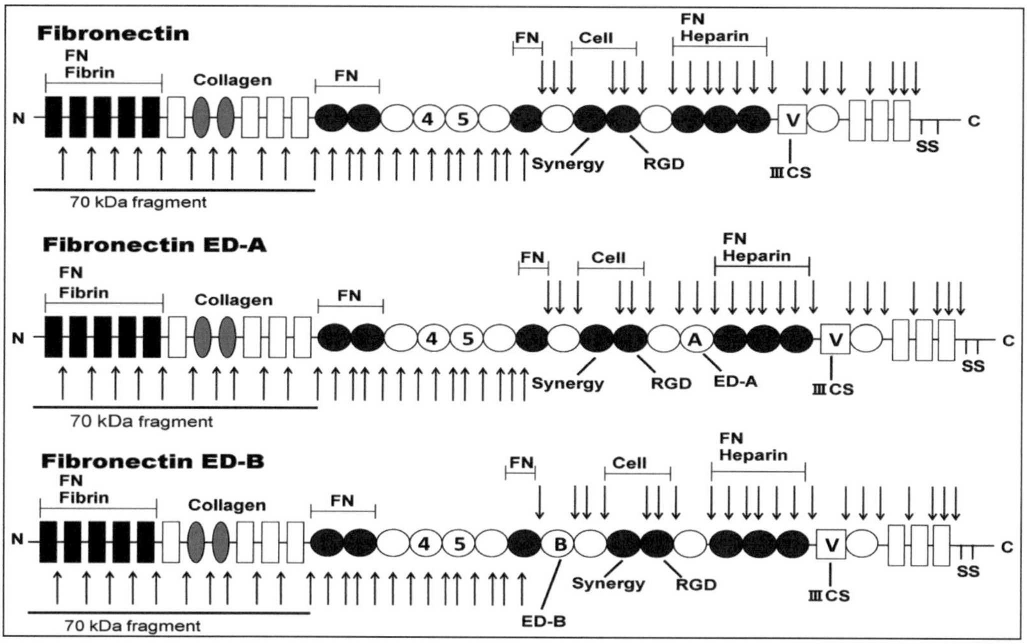

Fig. 1. The molecular structure of fibronectin ED-A and ED-B.

The fibronectin subunit is composed of three different repeating sequences: type I (rectangles), type II (ovals) and type III (circles). Sets of repeats constitute binding domains for fibrin, fibronectin (FN), collagen, cells and heparin as described. Sequence variations can occur in all three points of the fibronectin subunit: extra domains A and B (ED-A and ED-B, respectively) and the IIICS (Wierzbicka-Patynowski & Schwarzbauer, 2003). Allows indicate approximate intron positions determined in the murine gene.

2. Materials and methods

2.1 Materials

Porcine type I collagen solution was purchased from Nitta Gelatin (Osaka, Japan), recombinant human TGF-β_1 was purchased from R and D Systems (MN, USA), and the mouse monoclonal antibodies against α-SMA and ED-A were obtained from Sigma-Aldrich (MO, USA) and Abcam (Cambridge, UK), respectively. The fluorescein isothiocyanate (FITC)-conjugated goat anti-mouse IgG secondary antibody against these monoclonal antibodies was purchased from Caltag Laboratories (CA, USA). Rat type I collagen ELISA kits were obtained from Cusabio (Wuhan, China).

2.2 Cell culture

Normal rat kidney fibroblasts (NRK 49F cells) were obtained from the RIKEN Cell Bank (Tsukuba, Japan). The cells were maintained in Dulbecco's minimal essential medium (D-MEM) (Nissui Pharmaceutical, Tokyo, Japan) containing 100 IU ml^{-1} penicillin, 100 μg ml^{-1} streptomycin, and 10% fetal bovine serum (FBS) (JRH Biosciences, KS) at 37°C in a humidified, 5% CO_2 atmosphere. FBS had been heat-inactivated at 56°C for 30 min prior to use. Cells from passage 3 to passage 8 were used in the experiments described below.

Monolayer cultures of 2 X 10^4 cells ml^{-1} were grown on two-well Labtek Chamber Slides (AS ONE, Osaka, Japan). The cell cultures were divided into 4 groups: a control group, cultured with 0.5% FBS; a TGF-β_1 group, cultured with 0.5% FBS + 5 ng ml^{-1} TGF-β_1; an anti-ED-A antibody group, cultured with 0.5% FBS + 5 ng ml^{-1} TGF-β_1 + 10 μg ml^{-1} anti-ED-A antibody; an IgG group, cultured with 0.5%FBS + 5ng ml^{-1} TGF-β_1 + 10 μg ml^{-1} mouse IgG (negative control, R &D Systems, Inc., MN, USA). Furthermore, each group was sub-divided into two groups: the 1D (1 day) group, which was cultured for 24h after the initiation of culture; the 2D (2 day) group, which was cultured for 24h after refeeding the cells the same medium 24 h after culture initiation. The cells and the supernatants of all groups were subjected to immunofluorescence studies for fibronectin ED-A or α-SMA, and to an ELISA for type I collagen, respectively.

2.3 Immunofluorescence microscopy for fibronectin ED-A and α-SMA

The cells from monolayer cultures were fixed in 4% paraformaldehyde in 0.1 M phosphate-buffered saline (pH 7.4) for 10 min. After rinsing, the cells were permeabilized with 0.5% Triton X-100 for 20 min in order to identify α-SMA in the cells, this process was omitted in studies for detecting fibronectin ED-A. After washing, the cells were incubated with the primary antibody against α-SMA or fibronectin ED-A for 2 h at room temperature. After being rinsed, they were incubated with FITC-conjugated goat anti-mouse IgG secondary antibody for 1 h at room temperature. After staining, the cells were rinsed, observed and photographed using an Olympus BX 60 microscope equipped with epifluorescence optics. The assessment of the percentage of cells with α-SMA-positive stress fibers was performed as follows: when there were one or more stress fibers with α-SMA-positive staining in a cell, the cell was considered to be α-SMA-positive and was referred to as a "myofibroblast". The percentage of myofibroblasts was represented by counting the α-SMA-positive cells among 100 to 500 cells.

2.4 Gel contraction assay

A total of 7 ml of a collagen solution (3 mg/ml stock) was gently mixed with 2 ml of 5-fold-concentrated D-MEM on ice. The mixture was adjusted to pH 7.4 with 1 ml of 200 mM HEPES plus 2.2% $NaHCO_3$ in distilled water. This collagen mixture (0.3ml) was added to each well of a 24 well plate (Becton-Dickinson Labware, NJ). Then, the collagen gel was formed by the incubation of the mixture for 30 min at 37°C. After gelatinization, an NRK 49F cell suspension (2 X10^4 cells ml^{-1}) was poured on the gel in each well. Preincubation of the cell-populated collagen lattice was performed in D-MEM + 10% FBS for 24 h. Next, the gels were rinsed with serum-free D-MEM three times for 30 min. Then, the gel cultures were divided into 4 groups similar to the immunofluorescence studies: a control group, cultured in 0.5% FBS; a TGF-β_1 group, cultured in 0.5% FBS + 5 ng ml^{-1} TGF-β_1; an anti-ED-A antibody group, cultured in 0.5% FBS +5 ng ml^{-1} TGF-β_1+ 10 μg ml^{-1} anti-ED-A antibody and an IgG group, cultured in 0.5%FBS + 5ng ml^{-1} TGF-β_1 + 10 μg ml^{-1} mouse IgG. The gels were then detached from the lateral wall and bottom of each well with a microspatula and cultured for 48 h. After 48 h in culture, the diameter of each gel was measured with a ruler to assess the gel contraction after treatment with the reagents. In addition, to confirm that the shrinkage of the cell-populated collagen lattice occurred due to gel contraction, rather than gel digestion, another study was performed. For this study, after gelatinization, the

NRK49F cell suspension (5000 cells per 5μl) was placed in a very small area near the margin of the gel, and incubated for 1h at 37°C. Then, preincubation was done as above. After rinsing, the gels were cultured in the control medium and the medium with 5ng ml^{-1} TGF-β_1 for 48h at 37°C following gel detachment. After 48h, the shapes of the gels were observed.

2.5 Enzyme-linked immunosolvent assay for type I collagen accumulation in the supernatants of the cultures

The supernatants from monolayer cultures were added to the wells of 96 well plate, which were pre-coated with a mouse monoclonal antibody against rat type I collagen, and were incubated for 2 h at 37°C. After removing the liquid from each well, a biotin-conjugated anti-mouse IgG secondary antibody solution was added, and cells were incubated for 1 h at 37°C. After rinsing, each well was exposed to the horseradish peroxidase-avidin solution for 1 h at 37°C. After washing, the TMB substrate was added, and cells were incubated for 20 min at 37°C. Then, the stop solution was added to each well, while the optical density of each well was determined using a microplate reader, the Multiskan GO (Thermo Fisher Scientific, Yokohama, Japan), at 450 nm. The value of the optical density was converted to the type I collagen concentration in the supernatant of the monolayer culture.

2.6 Statistical analysis

The experimental data are presented as the means ±SD. The statistical analyses were performed using Student's *t*-test. Differences were considered to be statistically significant at $P<0.05$.

3. Results

3.1 TGF-β_1- induced the expression of ED-A and α-SMA

ED-A expression was induced in a dot or short linear pattern on the cell surface by TGF-β_1 by 24 h after initiation of culture (the 1D • TGF-β_1 group), and was further increased after the 48 h culture (the 2D • TGF-β_1 group) (Figs. 2c, 2d). On the other hand, the expression of intracellular α-SMA was not observed 24 h after the initiation of culture (the 1D • TGF-β_1 group), but was induced in stress fiber formations after 48 h in culture (the 2D • TGF-β_1 group) (Figs. 2g, 2h). The expression of ED-A and α-SMA was not observed in the cells cultured in the medium without TGF-β_1 (the 1D and 2D control groups) (Figs. 2a, 2b, 2e, 2f).

3.2 The effects of the anti-ED-A antibody on TGF-β_1- induced α-SMA expression

The TGF-β_1- induced α-SMA expression was markedly decreased by adding an anti-ED-A antibody to the medium (Fig. 3A). The rates of α-SMA-positive cells in stress fiber formations were as follows: the 2D control group (0%), the 2D TGF-β_1 group (97%), the 2D anti-ED-A antibody group (36%), and the 2D IgG group (95%) (Fig. 3B).

3.3 The characteristics of TGF-β_1-induced gel shrinkage

When the cells were ubiquitously poured on the gel, TGF-β_1-induced gel shrinkage occurred in the shape of a circle after culture for 48h (Fig. 4Aa). The diameters of gels were 99.4±1.0%

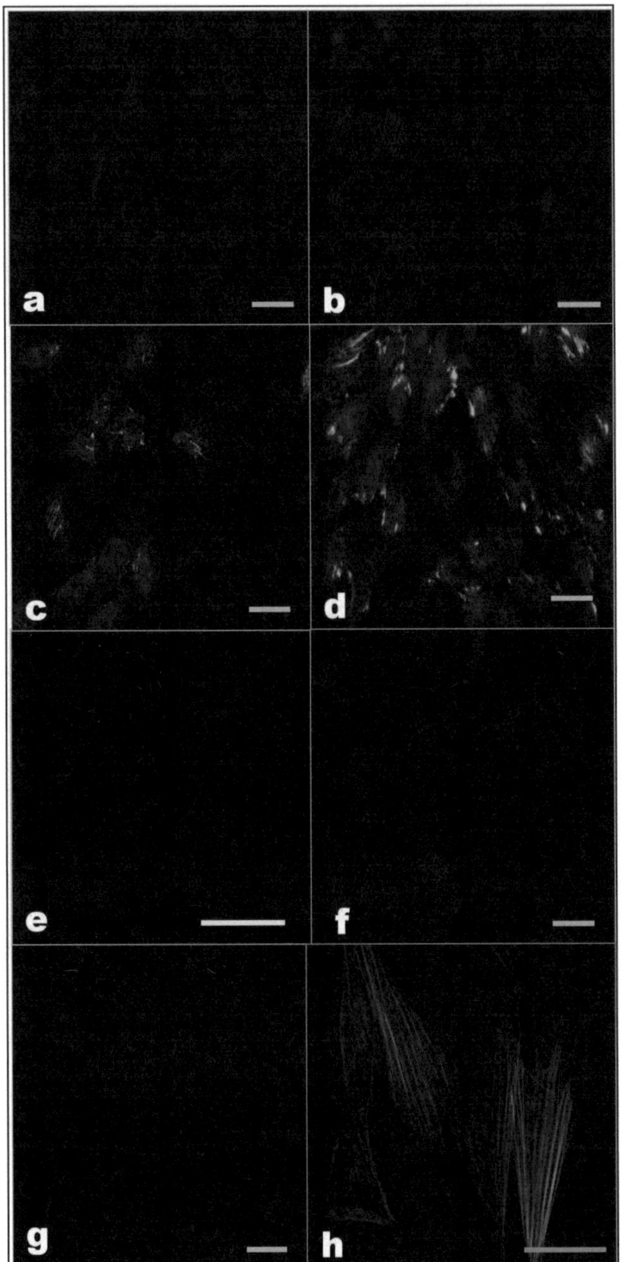

Fig. 2. Immunofluorescent staining for ED-A and α-SMA induced by TGF-β_1.
a, c, e, g, ID groups; b, d, f, h, 2D groups; a, b, c, d, Immunostaining for ED-A; e, f, g, h, Immunostaining for α-SMA; a, b, e, f, control groups; c, d, g, h, TGF-β_1 groups. a, No immunostaining. b, No immunostaining. c, Immunostaining for ED-A is shown by the dot or short linear pattern on the cell surface. d, Immunostaining for ED-A was increased. e, No immunostaining. f, No immunostaining, g, No immunostaining. h, Immunostaining for α-SMA is seen in the stress fiber formation in the cells. Bar, 10 μm.

in the control medium group and 86.4±1.7% in the TGF-β_1 group ($p<0.001$) (Fig. 4Ab). On the other hand, when the cells were placed in a small region close to the margin of the gel, the gel exhibited indentation toward the cell mass in response to TGF-β_1 (Fig. 4B). If gel shrinkage occurs due to gel digestion, the gel would reveal the features of digestion, such as the dissolution of the gel around the cell mass, and would form a thin layer or disappear. However, because the present study did not show these features, gel digestion was not considered to be responsible for the observed gel shrinkage. The observed indentation was thought to be caused by retraction of the gel resulting from cell contraction.

3.4 The effects of the anti-ED-A antibody on TGF-β_1-induced gel contraction

Gel contraction did not occur in the control medium throughout the experimental period. In addition, no gel contraction was observed in any of the 1D groups. In the 2D groups, TGF-β_1 remarkably evoked gel contraction. The treatment with the anti-ED-A antibody was shown to repress TGF-β_1-induced gel contraction. The diameters of the gels in the four groups were as follows: the 2D control group (100%), the 2D TGF-β_1 group (84.0±1.9%), the 2D anti-ED-A antibody group (89.5±1.9%, $p<0.05$ vs the 2D TGF-β_1 group), and the 2D IgG group (83.7±1.6%, $p<0.05$ vs the 2D anti-ED-A antibody group) (Fig. 5).

3.5 The effects of the anti-ED-A antibody on TGF-β_1-stimulated type I collagen accumulation in the supernatants of the cell cultures

There were no significant differences in the accumulation of type I collagen in the cell supernatants between the three 1D groups (the control group, 1420±200; the TGF-β_1 group, 1470±100; the anti-ED-A antibody group, 1510±160 ; the IgG group, 1513±26 pg ml^{-1}). In the 2D groups, the accumulation of type I collagen in the supernatant of the TGF-β_1 group was increased. The increased accumulation of collagen was repressed by addition of the anti-ED-A antibody to the medium with TGF-β_1 (Fig. 5). The concentrations of the supernatants in the four 2D groups (control, TGF-β_1, anti-ED-A antibody, IgG) were 1980±220, 2730±110, 2490±18, 2570±3 pg ml^{-1}, respectively ($p<0.001$, the control group vs the TGF-β_1 group; $p<0.05$, the TGF-β_1 group and the IgG group vs the anti-ED-A antibody group) (Fig. 6).

4. Discussion

Myofibroblasts expressing α-SMA have been shown to emerge in fibrotic diseases (Tomasek et al., 2002). In general, α-SMA is considered to be profoundly involved in the progression of fibrosis, but the detailed significance of α-SMA expression remains unresolved. For example, it is unclear whether myofibroblasts are really essential for fibrosis. In contrast to general considerations, there have been some reports indicating that myofibroblasts are not necessary for the progression of fibrosis. For example, Takeji et al. suggested that α-SMA expression provided benefits for fibrosis (Takeji et al., 2006). It was demonstrated that defects in α-SMA enhanced the progression of fibrosis by performing unilateral ureteral obstruction in a renal interstitial fibrosis model in an α-SMA knockout mouse. Furthermore, transfection of the α-SMA gene into α-SMA$^{-/-}$ myofibroblasts from these mice suppressed fibrosis. These results indicated that α-SMA expression suppresses, rather than accelerates, fibrosis. The α-SMA$^{-/-}$ myofibroblasts that were obtained possessed the ability to migrate, proliferate, and overproduced type I collagen. These cells did not express α-SMA, but did start to overexpress skeletal muscle α-actin, smooth muscle γ-actin, and related molecules.

These cells also overproduced type I collagen compared to conventional myofibroblasts expressing α-SMA. Because the cells which were established by transfection of the α-SMA gene into the α-SMA$^{-/-}$ cells failed to produce type I collagen, these cells might resemble smooth muscle cells. It is likely that myofibroblasts are an intermediate type of cells between α-SMA$^{-/-}$ cells and smooth muscle cells, given their ability to express α-SMA and produce type I collagen. Taken together, their report does not refute the generally accepted concept

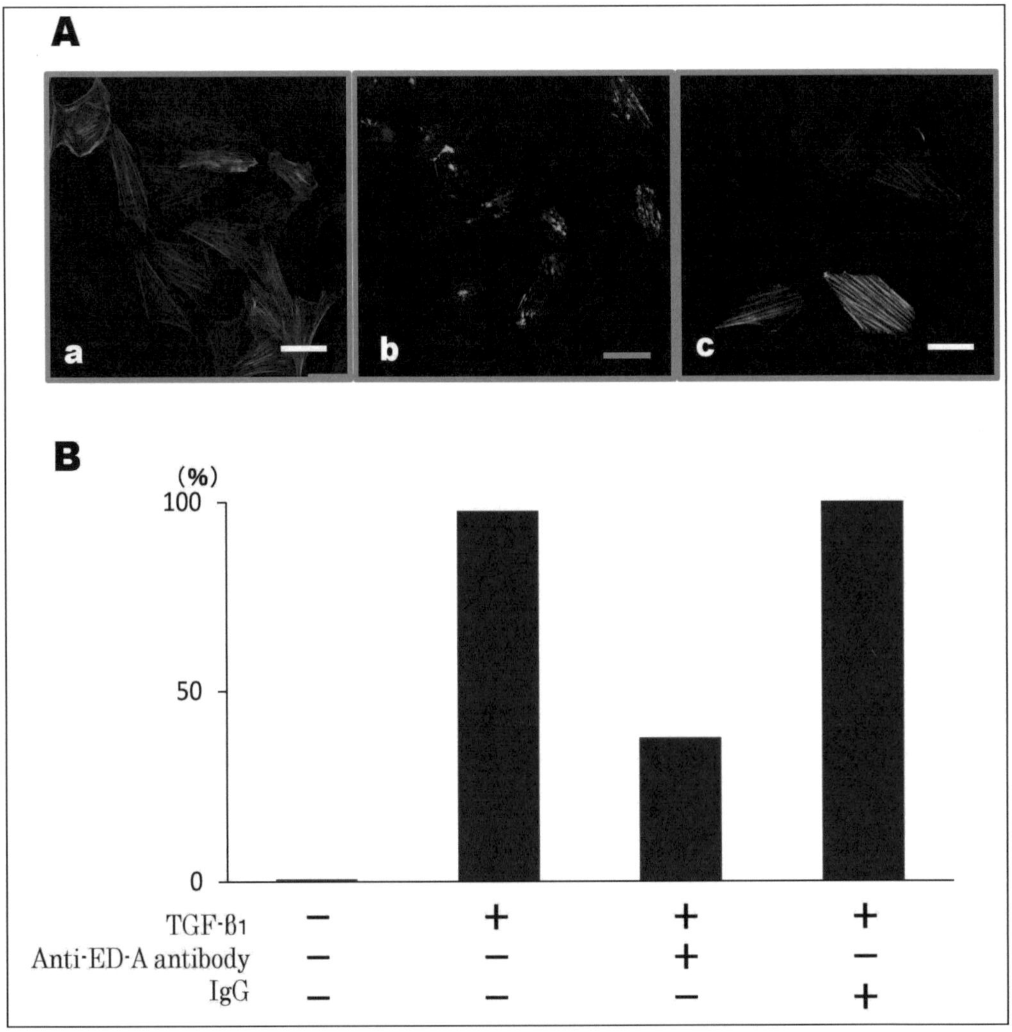

Fig. 3. Immunofluorescent staining for α-SMA was influenced by the anti-ED-A antibody Aa, the 2D TGF-β_1 group; b, the 2D anti-ED-A antibody group; c, the 2D IgG group; B, Counts of cells immunostained for α-SMA in the stress fiber formation. Aa and Ac, Immunostaining for α-SMA was shown in the stress fiber formation. Ab, Cells expressing α-SMA in the stress fiber formation were markedy decreased in number. Immunostaining for ED-A was seen in response to addition of the anti-ED-A antibody to the medium. B. Cells with α-SMA expression induced by TGF-β_1 were decreased in number in the anti-ED-A antibody group. Bar, 10 μm.

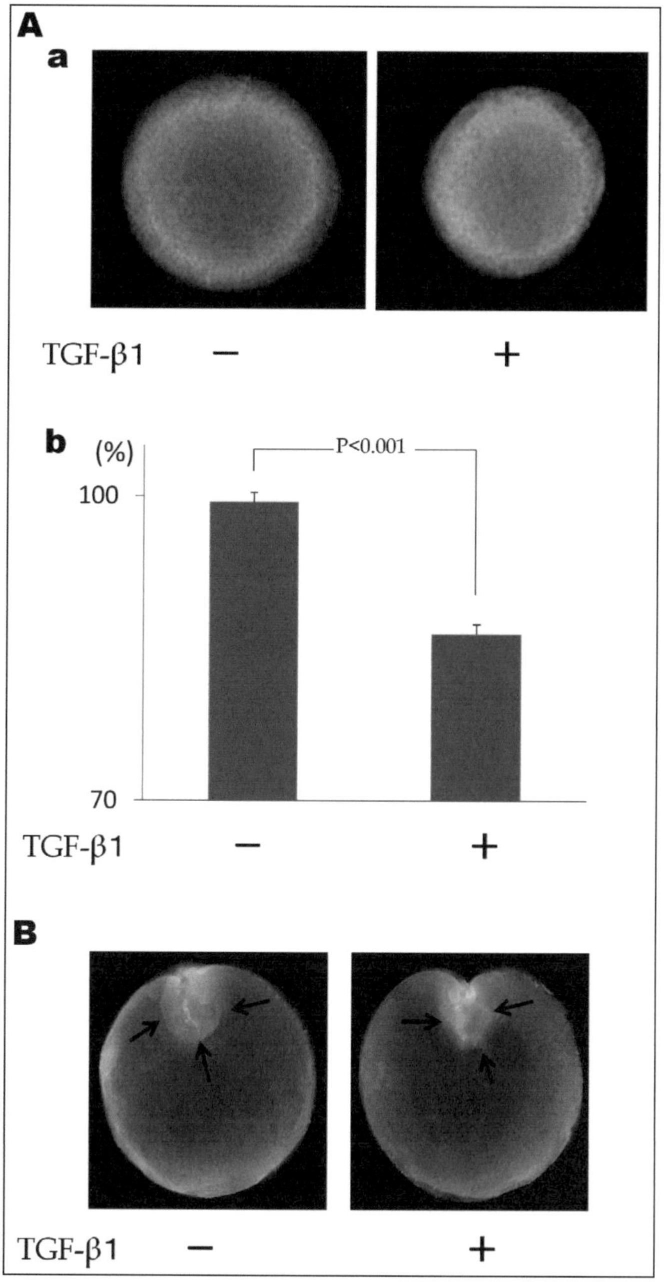

Fig. 4. Morphological alterations of gels in response to TGF-β_1 according to differences in the pouring methods.
A. Ubiquitous pouring of cells. a. The shape of the gel b. the diameters of the gels. B. Spot pouring of cells. Aa. The change in shape induced by TGF-β_1 is indicated by the circle. Ab. TGF-β_1 significantly induced gel shrinkage. The data represent the diameters of the gels compared to the well. B. The gel was deformed, as shown by the indentation torward the cell mass (arrows).

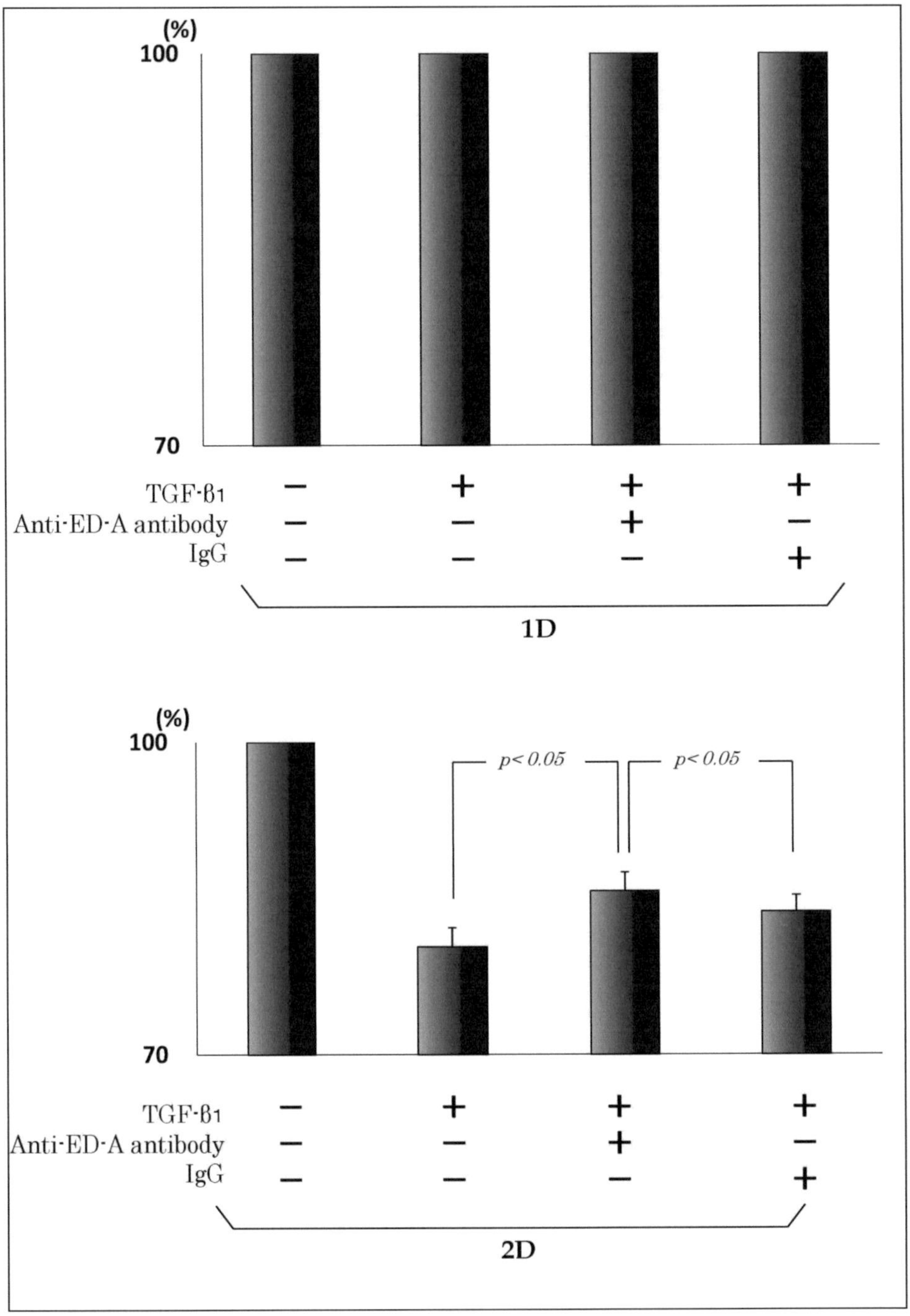

Fig. 5. Type I collagen gel contraction.
No gel contraction occurred in any of the 1D groups. TGF-β_1 was shown to evoke gel contraction in the 2D TGF-β_1 and IgG groups. TGF-β_1 -induced gel contraction was attenuated by adding the anti-ED-A antibody. The data represent the diameters of the gels compared to the well.

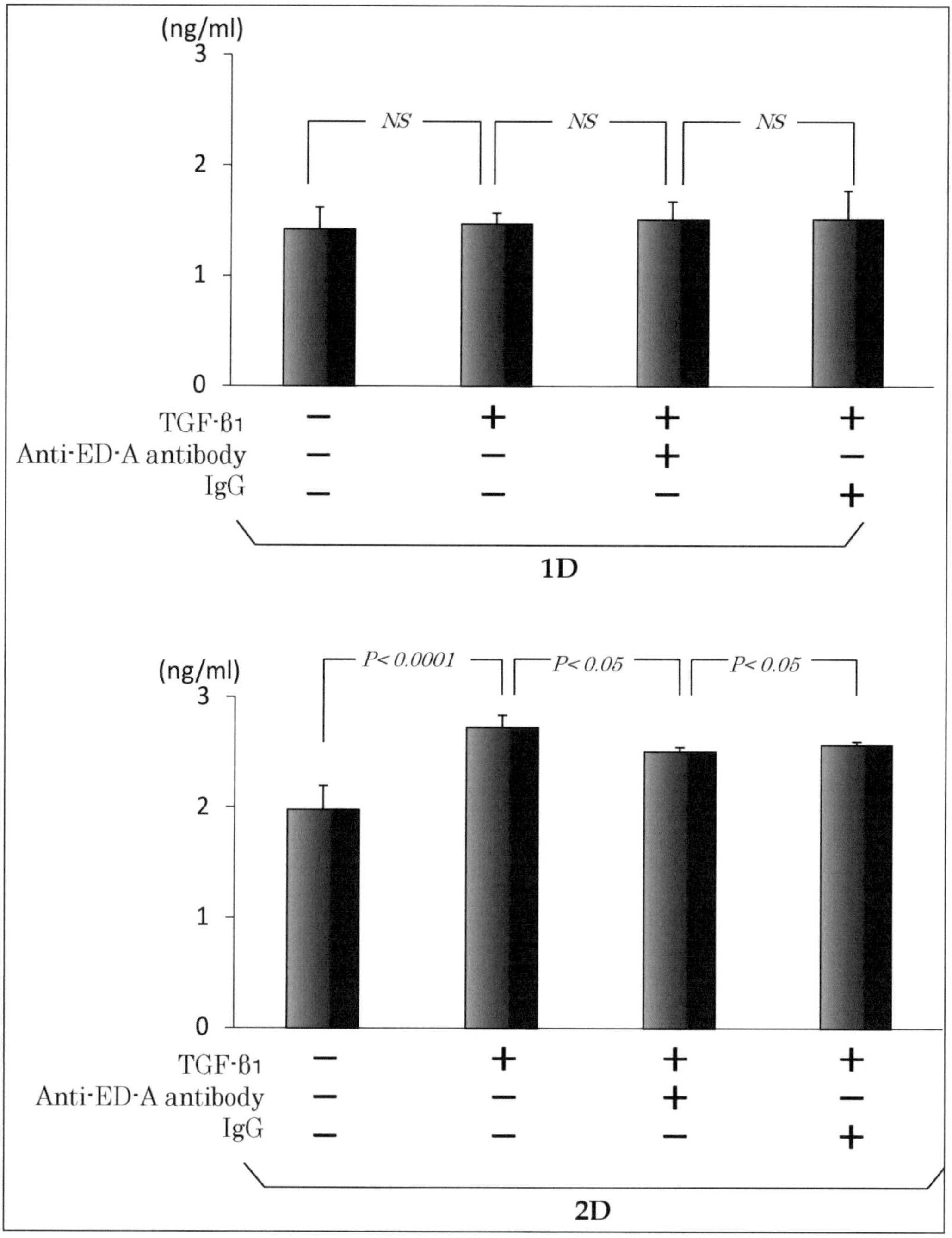

Fig. 6. Type I collagen accumulated in the supernatants of the monolayer cultures.
The TGF-β_1 and anti-ED-A antibodies do not influence the type I collagen accumulation in 1D groups. TGF-β_1 increased the type I collagen accumulation in the 2D TGF-β_1 and IgG groups. The TGF-β_1- accelerated collagen accumulation was repressed by the anti-ED-A antibody.

that α-SMA contributes to the progression of fibrosis, but do add an additional role for α-SMA producing cells. There was another report (Leemans et al., 2009) that suggested that renal fibrogenesis persists despite decreasing numbers of α-SMA$^+$ myofibroblasts. This also does not contradict the general consensus about the role of myofibroblasts, because it can be considered that after myofibroblasts induce the accumulation of collagen fibrils by forming rigid fibrils which are resistant to proteolysis by proteinases, they undergo apoptosis. Subsequently, the α-SMA$^-$ fibroblasts might add collagen fibers to these rigid fibers. In this case, myofibroblasts would make up the nucleus of the accumulated collagen fibrils.

In the present study, TGF-β_1 induced the production of fibronectin ED-A, which was anchored to kidney fibroblasts, and subsequently induced α-SMA expression in the stress fiber formations in cells. Stress fiber formation is involved in cell contraction, which results in gel contraction via the consecutive binding of α-SMA, focal adhesion, integrins, and type I collagen. In addition, the α-SMA expression was strongly inhibited by exposing the cells to an anti-ED-A antibody. Therefore, the TGF-β_1 -induced expression of α-SMA was considered to be, at least to a large extent, dependent on ED-A expression. This is compatible with the fact that the fibronectin ED-A isoform contributes to the transdifferentiation of a variety of cells into myofibroblasts with α-SMA (Bochaton-Piallat et al., 2000; Ffrench-Constant et al., 1989; Jamagin et al., 1994).

It was shown in the renal fibroblasts that the intracellular signaling pathways of TGF-β_1-induced fibronectin ED-A expression involves Smad 3 (Bondi et al., 2010). The pathways leading to α-SMA expression and myofibroblast transdifferentiation differed between reports. Our previous report suggested that the pathway of TGF-β_1-induced α-SMA expression involved p38 MAPK (Ina et al., 2011). This finding is consistent with a study by Miura et al. (Miura et al., 2006), in which retinal pigment epithelial cells were used. On the other hand, Masszi et al. (Masszi et al., 2003) have found that the activation of the Rho kinase pathway was involved in the α-SMA expression in renal tubular epithelial cells. The contrast between these findings might be due to the differences in the cells used. How ED-A expression activated the p38 MAPK pathway in the present study remains to be determined. However, ED-A has been identified as an endogenous ligand for Toll-like receptor-4 (Gondokaryono et al., 2007; Lefebvre et al., 2011; Ricupero et al., 2001) which is well known to be expressed in inflammatory cells such as macrophages, mast cells, and leukocytes, and is associated with innate immunity. Recently, it was demonstrated that Toll-like receptor 4 is also expressed in renal interstitial fibroblasts (Sorensen et al., 2011). Furthermore, the activation of Toll-like receptor 4 was reported to promote renal tubulointerstitial fibrosis (Campbell et al., 2011; Sorensen et al., 2011). It is therefore possible that ED-A binds to Toll-like receptor 4 and activates it, leading to stimulation of the related signaling pathways, eventually promoting the signaling by TGF-β_1 and stimulating α-SMA expression.

Because the immunostaining for fibronectin ED-A was positive in both conventional immunocytochemistry and in that without the first antibody (the anti-ED-A antibody) of the cells exposed to the antibody in culture, the epitope appears to be present in a region other than the receptor-binding site. In this case, the binding of the antibody to the epitope might cause alterations in the conformation of the receptor binding site, and inhibit the binding of ED-A to the receptor. In the current study, since contraction of the NRK49F cell-populated collagen lattice was suppressed by the adding anti-ED-A antibody, the ED-A expression was considered to be involved in TGF-β_1-induced gel contraction.

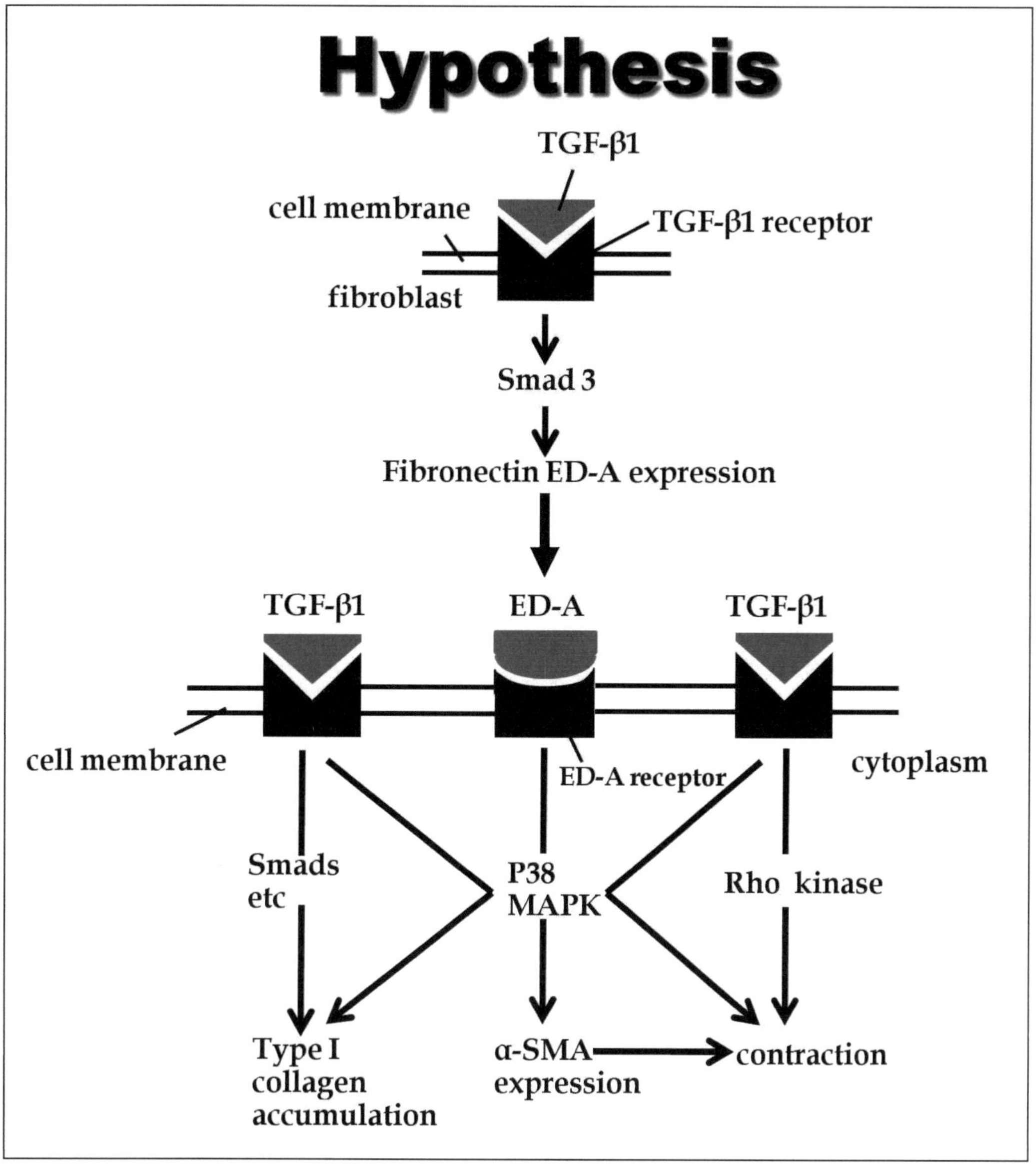

Fig. 7. The hypothesis: about the contribution of fibronectin ED-A expression to α-SMA expression and type I collagen accumulation.

We hypothesize the mechanism ad follows: TGF-β_1 induces ED-A domain expression through the pathway involving Smad 3 in the fibronectin molecule. The fibronectin ED-A is anchored to the cell via a combination of the cell-binding domain and the integrin on the cell. Subsequently, the ED-A domain binds to the receptor (the Toll-like receptor) and stimulates it. Furthermore, the signaling transfers to one of the TGF-β_1-activated pathways, which may be the p38 MAPK pathway. Finally, the ED-A-stimulated pathway induces α-SMA expression and type I collagen accumulation, which involves the increased synthesis of collagen and decreased degradation of collagen via the production of proteinase inhibitors, TIMPs and PAI-1.

The previous study demonstrated that TGF-β_1 caused the contraction of the fibroblast (without α-SMA expression)-populated collagen lattice in culture medium with 10% FBS. The TGF-β_1-induced gel contraction was accelerated by expressing α-SMA, which was induced by a low concentration of FBS and the addition of TGF-β_1 (Ina et al., 2011). Therefore, TGF-β_1 was suggested to exert distinct functions on α-SMA expression and gel contraction. In addition, it was shown that TGF-β_1-induced gel contraction occurred via the p38 MAPK pathway and the Rho kinase pathway (Ina et al., 2011). Taken together, since the p38 MARK pathway is involved in both α-SMA expression and gel contraction, it is likely that ED-A expression might stimulate the p38 MAPK pathway activated by TGF-β_1, followed by myofibroblast transdifferentiation and gel contraction.

These findings still have not clarified what gel contraction means in the fibrosis of diabetic nephropathy. We believe that it corresponds to the renal atrophy following fibrosis. However, it is also possible that gel contraction might reflect the shrinkage of collagen fibrils, allowing collagen molecules to become nearer to each other, followed by increased crosslinking, which leads to the formation of rigid fibrils. These are resistant to proteolysis by proteinases, thus leading to the accumulation of fibrils, and therefore, fibrosis.

In the present study, we also demonstrated that accumulation of type I collagen was, at least in part, dependent on ED-A expression. To our knowledge, this is the first report that ED-A mediates TGF-β_1-stimulated type I collagen accumulation, while there was a previous report that ED-A stimulated type I collagen mRNA expression (Serini et al., 1998). There are both Smad-dependent and independent pathways, including the p38 MAPK pathway, via which TGF-β_1 can stimulate the production of ECM containing type I collagen (Eickelberg, 2001). The observed α-SMA expression, gel contraction, and type I collagen accumulation are, at least in part, dependent on ED-A expression. The α-SMA expression was the most dependent of these events on ED-A. We therefore hypothesized that α-SMA expression is, to a large extent, dependent on ED-A expression via the p38 MAPK pathway. On the other hand, gel contraction and type I collagen accumulation were, to a lesser extent, dependent on ED-A expression, because they are comparatively mediated by pathways other than the p38 MAPK pathway. ED-A binds to Toll-like receptor-4 and activates it, followed by signaling via diverse pathways in inflammatory cells (Akira & Takeda, 2004). The p38 MAPK pathway is also included in these pathways. Thus, it is most likely that the α-SMA expression, gel contraction, and type I collagen accumulation induced by ED-A expression are mediated by activating the p38 MAPK pathway (Fig. 6). In other words, ED-A appears to enhance the activity of the p38 MARK pathway stimulated by TGF-β_1.

5. Conclusion

The TGF-β_1-induced α-SMA expression, followed by gel contraction and stimulated type I collagen accumulation, were, at least in part, dependent on fibronectin ED-A expression. These findings suggest that tubulointerstitial fibrosis associated with diabetic nephropathy and fibrotic tissue contraction leading to renal atrophy are partly mediated by TGF-β_1-induced fibronectin ED-A expression. In addition, since the fibronectin ED-A isoform is seldom found in normal adult subjects, the negative effects induced by inhibition of ED-A expression or activity would likely be minimal. Taken together, our findings and those of previous studies suggest that ED-A may be a target for treatment of diabetic nephropathy.

6. Acknowledgement

The authors thank Ms. Yukari Goto for her excellent secretarial assistance.

7. References

Akira, S., & Takeda, K. (2004) .Toll-like receptor signaling. *Nature Reviews*, Vol. 4, pp. 499-511, 1474-1733

Balza, E.L., Borsi, G., Allemmanni, G., & Zardi, L. (1988). Transforming growth factor β regulates the levels of different fibronectin isoforms in normal cultured fibroblasts. *FEBS Letters*, Vol. 228, pp. 42-44, 0014-5793

Bohle, A., Wehrmann, M., Bogenschtz, O., Batz, C., & Muller, G.A. (1991). The pathogenesis of chronic renal failure in diabetic nephropathy. *Pathology,Research and Practice*, Vol. 187, pp. 251-259, 0344-0338

Bochaton-Piallat, M.L., Kapetanios, A.D., Donati, G., Redard, M., Gabbiani, G., & Pournaras, C.J. (2000). TGF − β1,

TGF-β receptor II and ED-A fibronectin expression in myofibroblast of vitreoretinopathy. *Investigation Ophthalmology & Visual Science*, Vol. 41, No.8, pp. 2336-2342, 1552-5783

Bondi, C.D., Manickam, N., Lee, D.Y., Block, K., Gorin, Y., Abboud, H.E., & Barnes, J.L. (2010). NAD(P)H oxidase mediates TGF-β_1 -induced activation of kidney myofibroblasts. *Journal of the American Society of Nephrology*, Vol. 21, pp.93-102, 1046-6673

Borsi, L., Castellani, P., Risso, A.M., Leprini, A., & Zardi, L. (1990). Transforming growth factor *β* regulates the splicing pattern of fibronectin messenger RNA precursor. *FEBS Letters*, Vol. 261, pp. 175-178, 0014-5793

Campbell, M.T., Hile, K.L., Zhang, H., Asanuma, H., Vanderbrink, B.A., Rink, R.R., & Meldrum, K.K. (2011). Toll-like receptor 4: a novel signaling pathway during renal fibrogenesis. *Journal of Surgical Research*, Vol. 168, No. 1, pp. e61-e69, 0022-4804

Edwards, D.R., Murphy, G., Reynolds, J.J., Whitham, S.E., Docherty, A.J.P., Angel, P., & Heath, J.K. (1987). Transforming growth factor beta modulates the expression of collagenase and metalloprotease inhibitor. *EMBO Journal, Vol.* 6, pp. 1899-1904, 0261-4189

Eickelberg, O. (2001). Endless healing: TGF-β, SMADs, and fibrosis. *FEBS Letters*, Vol. 506, pp. 11-14, 0014-5793

Ffrench-Constant, C., Van, W.L., Dvorak, H.F., & Hynes, R.O. (1989). Reappearance of an embryonic pattern of fibronectin splicing during wound healing in the adult rat. *The Journal of Cell Biology*, Vol. 109, pp. 903-914, 0021-9525

Gabbiani, G. &, Ryan, G., & Majno, G. (1971). Presence of modified fibroblasts in granulation tissue and their possible in wound contraction. *Experientia,* Vol. 27, pp. 549-550, 0014-4754

Glukhova, M.A., Frid, M.G., Shekhomin, B.V., Vasilevskaya, T.D., Grunwald, J., Saginati, M., & Koteliansky, V.E. (1989). Expression of extra domain-A fibronectin sequence in vascular smooth muscle cells is phenotype dependent. *The Journal of Cell Biology,* Vol. 109, pp. 357-366, 0021-9525

Gondokaryono, S.P., Ushio, H., Niyonsaba, F., Hara, M., Takenaka, H., Jayawardana, S.T.M., Ikeda, S., Okumura, K., & Ogawa, H. (2007). The extra domain A of fibronectin stimulates murine mast cells via Toll-like receptor 4. *Journal of Leukocyte Biology,* Vol. 82, pp. 657-665, 1938-3673

Humphreys, B.D., Lin, S.L., Kobayashi, A., Hudson, T.E., Nowlin, B.T., Bonventre, J.V., Valerius, M.T., McMahon, A.P., & Duffield, J.S. (2010). Fate tracing reveals the pericyte and not epithelial origin of myofibroblasts in kidney fibrosis. *The American Journal of Pathology,* Vol. 176, pp. 85-97, 0002-9440

Ina, K., Kitamura, H., Tatsukawa, S., & Fujikura, Y. (2011). Significance of α-SMA in myofibroblasts emerging in renal tubulointerstitial fibrosis. *Histology and Histopathology,* Vol. 26, pp. 855-866, 1699-5848

Iwano, M., Plieth, D., Danoff, T.M., Xue, C., Okeda, H., & Neilson, E.G. (2002). Evidence that fibroblasts derive from epithelium during tissue fibrosis. *The Journal of Clinical Investigation,* Vol. 110, pp. 341-350, 0021-9738

Jamagin, W.R., Rockey, D.C., Koteliansky, V.E., Wang, S.S., & Bissel, D.M. (1994). Expression of variant fibronectins in wound healing: Cellular source and biological activity of the EIllA segment in rat hepatic fibrogenesis. *The Journal of Cell Biology,* Vol. 127, pp. 2037-2048, 0021-9525

Keeley, E.C., Mehrad, B., & Strieter, R.M. (2010). Fibrocytes: bringing new insights into mechanisms of inflammation and fibrosis. *The International Journal of Biochemistry & Cell Biology,* Vol. 42, pp. 535-542, 1357-2725

Laiho, M., Saksela, O., & Keski-Oja, J. (1987). Transforming growth factor-β induction of type-1 plasminogen activator inhibitor. *Journal of Biological Chemistry,* Vol. 262, pp. 17467-17474, 0021-9258

Leemans, J.C., Butter, L.M., Pulskens, W.P., Teske, G.J., Claessen, N., V.d.Poll, T., & Florequin, S. (2009). The role of Toll-like receptor 2 in inflammation and fibrosis during progressive renal injury. *PLoS ONE,* Vol. 4, pp. e5704, 1932-6203

Lefebvre, J.S., Lévesque, T., Picard, S., Paré, G., Gravel, A., Flamand, L., & Borgeat, P. (2011). Extra domain A of fibronectin primes leukotriene biosynthesis and stimulates neutrophil migration through activation of Toll-like receptor 4. *Arthritis & Rheumatism,* Vol. 63, No.6, pp. 1527-1533, 1529-0131

Magnusson, M.K., & Mosher. D.F. (1998). Fibronectin: Structure, assembly, and cardiovascular implications. *Arteriosclerosis, Thrombosis, and Vascular Biology,* Vol. 18, pp. 1363-1370, 0276-5047

Masszi, A., Ciano, C.D., Sirokmány, G., Arthur, W.T., Rotstein, O.D., Wang, J., McCulloch, C.A.G., Rosivall, L., Mucsi, I., & Kapus, A. (2003). Central role for Rho in TGF-β1-induced α-smooth muscle actin expression during epithelial-mesenchymal transition. *American Journal of Physiology-Renal Physiology*, Vol. 284, No. 5, pp. F911-F924, 1522-1466

Miura, M., Hata, H., Hirayama, K., Kita, T., Noda, Y., Fujisawa, K., Shimokawa, H., & Ishibashi, T. (2006). Critical role of the Rho-kinase pathway in TGF-β2-dependent collagen gel contraction by retinal pigment epithelial cells. *Experimental Eye Research*, Vol. 82, pp. 849-859, 0014-4835

Norton, P.A., & Hynes, R.O. (1987). Alternative splicing of chicken fibronectin in embryos and in normal and transformed cells. *Molecular and Cellular Biology*, Vol. 7, pp. 4297-4307

Petersen, T.E., Thogersen, H.C., Skorstengaard, K., Vibe-Pedersen, K., Sahi, P., Sottrup-Jensen, L., & Magnusson, S. (1983). Partial primary structure of bovine plasma fibronectin: Three types of internal homology. *Proceedings of the National Academy of Sciences of the United States of America*, Vol .80, pp. 137-141, 0027-8424

Ricupero, D.A., Poliks, C.F., Rishikof, D.C., Kuang, P-P., & Goldstein, R.H. (2001). Apigenin decreases expression of the myofibroblast phenotype. *FEBS Letters*, Vol. 506, pp. 15-21, I0014-5793

Serini, G., Bochaton-Piallat, M.L., Ropraz, P., Geinoz, A., Borsi, L., Zardi, L., & Gabbiani, G. (1998). The fibronectin domain ED-A is crucial for myofibroblastic phenotype induction by transforming growth factor-β1. *The Journal of Cell Biology*, Vol. 142, No.3, pp. 873-881, 0021-9525

Simonson, M.S. (2007). Phenotypic transitions and fibrosis in diabetic nephropathy. *Kidney International*, Vol. 71, pp. 846-854, 0085-2538

Sörensen, I., Susnik, N., Inhester, T., Degen, J.L., Melk, A., Haller, H., & Schmitt, R (2011). Fibrinogen, acting as a mitogen for tubulointerstitial fibroblasts, promotes renal fibrosis. *Kidney International*, [epub ahead of print], 0085-2539

Strutz, F., & Zeisberg, M. (2006). Renal fibroblasts and myofibroblasts in chronic kidney disease. *The Journal of American Society of Nephrology*, Vol. 17, pp. 2992-2998, 1046-6673

Takeji, M., Moriyama, T., Oseto, S., Kawada, N., Hori, M., Imai, E., & Miwa, T. (2006). Smooth muscle α-actin deficiency in myofibroblasts leads to enhanced renal tissue fibrosis. *Journal of Biological Chemistry*, Vol. 281, pp. 40193-40200, 1083-351X

Tomasek, J.J., Gabbiani, G., Hinz, B., Chaponnier, C., & Brown, R.A. (2002). Myofibroblasts and mechano-regulation of connective tissue remodeling. *National Reviews Molecular Cell Biology*, Vol. 3, No. 5, pp. 349-363, 1471-0072

Vartio, T., Laitinen, L., Narvanen, O., Cutolo, M., Thornell, L.E., Zardi, L., &Virtanen, I. (1987). Differential expression of the ED sequence-containing form of cellular fibronectin in embryonic and adult human tissues. *Journal of Cell Science*, Vol. 88, pp. 419-430, 1477-9137

Wierzbicka-Patynowski, I., & Schwarzbauer, J.E. (2003). The ins and outs of fibronectin matrix assembly. *Journal of cell Science*, Vol. 116, pp. 3269-3276, 1477-9137

Zeisberg, E.M., Potenta, S.E., Sugimono, H., Zeisberg, M., & Kalluri, R. (2008). Fibroblasts in kidney fibrosis emerge via endothelial-to-mesenchymal transition. *The Journal of American Society of Nephrology*, Vol. 19, pp. 2282-2287, 1046-6673

8

Immunoinflammation in Diabetic Nephropathy: Molecular Mechanisms and Therapeutic Options

Virginia Lopez-Parra, Beñat Mallavia,
Jesus Egido and Carmen Gomez-Guerrero
Renal and Vascular Inflammation, Nephrology Department,
IIS-Fundacion Jimenez Diaz, Autonoma University, Madrid
Spain

1. Introduction

The prevalence of diabetes mellitus, predominantly of type 2, has dramatically increased worldwide (Ritz et al., 2011). Diabetic nephropathy (DN) affects approximately one third of people with type 1 or type 2 diabetes mellitus (Reutens et al., 2011). In developed countries, the proportion of patients with diabetic kidney disease has stabilized despite increased use of glucose-lowering medications and renin-angiotensin-aldosterone system (RAAS) inhibitors (de Boer et al., 2011).

DN typically develops after many years of diabetes, and is usually manifested clinically by gradually worsening albuminuria, followed by a decline in glomerular filtration rate, which over years or decades leads to end-stage renal disease. DN is characterized by specific renal morphological and functional alterations. Features of early diabetic renal changes are glomerular hyperfiltration, glomerular and renal hypertrophy, increased urinary albumin excretion, increased basement membrane thickness, and mesangial expansion with the accumulation of extracellular matrix proteins such as collagens, fibronectin, and laminin. Pathologic alterations of the tubulointerstitium such as fibrosis and tubular atrophy are also closely linked to the deterioration of renal function in patients with diabetes of both types 1 and 2 (Wolf, 2000; Schrijvers et al., 2004).

Despite the modern therapies like antidiabetic, antihypertensive, and antioxidant drugs available to treat DN, most of patients continue to show progressive renal damage. It suggests that the key pathogenic mechanisms involved in the induction and progression of DN are still remaining active and unmodified by the present therapies (Balakumar et al., 2009). Many studies have attempted to elucidate the molecular signaling mechanisms that lead to DN so that effective therapies and preventive strategies might be developed. Through these efforts the general understanding of the pathogenic signaling factors that lead to progressive DN has expanded considerably during the past decade (Balakumar et al., 2009; Brosius et al., 2010).

In recent years, extensive research has elucidated several pathways involved in the development and progression of diabetic kidney disease beyond the relevant role of high blood glucose (Schrijvers et al., 2004). Our knowledge of the pathophysiological processes in

DN has notably improved on a genetic and molecular level. Thus, the classic view of metabolic and hemodynamic alterations as the main causes of renal injury in diabetes has been transformed significantly, with clear evidence indicating that these traditional factors are only a partial aspect of a much more complex picture. One of the most important changes is related to the participation of immune-mediated inflammatory processes in the pathophysiology of diabetes mellitus and its complications (Navarro-Gonzalez & Mora-Fernandez, 2008; Galkina & Ley, 2006; Shikata & Makino, 2001; Chow et al., 2004).

Although DN is traditionally considered a non-immune disease, accumulating evidence now indicates that immunologic and inflammatory mechanisms play a significant role in its development and progression. DN also includes a variety of inflammatory responses induced by hyperglycemic conditions. Furthermore, microinflammation is a common major mechanism for the progression of DN. This process is mediated by elements of the immune system, including lymphocytes and monocytes/macrophages, as well as cytokines, growth factors, chemokines, adhesion molecules, enzymes, and nuclear factors. In this review we summarized cell processes, mediators and intracellular pathways participating in the immune and inflammatory response during the development of diabetic renal damage.

2. Mechanisms of immune cell infiltration in the diabetic kidney

2.1 Immune cells

Yet, the molecular and cellular mechanisms of intrarenal inflammation in DN remain poorly characterized. Macrophages are the major inflammatory cells found in diabetic kidneys and their accumulation is a recognized feature in renal biopsies from diabetic patients (Xiao et al., 2009). In different experimental models of DN, renal macrophage accumulation correlates with the severity of glomerular and tubulointerstitial injury (Chow et al., 2004; Chow et al., 2005). However, it remains to be established whether macrophages are a major effector cell of diabetic renal damage, or merely recruited as a response to injury. Previous studies in diabetic animals reported the protective effect of mycophenolate or irradiation via reduction of renal macrophage infiltration (Wu et al., 2006). However, these treatments have additional effects on the kidney and immune system, and cannot be used for determining the long-term effects of macrophages on the progression of DN.

Macrophages mediate immunopathology and tissue remodeling in both non-renal and renal diseases, and blocking macrophage recruitment prevents the progression of many types of kidney disease models (Ricardo et al., 2008). There are at least two subtypes of resident macrophages in tissues: the M1 macrophages, classically activated by Th1 stimuli, that express proinflammatory cytokines and enhances tissue inflammatory response; and the M2 macrophages, alternatively activated by Th2 stimuli, that express antiinflammatory cytokines, and participate in the promotion of tissue repair, remodeling and vasculogenesis (Gordon, 2003). Obviously, modulating the macrophage phenotype is as important as reducing their overall number to prevent glomerular damage. The relative abundance of M1 and M2 macrophages in the injured kidney changes dynamically by recruitment of polarized monocytes or through the effects of local cytokines on macrophages. Different chemokines are able to recruit circulating monocytes to extravascular compartments such as the glomerulus. Classically activated M1 macrophages represent one end of the spectrum as they produce upon stimulation high amounts of reactive oxygen species (ROS), and proinflammatory cytokines, such as interleukins (ILs), tumor necrosis factor (TNF-α), and interferon-γ (IFN-γ), all of which exacerbate inflammation and tissue injury *in vivo* (Mantovani et al., 2004). Alternatively activated M2 macrophages represent the other end of the spectrum and they participate in the resolution of inflammation through the secretion of antiinflammatory factors such as IL-10 and transforming growth factor-β (TGF-β), as well as by inhibiting the production of proinflammatory cytokines, chemokines, and superoxide anion (Martinez et al., 2008; Ricardo et al., 2008). Recent studies demonstrated a reduction in the severity of glomerular inflammation with adoptive transfer of cytokine-programmed M2 macrophages (Ricardo et al., 2008). Furthermore, the antiinflammatory effects of statins (Fujita et al., 2010) and the angiotensin II type 1 receptor blocker olmesartan (Aki et al., 2010) in experimental glomerulonephritis are mediated through downregulation of M1 macrophage infiltration as well as augmentation of antiinflammatory M2 macrophages and cytokines. Based on this, strategies to control the dynamic balance of macrophage polarization could have therapeutic interests in DN, and future studies will determine the place of these novel approaches in diabetic patients.

T lymphocytes are known to play a significant role in renal injury induced by non-immune insults including ischaemia or toxins (e.g. adriamycin) (Lim et al., 2010). In patients with type 1 diabetes, the presence of nephropathy and proteinuria has been associated with increased activated peripheral blood T cells and also infiltration of T cells into the kidney (Xiao et al., 2009; Moriya et al., 2004; Ichinose et al., 2007), thus suggesting that lymphocyte activation may play a role in early DN. Activated T cells can cause injury directly through cytotoxic effects and indirectly by recruiting and activating macrophages. In addition, kidney autoantigens may develop during chronic diabetic renal injury and, if this occurs, B cells could present these antigens to T cells to promote their activation. Furthermore, diabetic patients have increased levels of serum immunoglobulins, which include antibodies (Abs) against proteins modified by glycoxidation or lipoxidation. These circulating Abs can form immune complexes (Atchley et al., 2002), which may deposit in glomeruli and promote activation of complement or macrophages via receptor interactions. Elements of the diabetic milieu can directly or indirectly activate T cells in diabetic kidneys. CD4+ T cells express the receptor for advanced glycation end products (AGEs) and can respond to AGEs by producing IFN-γ, which could exacerbate inflammation in the diabetic kidney. In addition, hyperglycemia induces macrophage production of IL-12, which can also stimulate CD4 cell production of IFN-γ (Wen et al., 2006; Lim et al., 2010). T lymphocyte-directed immunotherapies with anti-CD3 and anti-CD4 monoclonal Abs also induce disease remission in non-obese diabetic mice (Mehta et al., 2010). Some of them are currently in Phase III clinical trials for prevention of type 1 diabetes (Miller & St, 2011), although their renoprotective effects are not documented.

2.2 Inflammatory mediators

The infiltration of leukocytes into sites of inflammation is mediated by sequential binding to specific cell adhesion molecules and chemokine and cytokine release that together promote rolling, arrest, firm adhesion, transmigration, and activation (Hogg & Berlin, 1995). A large array of cell adhesion molecules, chemokines, and cytokines have been shown to be important in leukocyte accumulation and renal injury in models of non-diabetic and diabetic kidney damage, and some of these mediators are also found elevated in renal biopsies from diabetic patients (Navarro-Gonzalez & Mora-Fernandez, 2008; Galkina & Ley, 2006; Shikata

& Makino, 2001; Chow et al., 2004). The most representative members for each family are discussed below.

2.2.1 Adhesion molecules: ICAM-1

Intercellular adhesion molecule (ICAM)-1 is a 90-kD cell surface glycoprotein of the Ig superfamily involved in the firm attachment of leukocytes to endothelium (Staunton et al., 1988), which interacts with lymphocyte function-associated antigen (LFA)-1 (CD11a/CD18) and Mac-1 (CD11b/CD18) that are present on most leukocytes. ICAM-1 expression is upregulated and associated with leukocyte infiltration and disease progression in experimental models of type 1 and type 2 DN (Sugimoto et al., 1997; Coimbra et al., 2000) and also in diabetic patients (Rubio-Guerra et al., 2009). ICAM-1 is induced by factors common to both types of diabetes, such as hyperglycemia, AGEs, hyperfiltration, and oxidative stress, but it can also be increased by additional elements such as hyperlipidemia, hyperinsulinemia, and elevated levels of circulating TNF-α (Chow et al., 2006). Previous evidence from genetically deficient mice demonstrated that ICAM-1 is a critical mediator of macrophage accumulation in diabetic kidneys both in early and late stages of diabetes (Okada et al., 2003; Chow et al., 2005), while treatment with anti-ICAM-1 monoclonal Ab prevents mononuclear cell infiltration into diabetic glomeruli (Sugimoto et al., 1997). Furthermore, the reduced ICAM-1 overexpression is one of the renoprotective effecs of taurine treatment in streptozotocin-induced diabetic rats (Wang et al., 2008).

2.2.2 Chemokines: MCP-1

Monocyte chemotactic protein-1 (MCP-1) is a small cytokine belonging to the CC chemokine family that is also known as chemokine (C-C motif) ligand 2 (CCL2). MCP-1 recruits monocytes, T cells, macrophages and dendritic cells to sites of tissue injury, infection, and inflammation, and is gaining interest as a mediator of DN. MCP-1 is induced by high glucose concentrations, AGEs and cytokines in cultured renal cells (Chow et al., 2006), and its expression increases progressively in diabetic kidneys from different animal models. In diabetic patients, MCP-1 urinary levels correlate with albuminuria, therefore being considered a marker of renal function decline (Sayyed et al., 2011; Camilla et al., 2011).

MCP-1 is a potent chemokine involved in the accumulation and function of macrophages (Chow et al., 2006), thus playing a role in the inflammatory phase of DN. Renal cells like podocytes and mesangial cells are also able to produce MCP-1 in response to metabolic mediators, such as high glucose, and AGEs, and also by activation of RAAS and TGF-β (Yamagishi & Matsui, 2010). Renal cells are susceptible to paracrine and autocrine activation by MCP-1, through the interaction with CCR2, the main receptor of MCP-1 (Sayyed et al., 2011; Camilla et al., 2011). In fact, MCP-1/CCR2 system is involved in podocyte cytoskeleton reorganization and motility, and also in mesangial expression of fibronectin and type IV collagen (Lee et al., 2009; Park et al., 2008). Diabetic mice with gene deficiency in MCP-1 are protected from glomerular macrophage infiltration, renal injury, and development of albuminuria (Chow et al., 2006).

As upregulation of kidney MCP-1 is a feature of human diabetic renal injury associated with macrophage recruitment and disease progression, neutralizing MCP-1 activity should be viewed as an important therapeutic goal in the treatment of DN. Preclinical studies have demonstrated that blockade of MCP-1/CCR2 system with RO5234444, an orally active small-molecule CCR2 antagonist, reduced glomerular macrophage content, glomerulosclerosis, and albuminuria in diabetic mice, and also improved glomerular filtration rate (Sayyed et al., 2011; Camilla et al., 2011). Furthermore, the renoprotective effect of several compounds, including pioglitazone (Hu et al., 2010), clarithromycin (Tone et al., 2011), and exenatide (Wu et al., 2011) has been related to the local reduction of MCP-1 activity within the kidney. Furthermore, the indazolic derivative bindarit (AF-2838) is a potent antiinflammatory agent that inhibits chemokine synthesis, particularly MCP-1. Phase II trials in rheumatoid arthritis and lupus nephritis have shown that bindarit significantly reduced urinary MCP-1 and albumin excretion rate. A clinical trial aimed to reduce albuminuria and renal disease progression with bindarit added onto RAAS blockade therapy is ongoing in type 2 diabetic patients with micro- or macroalbuminuria (Cortinovis et al., 2008).

2.2.3 Cytokines: IL-1, IL-6, and TNF-α

There is growing support for the notion that circulating proinflammatory cytokines, such as ILs and TNF-α, are strongly associated with the risk of developing diabetic complications (Shikata & Makino, 2001). ILs comprise a large group of cytokines secreted by leukocytes and other body cells that can be classified as proinflammatory and antiinflammatory. In particular, the proinflammatory IL-1 increases the expression of chemotactic factors and adhesion molecules, enhances vascular endothelial permeability, and stimulates the proliferation of mesangial cells and matrix synthesis (Rivero et al., 2009). Renal IL-1 expression is found increased in diabetic animals and correlates with albuminuria and macrophage content (Hasegawa et al., 1991; Sassy-Prigent et al., 2000; Navarro et al., 2006). Specific blockade of IL-1 activity by the IL-1 receptor antagonist anakinra reduced the release of inflammatory cytokines and chemokines in pancreatic islet from diabetic rats, and also decreased hyperglycemia and improved insulin sensitivity (Ehses et al., 2009). In type 2 diabetic patients, anakinra improved glycemia and beta-cell secretory function and reduced markers of systemic inflammation (Larsen et al., 2007). Further studies are needed to demonstrate the biological effects of this compound on diabetic kidneys.

IL-6 is a pleiotropic cytokine secreted by renal cells in response to a diabetic milieu (Min et al., 2009; Tang et al., 2010a) that stimulates mesangial cell proliferation, affects extracellular matrix dynamics in renal cells, and enhances endothelial permeability (Navarro-Gonzalez & Mora-Fernandez, 2008; Galkina & Ley, 2006; Shikata & Makino, 2001; Chow et al., 2004). Serum IL-6 levels are significantly increased in patients with type 2 DN compared to levels observed in diabetic patients without nephropathy (Navarro-Gonzalez & Mora-Fernandez, 2008; Galkina & Ley, 2006; Dalla et al., 2005), and studies in renal biopsies revealed a significant association between the severity of diabetic glomerulopathy and the expression levels of IL-6 in glomerular cells (Suzuki et al., 1995), thus suggesting a role for IL-6 in the pathogenesis of DN. There are no direct data of treatment against elevated IL-6 levels in DN, however there are indirect evidences. In a recent study in patients with incipient and established DN, the treatment with pentoxyfylline, a methylxanthine derivate and nonselective phosphodiesterase inhibitor, caused a decrease in the urinary albumin excretion, and this renoprotective effect was attributable in part to reduced levels of IL-6 among other proinflammatory mediators (Hasegawa et al., 1991; Sassy-Prigent et al., 2000; Navarro et al., 2006).

TNF-α is a pleiotropic cytokine produced mainly by monocytes/macrophages that is involved in systemic inflammation (Sugimoto et al., 1999). TNF-α exerts cytotoxic effects on renal cells (McCarthy et al., 1998; Min et al., 2009), and it has been shown to participate in renal damage development in experimental models of renal disease including lupus nephritis, glomerulonephritis, nephropathy, hypertension, and diabetes (McCarthy et al., 1998; Elmarakby & Sullivan, 2010). A role for TNF-α in DN is supported by the finding that urinary albumin excretion significantly correlates with renal TNF-α levels and urinary TNF-α excretion in streptozotocin-induced diabetic rats (Navarro et al., 2005). TNF-α also contributes to sodium retention and renal hypertrophy, which are early characteristic signs of streptozotocin-induced DN (DiPetrillo et al., 2003). Renal TNF-α expression, particularly in the glomerulus and tubulointerestitium, is increased in streptozotocin diabetic rat kidneys, and serum TNF-α is increased in type 2 diabetic patients (Navarro et al., 2005). Therefore, TNF-α plays an important role in the incidence and progression of DN and renal TNF-α levels correlate with markers of DN.

Strategies to inhibit TNF-α have been successfully used in experimental diabetes. DiPetrillo et al. (DiPetrillo et al., 2003) reported that treatment of diabetic rats with the anti-TNF-α agent TNFR:Fc, a soluble TNF-α receptor fusion protein, reduced urinary TNF-α excretion and prevented sodium retention and renal hypertrophy. Similarly, TNF-α inhibition with infliximab, a chimeric monoclonal Ab directed against TNF-α, significantly reduced both albuminuria and urinary TNF-α in streptozotocin-induced diabetic rats (Moriwaki et al., 2007). Unfortunately, no other parameters such as structural changes or hemodynamics were studied. A recent retrospective study evaluated the effects of anti–TNF-α agents on control of type 2 diabetes in patients with rheumatoid arthritis and Crohn's disease. Anti-TNF treatment improved glucose tolerance and control, although future prospective studies are needed to solidify these results (Gupta-Ganguli et al., 2011).

3. Molecules involved in the progression of diabetic renal disease

3.1 Growth factors: TGF-β, CTGF, and VEGF

Hyperglycemia stimulates resident and non-resident renal cells to produce cytokines and growth factors that contribute to the development of renal injury. In particular, the expression of the profibrotic factor TGF-β is increased in both type 1 and type 2 diabetes (Cortinovis et al., 2008). Other growth factors are also implicated, including vascular endothelial growth factor (VEGF), connective tissue growth factor (CTGF), among others acting through several intracellular signaling pathways comprising protein kinases and transcription factors (Goh et al., 2008). Recently, specific Abs against different growth factors that might be useful for the treatment of chronic nephropathies, including DN, have been developed (Cortinovis et al., 2008).

3.1.1 TGF-β

TGF-β is a well-known profibrogenic factor which controls synthesis and degradation of extracellular matrix proteins by stimulating transcription of extracellular matrix genes in renal cells and reducing collagenase production, eventually inhibiting matrix turnover. Furthermore TGF-β is involved in tubuloglomerular sclerosis and podocyte apoptosis in diabetes. TGF-β gene and protein levels are significantly increased in glomeruli and tubulointerstitium of type 1 and 2 diabetic patients and animals (Yamagishi & Matsui, 2010; Goh et al., 2008). Factors that regulate TGF-β expression in renal cells include hyperglycemia, AGEs, endothelin, lipids and products of oxidative stress. TGF-β is also modulated by the RAAS (Goh et al., 2008). In fact, angiotensin II stimulates TGF-β and its receptors in the kidney by various mechanisms, and angiotensin converting enzyme (ACE) inhibition reduces serum and urinary levels of TGF-β (Wolf, 2006). In diabetic patients, treatment with the ACE inhibitor perindopril reduced the intrarenal TGF-β expression and activity (Langham et al., 2006). Furthermore, the antifibrotic agent N-acetyl-seryl-aspartyl-lysyl-proline, which reduced TGF-β-induced extracellular matrix production and prevented renal fibrosis and albuminuria in diabetic db/db mice, conferred an additional renoprotective effect when combined with the angiotensin II receptor antagonist losartan (Sugaru et al., 2006).

A range of novel compounds has been recently examined to inhibit TGF-β and TGF-β-dependent pathways in diabetes. Several blocking Abs against TGF-β effectively reduce mesangial matrix accumulation and glomerulosclerosis in diabetic mouse models (Ziyadeh et al., 2000; Goh et al., 2008), and particularly the TGF-AY1 Ab is in clinical development for the treatment of chronic kidney disease, with focus on DN (Cortinovis et al., 2008). In addition, the soluble human TGF-β type II receptor (sT β RII-Fc), a high-affinity TGF-β1 binding molecule, has been proposed as a potential new agent for the treatment of fibrosis and albuminuria in DN (Russo et al., 2007).

A potential therapeutic approach is the use of micro RNA (miRNA)-based strategies. The miRNAs are short noncoding nucleotides that regulate target messenger RNAs at the post-transcriptional level and are involved in many biological processes (Lorenzen et al., 2011). Recent studies have identified miRNA-mediated circuits controlling auto-upregulation of TGF-β1 and amplification of TGF-β1 signaling that accelerate chronic fibrotic kidney diseases including DN (Kato et al., 2011). In particular, miRNA-92c and miRNA-192 are induced in renal cells by high glucose and TGF-β, and mediate cell apoptosis and extracellular matrix accumulation (Kato et al., 2011; Long et al., 2011). Renal expression of these miRNAs increased in type 1 and type 2 diabetic animals, and *in vivo* knockdown prevented progression of DN. Their widespread and distinct expression patterns under normal and disease states make miRNAs attractive molecular therapeutic targets for human diseases. In fact, different miRNA modulators (such as antagomirs and locked nucleic acid antimiRs) have been developed for specific targeting of miRNAs and respective downstream gene networks (Lorenzen et al., 2011). The therapeutic potential of miRNA-based treatment in DN requires further study.

3.1.2 CTGF

Several reports have described an increased expression of CTGF in diabetic kidneys, that is therefore being considered a marker and a mediator of disease. Synthesis of CTGF is stimulated by TGF-β, hyperglycemia and AGEs, as well as CTGF itself. CTGF induces mesangial cell hypertrophy and cytoskeletal disassembling, upregulates cell production of fibronectin and collagens, and is also involved in epithelial-to-mesenchymal transition of tubular cells (Twigg, 2010; Connolly et al., 2003).

CTGF is also an important downstream mediator of the profibrotic activity of TGF-β. But in contrast to TGF-β, CTGF is not centrally involved in the modulation of inflammation or immune reactions (Goldschmeding et al., 2000) and thus this profibrotic factor may be a more attractive target for new renoprotective therapies. In fact, decreased CTGF expression in the kidney has been suggested as the mechanism involved in the inhibition of diabetic renal damage by different agents including the AGE inhibitors aminoguanidine (Twigg &

Cooper, 2004) and XLF-III-43 (Li et al., 2010), the aldosterone receptor blocker spironolactone (Han et al., 2006), and the flavonoid compound astilbin (Li et al., 2009). More specific therapies include FG-3019, a humanized monoclonal Ab that neutralizes the effects of CTGF in diabetic animals (Cortinovis et al., 2008). FG-3019 is currently under development for idiopathic pulmonary fibrosis, pancreatic cancer and diabetes. In an open-label, dose-escalation Phase Ib trial in type 1 or 2 diabetic patients with incipient nephropathy, FG-3019 effectively decreased albuminuria (Adler et al., 2010), although further validation in a prospective, randomized, blinded study is required.

3.1.3 VEGF

VEGF is a potent inducer of vasopermeability and angiogenesis that plays a major pathophysiological role in DN, despite VEGF exhibiting protective roles in non-diabetic renal disease. Serum levels of VEGF correlate with albuminuria and increase with DN stage in patients with type 1 and 2 diabetes (Hovind et al., 2000). Several experimental model studies have demonstrated that VEGF may contribute to some of the hemodynamic changes in DN, including hyperfiltration and albuminuria. Expression of VEGF and its receptors are modulated by high glucose, endothelin 1, AGEs, angiotensin II, stretch and TGF-β, and their renal expression is increased in diabetic kidneys (Chen & Ziyadeh, 2008; Cooper et al., 1999). Furthermore, VEGF is a trophic factor for glomerular endothelial cells, affects podocyte function, and is also involved in macrophage influx during early DN (Chen & Ziyadeh, 2008).

Since VEGF levels are elevated in patients and animal models of DN, a number of studies have examined the effect of inhibition of VEGF receptor binding or activation. Antagonism of VEGF using a variety of different strategies has been reported to improve the outcome in experimental nephropathies of various origins, including DN. Neutralizing VEGF Abs ameliorate early and long-term renal changes in diabetic animals (De Vriese et al., 2001; Schrijvers et al., 2006), while treatment with the pan-VEGF receptor tyrosine kinase inhibitor SU5416 ameliorates diabetic albuminuria in mice (Sung et al., 2006). Several clinical studies have evaluated the beneficial effect of these anti-VEGF agents in the treatment of diabetic retinopathy, but more studies are needed to determine the viability of such strategy in diabetic renal disease.

3.2 Oxidative stress

Oxidative stress defined as an excessive production of ROS surpassing existing antioxidative defense mechanisms plays a critical role in the pathogenesis of diabetes, and more importantly in the development of diabetic complications, including DN. Free radicals are capable of disturb physiological cell function both directly, by damaging cellular macromolecules such as DNA, proteins, and lipids, and indirectly through the stimulation of multiple pathways, such as protein kinases, polyol and hexosamine pathways and AGEs formation. In addition, low antioxidant bioavailability promotes cellular oxidative stress leading to additional cellular damage (Forbes et al., 2008; Elmarakby & Sullivan, 2010; Noh & Ha, 2011).

Overproduction of ROS in the diabetic milieu is both a direct consequence of hyperglycemia and an indirect consequence through AGEs or mediators of glucotoxicity such as cytokines and growth factors (Noh & Ha, 2011; Forbes et al., 2008). The effects of ROS in renal cells comprise mesangial cell proliferation, expression of growth factors, extracellular matrix accumulation, RAAS activation and induction of epithelial-mesenchymal transition (Noh &

Ha, 2011; Elmarakby & Sullivan, 2010). Among many pathways, nicotinamide adenosine dinucleotide phosphate (NADPH) oxidase and mitochondrial dysfunction have been recognized as two major sources of ROS generation in diabetic kidneys, and NADPH oxidase-derived ROS has been shown to facilitate renal mitochondrial superoxide production in hyperglycemia (Tojo et al., 2007).

Inhibition of ROS production and their activity has been demonstrated to be effective in preventing the development and progression of experimental diabetes. Different approaches including oral administration of resveratrol (Palsamy & Subramanian, 2011) and dietary antioxidant supplementation with N-acetylcysteine, vitamins C and E (Park et al., 2011) and curcuminoids (Sharma et al., 2006) have been shown to reduce oxidative stress and renal inflammation in diabetic animals. Clinical observations have also revealed a positive effect on oxidative stress in diabetic patients (Gupta et al., 2011). Alternative strategies based on upregulation of antioxidant proteins, such as superoxide dismutase, heme oxygenase-1, and catalase, have also been proven to diminish high glucose-induced ROS in cell cultures and animal models (Li et al., 2011). A recent study in diabetic animals reported the renoprotective effects of luteolin (Wang et al., 2011), a plant-derived flavonoid with antiinflammatory and antitumorigenic properties (Lopez-Lazaro, 2009). The improvement of renal function in luteolin treated animals was associated with changes in superoxide dismutase activity, malondialdehyde content and expression of heme oxygenase-1 expression (Wang et al., 2011). New strategies targeting NF-E2-related factor 2, the transcription factor that controls antioxidant protein expression, mitochondrial dysfunction, and NADPH oxidase might provide a potential approach for the prevention and treatment of DN (Noh & Ha, 2011). Presently, designing new antioxidant therapies focus on effective, cell compartment-specific agents that would improve renoprotection in combination with current therapies (Forbes et al., 2008). Reports on their efficacy in clinical trials for inflammatory-associated pathologies, including diabetes, have yet to be published.

4. Intracellular pathways activated in diabetic kidney

Intense investigation revealed that numerous inflammatory signaling pathways such as phospholipases, protein kinase cascades and transcription factors, are implicated in the pathogenesis of DN, from early phase to the progression and final complications. Among them, nuclear factor-κB (NF-κB) and janus kinase/signal transducers and activators of transcription (JAK/STAT) have a relevant role in the control of immunoinflammatory responses in the diabetic kidney. Mechanisms of action and therapeutic opportunities are discussed.

4.1 NF-κB

The transcription factor NF-κB is induced by various cell stress-associated stimuli including growth factors, vasoactive agents, cytokines, and oxidative stress. NF-κB in turn controls the regulation of numerous genes activated during inflammation, such as cytokines, chemokines, growth factors, cellular ligands, and adhesion molecules (Karin & Greten, 2005). The activation and nuclear translocation of NF-κB has been demonstrated in diabetic kidneys from human and rodents (Mezzano et al., 2004; Liu et al., 2010), and also in proximal tubular cells in the urinary sediment of patients with type 2 diabetes (Brosius et al., 2010). Furthermore, a study integrating gene-expression profiling in human renal biopsies with promoter modeling has identified the specific set of target genes, especially chemokines, containing a specific NF-κB promoter module (NFKB_IRFF_01) with a NF-κB binding site, that were activated in progressive DN (Schmid et al., 2006). These findings emphasize the NF-κB proinflammatory pathway as potentially a major upstream target for developing new renoprotective agents in diabetes. There is a raising number of reported inhibitors of NF-κB pathway with potential benefits for future therapies in humans. Inhibitors can be divided into basic categories according to the step at which NF-κB is blocked: 1) upstream of IκB kinase complex; 2) IκB phosphorylation/degradation; 3) nuclear translocation; 4) DNA binding; and 5) gene transactivation (Gomez-Guerrero et al., 2011). Some of these compounds are in clinical development against various inflammatory diseases, but studies in diabetic patients are scarce.

It has been suggested that the preventive effects of thiazolidinedione, a ligand for peroxisome proliferator-activated receptor-γ, are mediated by its antiinflammatory actions, including inhibition of NF-κB. Thiazolidinedione caused a reduction in intranuclear NF-κB binding activity in type 2 diabetic patients with obesity (Aljada et al., 2001), and ameliorated renal injury in experimental diabetic rats through NF-κB inhibition (Ohga et al., 2007). Other studies demonstrated that 1,25-dihydroxyvitamin D3 suppresses hyperglycemia-induced gene expression by blocking NF-κB activation in mesangial cells (Zhang et al., 2007). Statins and fenofibrate also exhibit a downregulating effect on NF-κB pathway in kidneys from diabetic rats (Usui et al., 2003; Chen et al., 2008). In the same way, a recent report demonstrates that the ameliorative effects of the plant alkaloid berberine on renal dysfunction in diabetic rats is associated with its inhibitory function on NF-κB signal pathway in the kidney (Liu et al., 2010).

NF-κB is modulated by upstream enzymes like poly(ADP-ribose) polymerase (PARP). Increased PARP activity has been shown to participate in the pathogenesis of diabetic complications. Pharmacological inhibition of PARP by two different inhibitors (PJ-34 and INO-1001) decreased kidney hypertrophy in type 1 diabetic mice (Drel et al., 2011) and this effect was associated with a decrease in NF-κB p50 nuclear translocation (Goh et al., 2008). This provides rationale reasons for development and further studies of PARP inhibitors as promising approaches to DN. In fact, PARP inhibitors are currently being tested in clinical trials for cancer.

4.2 JAK/STAT

The Janus kinase/signal transducers and activators of transcription (JAK/STAT) pathway is an essential intracellular mechanism of cytokines and other stimuli that regulates gene expression and cellular activation, proliferation, and differentiation. Members of the JAK/STAT pathway have been claimed as new molecular targets of antiinflammatory treatment in acute and chronic inflammatory diseases (de Prati et al., 2005; Marrero et al., 2006), and their activation is involved in the development of the diabetes complications. A recent report using a transcriptomic approach documented enhanced expression of a large number of JAK/STAT mRNAs and JAK2 protein in glomerular and tubulointerstitial regions from patients with both early and progressive DN (Berthier et al., 2009).

JAK/STAT pathway, especially the JAK2/STAT1/STAT3-dependent axis, contributes to high glucose mediated renal cell responses, including enhanced expression of genes involved in leukocyte infiltration, cell growth, and fibrosis (Brosius et al., 2010; Brosius, III,

2008; Amiri et al., 2002; de Prati et al., 2005; Lu et al., 2009). JAK/STAT also mediates the mitogenic and fibrotic actions of cytokines and angiotensin II in the kidney (Marrero et al., 2006), suggesting that modulation of this pathway may prevent diabetic renal disease. Importantly, studies in experimental models of diabetes suggest that the renal protective effects of current drugs like captopril, statins and rosiglitazone (Banes et al., 2004; Shi et al., 2007; Tang et al., 2010b) could be partially attributed to a modulation in JAK/STAT phosphorylation. More selective therapies, such as inhibitors of JAK2 and JAK3, and STAT1 antisense oligonucleotides have been proven to counteract the harmful effects of JAK/STAT activation in cultured renal cells and in experimental models of DN (Wang et al., 2002; Shi et al., 2007; de Prati et al., 2005).

The JAK/STAT pathway is controlled through different mechanisms: 1) receptor internalization; 2) protein tyrosine phosphatases; 3) protein inhibitors of activated STAT; and 4) suppressors of cytokine signaling (SOCS). In particular, SOCS family of intracellular proteins has emerged as a potential target to modulate the magnitude and duration of JAK/STAT signaling (Yoshimura et al., 2007). SOCS are induced by many pathologic stimuli (*e.g.*, cytokines, angiotensin II, chemokines, insulin, immunoglobulins, and lipoproteins) thus indicating their involvement in many biologic processes (Ortiz-Munoz et al., 2009; Yoshimura et al., 2007; Hernandez-Vargas et al., 2005; Gomez-Guerrero et al., 2004). Our group has recently reported an increased expression of SOCS proteins in renal samples from patients with progressive DN and diabetic animals (Ortiz-Munoz et al., 2010). *In vitro*, SOCS induction prevented the expression of STAT-dependent genes including adhesion molecules, chemokines, and cytokines. *In vivo* gene therapy with SOCS-expressing adenovirus reduced JAK/STAT activation and ameliorated the early renal changes in diabetic rats. Further research into inducers of SOCS expression or SOCS mimetics could have therapeutic value to prevent or retard the progression of diabetic complications.

5. Conclusion

The current knowledge of the cellular and molecular processes involved in the initiation and progression of diabetic renal injury continues to expand (Figure 1). Inflammation is now recognized as an important player in the pathogenesis of DN, and a number of studies have been designed to address whether blockade or modulation of specific inflammatory molecules can be beneficial for this disease. Furthermore, the increased understanding of the functionality of signal transduction pathways will lead to identification of therapeutic targets able to specifically downregulate proinflammatory responses and mediators, potentially even harnessing some of the sophisticated regulatory systems designed to normally limit the inflammatory response. Nevertheless, because of multiple molecular links between inflammation, immune response and diabetes complications, it seems unlikely that suppressing one single specific effector molecule could be sufficient to produce clinically relevant benefit. Effective treatment and/or prevention of diabetic renal disease will therefore require an integrated approach combining multiple strategies to target the underlying inflammatory processes. In addition, as diabetes complications require chronic treatment, long-term antiinflammatory therapies could potentially have other side effects despite improving renal function. Future research will provide answers to these uncertainties regarding multiple and long-term interventional therapies based on modulation of immunoinflammatory responses. In fact, progress towards therapeutics designed to target specific cytokines, chemokines, growth factors and even transcription factors is already well underway. Besides the assessment of pharmacological safety, bioavailability, and efficacy *in vivo*, more clinical studies will further support the potential of such strategies to be used in diabetes therapy.

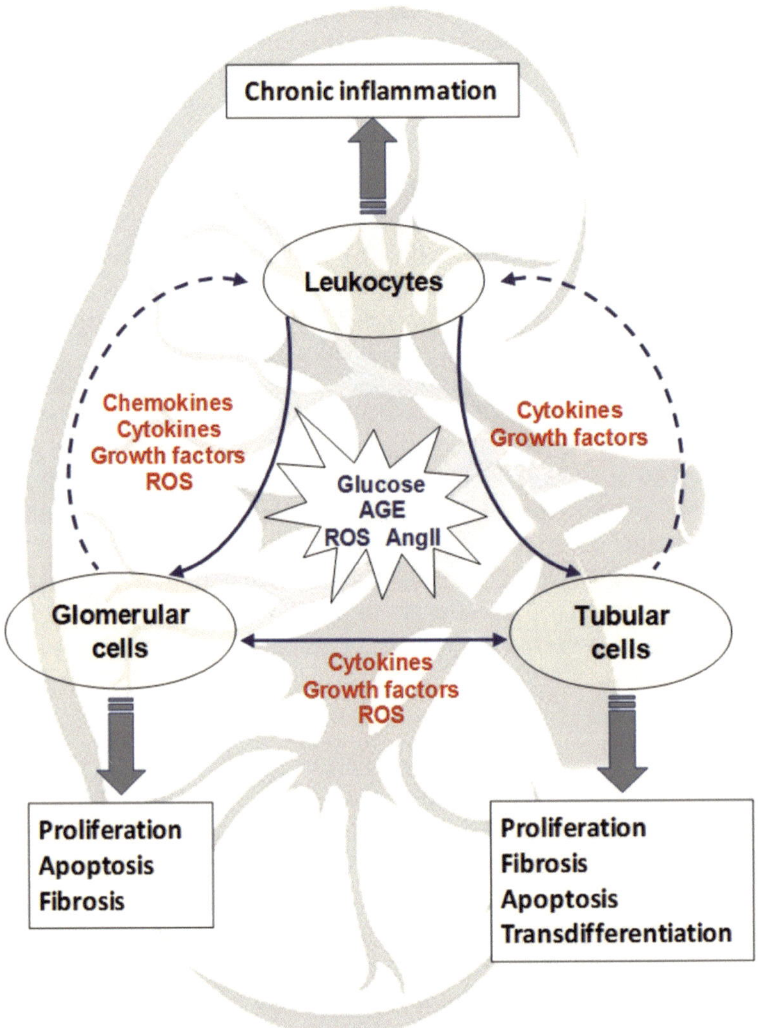

Fig. 1. Immunoinflammatory mechanisms in DN. Elements of the diabetic milieu (high glucose, AGEs, angiotensin, and oxidative stress) induce the expression of chemokines and adhesion molecules by renal cells, which favours leukocyte infiltration into the kidney. Further exposure of kidney macrophages and resident cells to diabetic milieu promotes cell activation, with the subsequent release of proinflammatory cytokines (e.g. IL-1, IL-6, TNF-α), ROS, and profibrotic growth factors (e.g. TGF-β). The initial inflammatory response is self-amplified then causing renal injury and cell death. Furthermore, the fibrotic response induces proliferation and extracellular matrix accumulation in mesangial and tubular cells. Diabetic renal injury then progresses to glomerulosclerosis and tubulointerstitial fibrosis.

6. Acknowledgment

The authors have been granted by Ministry of Science (SAF2007/63648 and SAF2009/11794), Ministry of Health (Instituto de Salud Carlos III, Red RECAVA RD06/0014/0035), Ramon Areces Foundation, and Comunidad de Madrid (S2006/GEN-0247).

7. References

Adler SG, Schwartz S, Williams ME, Arauz-Pacheco C, Bolton WK, Lee T, Li D, Neff TB, Urquilla PR, & Sewell KL. (2010). Phase 1 study of anti-CTGF monoclonal antibody in patients with diabetes and microalbuminuria. *Clin. J. Am. Soc. Nephrol.*, Vol.5, No.8, pp.1420-1428

Aki K, Shimizu A, Masuda Y, Kuwahara N, Arai T, Ishikawa A, Fujita E, Mii A, Natori Y, Fukunaga Y, & Fukuda Y. (2010). ANG II receptor blockade enhances anti-inflammatory macrophages in anti-glomerular basement membrane glomerulonephritis. *Am. J. Physiol Renal Physiol,* Vol.298, No.4, pp.F870-F882

Aljada A, Garg R, Ghanim H, Mohanty P, Hamouda W, Assian E, & Dandona P. (2001). Nuclear factor-kappaB suppressive and inhibitor-kappaB stimulatory effects of troglitazone in obese patients with type 2 diabetes: evidence of an antiinflammatory action? *J. Clin. Endocrinol. Metab,* Vol.86, No.7, pp.3250-3256

Amiri F, Shaw S, Wang X, Tang J, Waller JL, Eaton DC, & Marrero MB. (2002). Angiotensin II activation of the JAK/STAT pathway in mesangial cells is altered by high glucose. *Kidney Int.,* Vol.61, No.5, pp.1605-1616

Atchley DH, Lopes-Virella MF, Zheng D, Kenny D, & Virella G. (2002). Oxidized LDL-anti-oxidized LDL immune complexes and diabetic nephropathy. *Diabetologia,* Vol.45, No.11, pp.1562-1571

Balakumar P, Arora MK, Reddy J, & Anand-Srivastava MB. (2009). Pathophysiology of diabetic nephropathy: involvement of multifaceted signalling mechanism. *J. Cardiovasc. Pharmacol.,* Vol.54, No.2, pp.129-138

Banes AK, Shaw S, Jenkins J, Redd H, Amiri F, Pollock DM, & Marrero MB. (2004). Angiotensin II blockade prevents hyperglycemia-induced activation of JAK and STAT proteins in diabetic rat kidney glomeruli. *Am. J. Physiol Renal Physiol,* Vol.286, No.4, pp.F653-F659

Berthier CC, Zhang H, Schin M, Henger A, Nelson RG, Yee B, Boucherot A, Neusser MA, Cohen CD, Carter-Su C, Argetsinger LS, Rastaldi MP, Brosius FC, & Kretzler M. (2009). Enhanced expression of Janus kinase-signal transducer and activator of transcription pathway members in human diabetic nephropathy. *Diabetes,* Vol.58, No.2, pp.469-477

Brosius FC, III. (2008). New insights into the mechanisms of fibrosis and sclerosis in diabetic nephropathy. *Rev. Endocr. Metab Disord.,* Vol.9, No.4, pp.245-254

Brosius FC, Khoury CC, Buller CL, & Chen S. (2010). Abnormalities in signaling pathways in diabetic nephropathy. *Expert. Rev. Endocrinol. Metab,* Vol.5, No.1, pp.51-64

Camilla R, Brachemi S, Pichette V, Cartier P, Laforest-Renald A, MacRae T, Madore F, & Troyanov S. (2011). Urinary monocyte chemotactic protein 1: marker of renal function decline in diabetic and nondiabetic proteinuric renal disease. *J. Nephrol.,* Vol.24, No.1, pp.60-67

Chen L, Zhang J, Zhang Y, Wang Y, & Wang B. (2008). Improvement of inflammatory responses associated with NF-kappa B pathway in kidneys from diabetic rats. *Inflamm. Res.*, Vol.57, No.5, pp.199-204

Chen S & Ziyadeh FN. (2008). Vascular endothelial growth factor and diabetic nephropathy. *Curr. Diab. Rep.*, Vol.8, No.6, pp.470-476

Chow F, Ozols E, Nikolic-Paterson DJ, Atkins RC, & Tesch GH. (2004). Macrophages in mouse type 2 diabetic nephropathy: correlation with diabetic state and progressive renal injury. *Kidney Int.*, Vol.65, No.1, pp.116-128

Chow FY, Nikolic-Paterson DJ, Ozols E, Atkins RC, Rollin BJ, & Tesch GH. (2006). Monocyte chemoattractant protein-1 promotes the development of diabetic renal injury in streptozotocin-treated mice. *Kidney Int.*, Vol.69, No.1, pp.73-80

Chow FY, Nikolic-Paterson DJ, Ozols E, Atkins RC, & Tesch GH. (2005). Intercellular adhesion molecule-1 deficiency is protective against nephropathy in type 2 diabetic db/db mice. *J. Am. Soc. Nephrol.*, Vol.16, No.6, pp.1711-1722

Coimbra TM, Janssen U, Grone HJ, Ostendorf T, Kunter U, Schmidt H, Brabant G, & Floege J. (2000). Early events leading to renal injury in obese Zucker (fatty) rats with type II diabetes. *Kidney Int.*, Vol.57, No.1, pp.167-182

Connolly SB, Sadlier D, Kieran NE, Doran P, & Brady HR. (2003). Transcriptome profiling and the pathogenesis of diabetic complications. *J. Am. Soc. Nephrol.*, Vol.14, No.8 Suppl 3, pp.S279-S283

Cooper ME, Vranes D, Youssef S, Stacker SA, Cox AJ, Rizkalla B, Casley DJ, Bach LA, Kelly DJ, & Gilbert RE. (1999). Increased renal expression of vascular endothelial growth factor (VEGF) and its receptor VEGFR-2 in experimental diabetes. *Diabetes*, Vol.48, No.11, pp.2229-2239

Cortinovis M, Cattaneo D, Perico N, & Remuzzi G. (2008). Investigational drugs for diabetic nephropathy. *Expert. Opin. Investig. Drugs*, Vol.17, No.10, pp.1487-1500

Dalla VM, Mussap M, Gallina P, Bruseghin M, Cernigoi AM, Saller A, Plebani M, & Fioretto P. (2005). Acute-phase markers of inflammation and glomerular structure in patients with type 2 diabetes. *J. Am. Soc. Nephrol.*, Vol.16 Suppl 1, No., pp.S78-S82

de Boer IH, Rue TC, Hall YN, Heagerty PJ, Weiss NS, & Himmelfarb J. (2011). Temporal trends in the prevalence of diabetic kidney disease in the United States. *JAMA.*, Jun 22;Vol.305, No.24, pp.2532-2539

de Prati AC, Ciampa AR, Cavalieri E, Zaffini R, Darra E, Menegazzi M, Suzuki H, & Mariotto S. (2005). STAT1 as a new molecular target of anti-inflammatory treatment. *Curr. Med. Chem.*, Vol.12, No.16, pp.1819-1828

De Vriese AS, Tilton RG, Elger M, Stephan CC, Kriz W, & Lameire NH. (2001). Antibodies against vascular endothelial growth factor improve early renal dysfunction in experimental diabetes. *J. Am. Soc. Nephrol.*, Vol.12, No.5, pp.993-1000

DiPetrillo K, Coutermarsh B, & Gesek FA. (2003). Urinary tumor necrosis factor contributes to sodium retention and renal hypertrophy during diabetes. *Am. J. Physiol Renal Physiol*, Vol.284, No.1, pp.F113-F121

Drel VR, Pacher P, Stavniichuk R, Xu W, Zhang J, Kuchmerovska TM, Slusher B, & Obrosova IG. (2011). Poly(ADP-ribose)polymerase inhibition counteracts renal hypertrophy and multiple manifestations of peripheral neuropathy in diabetic Akita mice. *Int. J. Mol. Med.*, Vol.28, No.4, pp.629-635

Ehses JA, Lacraz G, Giroix MH, Schmidlin F, Coulaud J, Kassis N, Irminger JC, Kergoat M, Portha B, Homo-Delarche F, & Donath MY. (2009). IL-1 antagonism reduces hyperglycemia and tissue inflammation in the type 2 diabetic GK rat. *Proc. Natl. Acad. Sci. U. S. A*, Vol.106, No.33, pp.13998-14003

Elmarakby AA & Sullivan JC. (2010). Relationship between Oxidative Stress and Inflammatory Cytokines in Diabetic Nephropathy. *Cardiovasc. Ther.*,

Forbes JM, Coughlan MT, & Cooper ME. (2008). Oxidative stress as a major culprit in kidney disease in diabetes. *Diabetes*, Vol.57, No.6, pp.1446-1454

Fujita E, Shimizu A, Masuda Y, Kuwahara N, Arai T, Nagasaka S, Aki K, Mii A, Natori Y, Iino Y, Katayama Y, & Fukuda Y. (2010). Statin attenuates experimental anti-glomerular basement membrane glomerulonephritis together with the augmentation of alternatively activated macrophages. *Am. J. Pathol.*, Vol.177, No.3, pp.1143-1154

Galkina E & Ley K. (2006). Leukocyte recruitment and vascular injury in diabetic nephropathy. *J. Am. Soc. Nephrol.*, Vol.17, No.2, pp.368-377

Goh SY, Jasik M, & Cooper ME. (2008). Agents in development for the treatment of diabetic nephropathy. *Expert. Opin. Emerg. Drugs*, Vol.13, No.3, pp.447-463

Goldschmeding R, Aten J, Ito Y, Blom I, Rabelink T, & Weening JJ. (2000). Connective tissue growth factor: just another factor in renal fibrosis? *Nephrol. Dial. Transplant.*, Vol.15, No.3, pp.296-299

Gomez-Guerrero C, Lopez-Franco O, Sanjuan G, Hernandez-Vargas P, Suzuki Y, Ortiz-Munoz G, Blanco J, & Egido J. (2004). Suppressors of cytokine signaling regulate Fc receptor signaling and cell activation during immune renal injury. *J. Immunol.*, Vol.172, No.11, pp.6969-6977

Gomez-Guerrero C, Mallavia B, & Egido J. (2011). Targeting Inflammation in Cardiovascular Diseases. Still a Neglected field? *Cardiovasc. Ther.*,

Gordon S. (2003). Alternative activation of macrophages. *Nat. Rev. Immunol.*, Vol.3, pp.23-35

Gupta S, Sharma TK, Kaushik GG, & Shekhawat VP. (2011). Vitamin E supplementation may ameliorate oxidative stress in type 1 diabetes mellitus patients. *Clin. Lab*, Vol.57, No.5-6, pp.379-386

Gupta-Ganguli M, Cox K, Means B, Gerling I, & Solomon SS. (2011). Does therapy with anti-TNF-alpha improve glucose tolerance and control in patients with type 2 diabetes? *Diabetes Care*, Vol.34, No.7, pp.e121

Han KH, Kang YS, Han SY, Jee YH, Lee MH, Han JY, Kim HK, Kim YS, & Cha DR. (2006). Spironolactone ameliorates renal injury and connective tissue growth factor expression in type II diabetic rats. *Kidney Int.*, Vol.70, No.1, pp.111-120

Hasegawa G, Nakano K, Sawada M, Uno K, Shibayama Y, Ienaga K, & Kondo M. (1991). Possible role of tumor necrosis factor and interleukin-1 in the development of diabetic nephropathy. *Kidney Int.*, Vol.40, No.6, pp.1007-1012

Hernandez-Vargas P, Lopez-Franco O, Sanjuan G, Ruperez M, Ortiz-Munoz G, Suzuki Y, Aguado-Roncero P, Perez-Tejerizo G, Blanco J, Egido J, Ruiz-Ortega M, & Gomez-Guerrero C. (2005). Suppressors of cytokine signaling regulate angiotensin II-activated Janus kinase-signal transducers and activators of transcription pathway in renal cells. *J. Am. Soc. Nephrol.*, Vol.16, No.6, pp.1673-1683

Hogg N & Berlin C. (1995). Structure and function of adhesion receptors in leukocyte trafficking. *Immunol. Today*, Vol.16, No.7, pp.327-330

Hovind P, Tarnow L, Oestergaard PB, & Parving HH. (2000). Elevated vascular endothelial growth factor in type 1 diabetic patients with diabetic nephropathy. *Kidney Int. Suppl*, Vol.75, No., pp.S56-S61

Hu YY, Ye SD, Zhao LL, Zheng M, Wu FZ, & Chen Y. (2010). Hydrochloride pioglitazone decreases urinary cytokines excretion in type 2 diabetes. *Clin. Endocrinol. (Oxf),* Vol.73, No.6, pp.739-743

Ichinose K, Kawasaki E, & Eguchi K. (2007). Recent advancement of understanding pathogenesis of type 1 diabetes and potential relevance to diabetic nephropathy. *Am. J. Nephrol.,* Vol.27, No.6, pp.554-564

Karin M & Greten FR. (2005). NF-kappaB: linking inflammation and immunity to cancer development and progression. *Nat. Rev. Immunol.,* Vol.5, No.10, pp.749-759

Kato M, Arce L, Wang M, Putta S, Lanting L, & Natarajan R. (2011). A microRNA circuit mediates transforming growth factor-beta1 autoregulation in renal glomerular mesangial cells. *Kidney Int.,* Vol.80, No.4, pp.358-368

Langham RG, Kelly DJ, Gow RM, Zhang Y, Cordonnier DJ, Pinel N, Zaoui P, & Gilbert RE. (2006). Transforming growth factor-beta in human diabetic nephropathy: effects of ACE inhibition. *Diabetes Care,* Vol.29, No.12, pp.2670-2675

Larsen CM, Faulenbach M, Vaag A, Volund A, Ehses JA, Seifert B, Mandrup-Poulsen T, & Donath MY. (2007). Interleukin-1-receptor antagonist in type 2 diabetes mellitus. *N. Engl. J. Med.,* Vol.356, No.15, pp.1517-1526

Lee EY, Chung CH, Khoury CC, Yeo TK, Pyagay PE, Wang A, & Chen S. (2009). The monocyte chemoattractant protein-1/CCR2 loop, inducible by TGF-beta, increases podocyte motility and albumin permeability. *Am. J. Physiol Renal Physiol,* Vol.297, No.1, pp.F85-F94

Li GS, Jiang WL, Yue XD, Qu GW, Tian JW, Wu J, & Fu FH. (2009). Effect of astilbin on experimental diabetic nephropathy in vivo and in vitro. *Planta Med.,* Vol.75, No.14, pp.1470-1475

Li H, Wang F, Zhang L, Cao Y, Liu W, Hao J, Liu Q, & Duan H. (2011). Modulation of Nrf2 expression alters high glucose-induced oxidative stress and antioxidant gene expression in mouse mesangial cells. *Cell Signal.,* Vol.23, No.10, pp.1625-1632

Li H, Zheng X, Wang H, Zhang Y, Xin H, & Chen X. (2010). XLF-III-43, a novel coumarin-aspirin compound, prevents diabetic nephropathy in rats via inhibiting advanced glycation end products. *Eur. J. Pharmacol.,* Vol.627, No.1-3, pp.340-347

Lim AK, Ma FY, Nikolic-Paterson DJ, Kitching AR, Thomas MC, & Tesch GH. (2010). Lymphocytes promote albuminuria, but not renal dysfunction or histological damage in a mouse model of diabetic renal injury. *Diabetologia,* Vol.53, No.8, pp.1772-1782

Liu W, Zhang X, Liu P, Shen X, Lan T, Li W, Jiang Q, Xie X, & Huang H. (2010). Effects of berberine on matrix accumulation and NF-kappa B signal pathway in alloxan-induced diabetic mice with renal injury. *Eur. J. Pharmacol.,* Vol.638, No.1-3, pp.150-155

Long J, Wang Y, Wang W, Chang BH, & Danesh FR. (2011). MicroRNA-29c is a signature microRNA under high glucose conditions that targets Sprouty homolog 1, and its in vivo knockdown prevents progression of diabetic nephropathy. *J. Biol. Chem.,* Vol.286, No.13, pp.11837-11848

Lopez-Lazaro M. (2009). Distribution and biological activities of the flavonoid luteolin. *Mini. Rev. Med. Chem.,* Vol.9, No.1, pp.31-59

Lorenzen JM, Haller H, & Thum T. (2011). MicroRNAs as mediators and therapeutic targets in chronic kidney disease. *Nat. Rev. Nephrol.,* Vol.7, No.5, pp.286-294

Lu TC, Wang ZH, Feng X, Chuang PY, Fang W, Shen Y, Levy DE, Xiong H, Chen N, & He JC. (2009). Knockdown of Stat3 activity in vivo prevents diabetic glomerulopathy. *Kidney Int.,* Vol.76, No.1, pp.63-71

Mantovani A, Sica A, Sozzani S, Allavena P, Vecchi A, & Locati M. (2004). The chemokine system in diverse forms of macrophage activation and polarization. *Trends Immunol.*, Vol.25, No.12, pp.677-686

Marrero MB, Banes-Berceli AK, Stern DM, & Eaton DC. (2006). Role of the JAK/STAT signaling pathway in diabetic nephropathy. *Am. J. Physiol Renal Physiol,* Vol.290, No.4, pp.F762-F768

Martinez FO, Sica A, Mantovani A, & Locati M. (2008). Macrophage activation and polarization. *Front Biosci.*, Vol.13, No., pp.453-461

McCarthy ET, Sharma R, Sharma M, Li JZ, Ge XL, Dileepan KN, & Savin VJ. (1998). TNF-alpha increases albumin permeability of isolated rat glomeruli through the generation of superoxide. *J. Am. Soc. Nephrol.*, Vol.9, No.3, pp.433-438

Mehta DS, Christmas RA, Waldmann H, & Rosenzweig M. (2010). Partial and transient modulation of the CD3-T-cell receptor complex, elicited by low-dose regimens of monoclonal anti-CD3, is sufficient to induce disease remission in non-obese diabetic mice. *Immunology,* Vol.130, No.1, pp.103-113

Mezzano S, Aros C, Droguett A, Burgos ME, Ardiles L, Flores C, Schneider H, Ruiz-Ortega M, & Egido J. (2004). NF-kappaB activation and overexpression of regulated genes in human diabetic nephropathy. *Nephrol. Dial. Transplant.*, Vol.19, No.10, pp.2505-2512

Miller SA & St OE. (2011). Otelixizumab: a novel agent for the prevention of type 1 diabetes mellitus. *Expert. Opin. Biol. Ther.,*

Min D, Lyons JG, Bonner J, Twigg SM, Yue DK, & MCLennan SV. (2009). Mesangial cell-derived factors alter monocyte activation and function through inflammatory pathways: possible pathogenic role in diabetic nephropathy. *Am. J. Physiol Renal Physiol,* Vol.297, No.5, pp.F1229-F1237

Moriwaki Y, Inokuchi T, Yamamoto A, Ka T, Tsutsumi Z, Takahashi S, & Yamamoto T. (2007). Effect of TNF-alpha inhibition on urinary albumin excretion in experimental diabetic rats. *Acta Diabetol.*, Vol.44, No.4, pp.215-218

Moriya R, Manivel JC, & Mauer M. (2004). Juxtaglomerular apparatus T-cell infiltration affects glomerular structure in Type 1 diabetic patients. *Diabetologia,* Vol.47, No.1, pp.82-88

Navarro JF, Milena FJ, Mora C, Leon C, Claverie F, Flores C, & Garcia J. (2005). Tumor necrosis factor-alpha gene expression in diabetic nephropathy: relationship with urinary albumin excretion and effect of angiotensin-converting enzyme inhibition. *Kidney Int. Suppl,*99, pp.S98-102

Navarro JF, Milena FJ, Mora C, Leon C, & Garcia J. (2006). Renal pro-inflammatory cytokine gene expression in diabetic nephropathy: effect of angiotensin-converting enzyme inhibition and pentoxifylline administration. *Am. J. Nephrol.*, Vol.26, No.6, pp.562-570

Navarro-Gonzalez JF & Mora-Fernandez C. (2008). The role of inflammatory cytokines in diabetic nephropathy. *J. Am. Soc. Nephrol.*, Vol.19, No.3, pp.433-442

Noh H & Ha H. (2011). Reactive oxygen species and oxidative stress. *Contrib. Nephrol.*, Vol.170, No., pp.102-112

Ohga S, Shikata K, Yozai K, Okada S, Ogawa D, Usui H, Wada J, Shikata Y, & Makino H. (2007). Thiazolidinedione ameliorates renal injury in experimental diabetic rats through anti-inflammatory effects mediated by inhibition of NF-kappaB activation. *Am. J. Physiol Renal Physiol,* Vol.292, No.4, pp.F1141-F1150

Okada S, Shikata K, Matsuda M, Ogawa D, Usui H, Kido Y, Nagase R, Wada J, Shikata Y, & Makino H. (2003). Intercellular adhesion molecule-1-deficient mice are resistant against renal injury after induction of diabetes. *Diabetes,* Vol.52, No.10, pp.2586-2593

Ortiz-Munoz G, Lopez-Parra V, Lopez-Franco O, Fernandez-Vizarra P, Mallavia B, Flores C, Sanz A, Blanco J, Mezzano S, Ortiz A, Egido J, & Gomez-Guerrero C. (2010). Suppressors of cytokine signaling abrogate diabetic nephropathy. *J. Am. Soc. Nephrol.*, Vol.21, No.5, pp.763-772

Ortiz-Munoz G, Martin-Ventura JL, Hernandez-Vargas P, Mallavia B, Lopez-Parra V, Lopez-Franco O, Munoz-Garcia B, Fernandez-Vizarra P, Ortega L, Egido J, & Gomez-Guerrero C. (2009). Suppressors of cytokine signaling modulate JAK/STAT-mediated cell responses during atherosclerosis. *Arterioscler. Thromb. Vasc. Biol.*, Vol.29, No.4, pp.525-531

Palsamy P & Subramanian S. (2011). Resveratrol protects diabetic kidney by attenuating hyperglycemia-mediated oxidative stress and renal inflammatory cytokines via Nrf2-Keap1 signaling. *Biochim. Biophys. Acta,* Vol.1812, No.7, pp.719-731

Park J, Ryu DR, Li JJ, Jung DS, Kwak SJ, Lee SH, Yoo TH, Han SH, Lee JE, Kim DK, Moon SJ, Kim K, Han DS, & Kang SW. (2008). MCP-1/CCR2 system is involved in high glucose-induced fibronectin and type IV collagen expression in cultured mesangial cells. *Am. J. Physiol Renal Physiol,* Vol.295, No.3, pp.F749-F757

Park NY, Park SK, & Lim Y. (2011). Long-term dietary antioxidant cocktail supplementation effectively reduces renal inflammation in diabetic mice. *Br. J. Nutr.*, pp.1-8

Reutens AT, & Atkins RC. (2011). Epidemiology of diabetic nephropathy. *Contrib Nephrol.*, Vol.170, pp.1-7

Ricardo SD, van GH, & Eddy AA. (2008). Macrophage diversity in renal injury and repair. *J. Clin. Invest,* Vol.118, No.11, pp.3522-3530

Ritz E, Zeng XX, & Rychlík I. (2011). Clinical manifestation and natural history of diabetic nephropathy. *Contrib Nephrol,* Vol.170, pp.19-27

Rivero A, Mora C, Muros M, Garcia J, Herrera H, & Navarro-Gonzalez JF. (2009). Pathogenic perspectives for the role of inflammation in diabetic nephropathy. *Clin. Sci. (Lond),* Vol.116, No.6, pp.479-492

Rubio-Guerra AF, Vargas-Robles H, Lozano Nuevo JJ, & Escalante-Acosta BA. (2009). Correlation between circulating adhesion molecule levels and albuminuria in type-2 diabetic hypertensive patients. *Kidney Blood Press Res.*, Vol.32, No.2, pp.106-109

Russo LM, del RE, Brown D, & Lin HY. (2007). Evidence for a role of transforming growth factor (TGF)-beta1 in the induction of postglomerular albuminuria in diabetic nephropathy: amelioration by soluble TGF-beta type II receptor. *Diabetes,* Vol.56, No.2, pp.380-388

Sassy-Prigent C, Heudes D, Mandet C, Belair MF, Michel O, Perdereau B, Bariety J, & Bruneval P. (2000). Early glomerular macrophage recruitment in streptozotocin-induced diabetic rats. *Diabetes,* Vol.49, No.3, pp.466-475

Sayyed SG, Ryu M, Kulkarni OP, Schmid H, Lichtnekert J, Gruner S, Green L, Mattei P, Hartmann G, & Anders HJ. (2011). An orally active chemokine receptor CCR2 antagonist prevents glomerulosclerosis and renal failure in type 2 diabetes. *Kidney Int.*, Vol.80, No.1, pp.68-78

Schmid H, Boucherot A, Yasuda Y, Henger A, Brunner B, Eichinger F, Nitsche A, Kiss E, Bleich M, Grone HJ, Nelson PJ, Schlondorff D, Cohen CD, & Kretzler M. (2006). Modular activation of nuclear factor-kappaB transcriptional programs in human diabetic nephropathy. *Diabetes,* Vol.55, No.11, pp.2993-3003

Schrijvers BF, De Vriese AS, & Flyvbjerg A. (2004). From hyperglycemia to diabetic kidney disease: the role of metabolic, hemodynamic, intracellular factors and growth factors/cytokines. *Endocr. Rev.*, Vol.25, No.6, pp.971-1010

Schrijvers BF, Flyvbjerg A, Tilton RG, Lameire NH, & De Vriese AS. (2006). A neutralizing VEGF antibody prevents glomerular hypertrophy in a model of obese type 2 diabetes, the Zucker diabetic fatty rat. *Nephrol. Dial. Transplant.*, Vol.21, No.2, pp.324-329

Sharma S, Kulkarni SK, & Chopra K. (2006). Curcumin, the active principle of turmeric (Curcuma longa), ameliorates diabetic nephropathy in rats. *Clin. Exp. Pharmacol. Physiol*, Vol.33, No.10, pp.940-945

Shi YH, Zhao S, Wang C, Li Y, & Duan HJ. (2007). Fluvastatin inhibits activation of JAK and STAT proteins in diabetic rat glomeruli and mesangial cells under high glucose conditions. *Acta Pharmacol. Sin.*, Vol.28, No.12, pp.1938-1946

Shikata K & Makino H. (2001). Role of macrophages in the pathogenesis of diabetic nephropathy. *Contrib. Nephrol.*,134, pp.46-54

Staunton DE, Marlin SD, Stratowa C, Dustin ML, & Springer TA. (1988). Primary structure of ICAM-1 demonstrates interaction between members of the immunoglobulin and integrin supergene families. *Cell*, Vol.52, No.6, pp.925-933

Sugaru E, Nakagawa T, Ono-Kishino M, Nagamine J, Tokunaga T, Kitoh M, Hume WE, Nagata R, & Taiji M. (2006). Enhanced effect of combined treatment with SMP-534 (antifibrotic agent) and losartan in diabetic nephropathy. *Am. J. Nephrol.*, Vol.26, No.1, pp.50-58

Sugimoto H, Shikata K, Hirata K, Akiyama K, Matsuda M, Kushiro M, Shikata Y, Miyatake N, Miyasaka M, & Makino H. (1997). Increased expression of intercellular adhesion molecule-1 (ICAM-1) in diabetic rat glomeruli: glomerular hyperfiltration is a potential mechanism of ICAM-1 upregulation. *Diabetes*, Vol.46, No.12, pp.2075-2081

Sugimoto H, Shikata K, Wada J, Horiuchi S, & Makino H. (1999). Advanced glycation end products-cytokine-nitric oxide sequence pathway in the development of diabetic nephropathy: aminoguanidine ameliorates the overexpression of tumour necrosis factor-alpha and inducible nitric oxide synthase in diabetic rat glomeruli. *Diabetologia*, Vol.42, No.7, pp.878-886

Sung SH, Ziyadeh FN, Wang A, Pyagay PE, Kanwar YS, & Chen S. (2006). Blockade of vascular endothelial growth factor signaling ameliorates diabetic albuminuria in mice. *J. Am. Soc. Nephrol.*, Vol.17, No.11, pp.3093-3104

Suzuki D, Miyazaki M, Naka R, Koji T, Yagame M, Jinde K, Endoh M, Nomoto Y, & Sakai H. (1995). In situ hybridization of interleukin 6 in diabetic nephropathy. *Diabetes*, Vol.44, No.10, pp.1233-1238

Tang SC, Chan LY, Leung JC, Cheng AS, Chan KW, Lan HY, & Lai KN. (2010a). Bradykinin and high glucose promote renal tubular inflammation. *Nephrol. Dial. Transplant.*, Vol.25, No.3, pp.698-710

Tang SC, Leung JC, Chan LY, Cheng AS, Lan HY, & Lai KN. (2010b). Renoprotection by rosiglitazone in accelerated type 2 diabetic nephropathy: Role of STAT1 inhibition and nephrin restoration. *Am. J. Nephrol.*, Vol.32, No.2, pp.145-155

Tojo A, Asaba K, & Onozato ML. (2007). Suppressing renal NADPH oxidase to treat diabetic nephropathy. *Expert. Opin. Ther. Targets.*, Vol.11, No.8, pp.1011-1018

Tone A, Shikata K, Nakagawa K, Hashimoto M, & Makino H. (2011). Renoprotective effects of clarithromycin via reduction of urinary MCP-1 levels in type 2 diabetic patients. *Clin. Exp. Nephrol.*, Vol.15, No.1, pp.79-85

Twigg SM. (2010). Mastering a mediator: blockade of CCN-2 shows early promise in human diabetic kidney disease. *J. Cell Commun. Signal.*, Vol.4, No.4, pp.189-196

Twigg SM & Cooper ME. (2004). The time has come to target connective tissue growth factor in diabetic complications. *Diabetologia*, Vol.47, No.6, pp.965-968

Usui H, Shikata K, Matsuda M, Okada S, Ogawa D, Yamashita T, Hida K, Satoh M, Wada J, & Makino H. (2003). HMG-CoA reductase inhibitor ameliorates diabetic nephropathy by its pleiotropic effects in rats. *Nephrol. Dial. Transplant.*, Vol.18, No.2, pp.265-272

Wang GG, Lu XH, Li W, Zhao X, & Zhang C. (2011). Protective Effects of Luteolin on Diabetic Nephropathy in STZ-Induced Diabetic Rats. *Evid. Based. Complement Alternat. Med.*, Vol.2011, No., pp.323171

Wang L, Zhang L, Yu Y, Wang Y, & Niu N. (2008). The protective effects of taurine against early renal injury in STZ-induced diabetic rats, correlated with inhibition of renal LOX-1-mediated ICAM-1 expression. *Ren Fail.*, Vol.30, No.8, pp.763-771

Wang X, Shaw S, Amiri F, Eaton DC, & Marrero MB. (2002). Inhibition of the Jak/STAT signaling pathway prevents the high glucose-induced increase in tgf-beta and fibronectin synthesis in mesangial cells. *Diabetes,* Vol.51, No.12, pp.3505-3509

Wen Y, Gu J, Li SL, Reddy MA, Natarajan R, & Nadler JL. (2006). Elevated glucose and diabetes promote interleukin-12 cytokine gene expression in mouse macrophages. *Endocrinology,* Vol.147, No.5, pp.2518-2525

Wolf G. (2000). Cell cycle regulation in diabetic nephropathy. *Kidney Int. Suppl,* Vol.77, No., pp.S59-S66

Wolf G. (2006). Renal injury due to renin-angiotensin-aldosterone system activation of the transforming growth factor-beta pathway. *Kidney Int.,* Vol.70, No.11, pp.1914-1919

Wu JD, Xu XH, Zhu J, Ding B, Du TX, Gao G, Mao XM, Ye L, Lee KO, & Ma JH. (2011). Effect of exenatide on inflammatory and oxidative stress markers in patients with type 2 diabetes mellitus. *Diabetes Technol. Ther.*, Vol.13, No.2, pp.143-148

Wu YG, Lin H, Qi XM, Wu GZ, Qian H, Zhao M, Shen JJ, & Lin ST. (2006). Prevention of early renal injury by mycophenolate mofetil and its mechanism in experimental diabetes. *Int. Immunopharmacol.*, Vol.6, No.3, pp.445-453

Xiao X, Ma B, Dong B, Zhao P, Tai N, Chen L, Wong FS, & Wen L. (2009). Cellular and humoral immune responses in the early stages of diabetic nephropathy in NOD mice. *J. Autoimmun.*, Vol.32, No.2, pp.85-93

Yamagishi S & Matsui T. (2010). Advanced glycation end products, oxidative stress and diabetic nephropathy. *Oxid. Med. Cell Longev.*, Vol.3, No.2, pp.101-108

Yoshimura A, Naka T, & Kubo M. (2007). SOCS proteins, cytokine signalling and immune regulation. *Nat. Rev. Immunol.*, Vol.7, No.6, pp.454-465

Zhang Z, Yuan W, Sun L, Szeto FL, Wong KE, Li X, Kong J, & Li YC. (2007). 1,25-Dihydroxyvitamin D3 targeting of NF-kappaB suppresses high glucose-induced MCP-1 expression in mesangial cells. *Kidney Int.*, Vol.72, No.2, pp.193-201

Ziyadeh FN, Hoffman BB, Han DC, Iglesias-de la Cruz MC, Hong SW, Isono M, Chen S, McGowan TA, & Sharma K. (2000). Long-term prevention of renal insufficiency, excess matrix gene expression, and glomerular mesangial matrix expansion by treatment with monoclonal antitransforming growth factor-beta antibody in db/db diabetic mice. *Proc. Natl. Acad. Sci. U. S. A,* Vol.97, No.14, pp.8015-8020

9

Study of Diabetic Hypertensive Nephropathy in the Local Population of Pakistan

Samreen Riaz and Saadia Shahzad Alam
University of the Punjab, Lahore, Pakistan and FPGMI, Shaikh Zayed Hospital Lahore Pakistan

1. Introduction

Diabetes mellitus is a metabolic disorder that is characterized by high blood sugar and it is because of either problem in insulin secretion (type 1-β cell destruction) or either because of combination of insulin resistance or improper insulin secretion to compensate (type 2). (Riaz, S. 2009)

2. Mechanism of action

Despite ingestion of dietary carbohydrates, serum glucose level remain relatively steady throughout the day. This requires the concerted actions of several different tissues. Pancreatic β-cells, for example, secrete insulin in response to the elevation in glucose that occur after eating. Insulin promotes glucose disposal in adipose tissue and muscle, and also prevents the liver from producing more glucose by suppressing glycogenolysis and gluconeogenesis. In the fasting state, low insulin levels combined with elevated counter-regulatory hormones such as glucagon, adrenaline and corticosteroids promote hepatic glucose production. Recently, evidence has emerged that the brain coordinates many of these effects as well, through direct and indirect glucose sensing and neural outputs to peripheral organs.

Diabetes results from the dysregulation of multiple glucoregulatory hormones that normally acto to maintain glucose homeostasis. For example any defect in insulin production lead to improper regulation of glucose in the blood and result in diabetes. Similarly in patients with type1 and type 2 diabetes, post prandial glucagon secretion is abnormally elevated. This inappropriate secretion of glucagon leads to excess hepatic glucose production and is important contributor to postprandial hyperglycemia in patients with diabetes.

3. Insulin resistance

Deficient insulin action results from inadequate insulin secretion or decrease the tissue response.Insulin resistance is define as lack of sufficient insulin receptors, in target tissue, defect in intracellular transport of glucose and or an altered insulin secondary pattern that is dys-synchronization between pancreatic β cell release of insulin and the body's insulin requirement.(Defronzo, R.A., 1992)

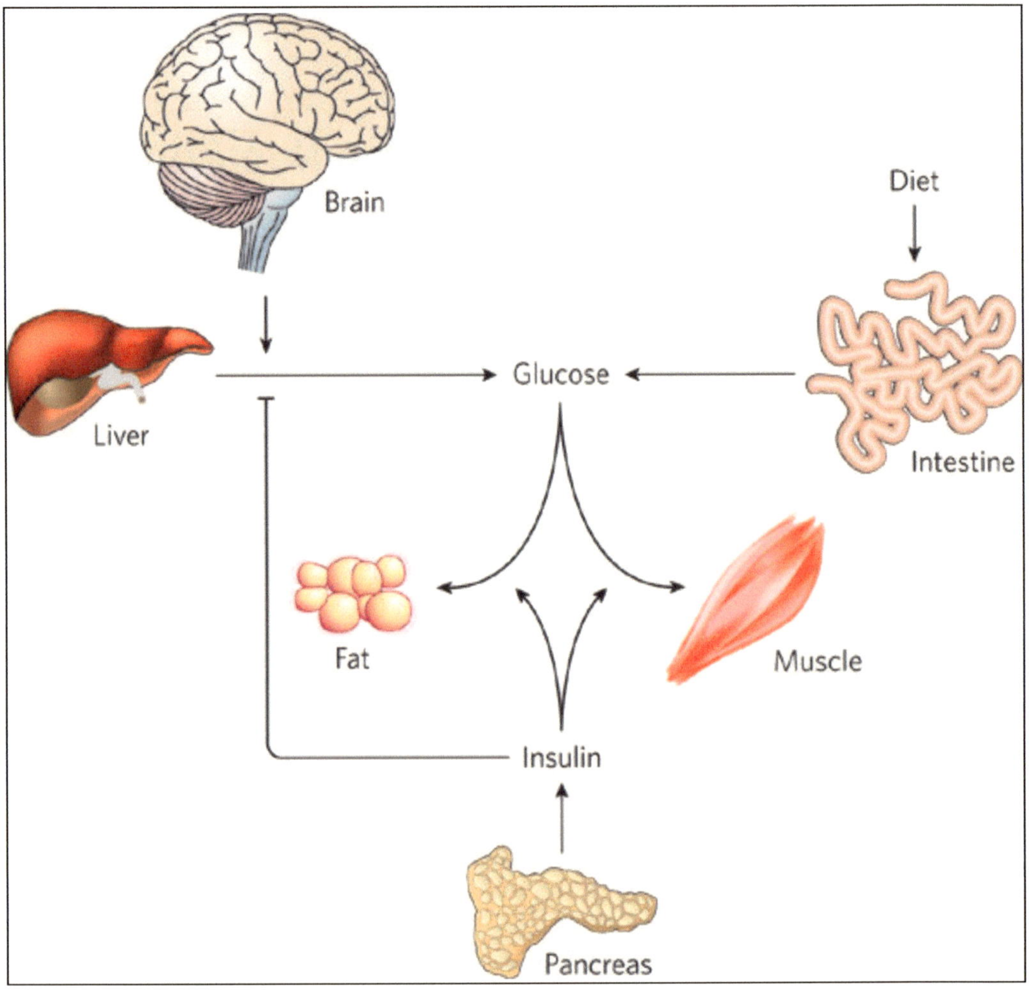

Fig. 1. Glucose homeostasis

4. Prevalence of diabetes

As the prevalence of diabetes is exponentially increasing in many parts of world. It is estimated by WHO that until 2025 there will be 300 million diabetics from which 75% will be from developing countries.

In terms of number of people with diabetes mellitus by the year 2025 USA will be most leading country while Pakistan will be at forth country in the list after China and USA. (Jawaid, S. A., 2002). According to a new publication released by World Health Organization (WHO) and International Diabetes Federation (IDF) 3.2million deaths occur because of diabetes. (Launch of "Diabetes action Now" 5May 2004Igeneva) And it is six leading cause of death by disease world wide.

There are several factors that contribute in increasing the prevalence of diabetes thy include:

- Increase population growth
- Aging
- Urbanization
- Increasing prevalence of obesity
- Increasing prevalence of physical inactivity. (King, H., and Rewers, M., 1993.)

5. Etiologic classification of diabetes mellitus

The World Health Organization (WHO) Expert Committee on diabetes in 1980 and later WHO study group on diabetes mellitus approve the recommendation of National Diabetes Data Group (NDDG). (Report of a WHO Study Group1985) They divide diabetes mellitus into 4 different types :

1. Insulin dependant diabetes mellitus(IDDM)
2. Non-insulin dependant diabetes mellitus(NIDDM)
3. Gestational diabetes mellitus(GDM)
4. Other types

5.1 Type 1 diabetes

5.1.1 Immune mediated diabetes

This is also called as insulin dependand diabetes or juvenile onset diabetes. In this type autoimmunity cause the destruction of β-cells of pancreas. Marker for immune mediated diabetes include islet cell autoantibodies (ICAs), autoantibodies to insulin (IAA), autoantibodies to glutamic acid decarboxylase(GAD65) and autoantibodies to tyrosine phosphatase 1A-2 and 1A-2β. For survival these patients are insulin dependant.

5.1.2 Idiopathic diabetes

In this case there is no known reason and these patients have mostly African or Asian origin. This is strongly inherited but not HLA associated. They are also insulin dependant.

5.2 Type 2 diabetes

This is also known as non-insulin dependant diabetes mellitus or adult onset diabetes. For survival of these patients insulin is not necessary.In these patients obesity is a major cause of insulin resistance while increase age and physical inactivity are also important factors.Ketoacidosis occur because of stress of other infection. it has strong genetic predisposition (Riaz, S. 2009).

5.3 Other specific types of diabetes

5.3.1 Genetic defect of β cell

This is also called as maturity onset diabetes of young (MODY), as it appears before age 25 years and it is characterized by defect in β cell function. In some families inabilityto convert proinsulin to insulin while in some cases mature insulin molecule production.

5.3.2 Genetic defect in insulin action

Metabolic abnormalities cause the mutations in insulin receptor. For example in type A insulin resistance, leprechaunism, Rabson, Mendenhall syndrome are two pediatric syndromes that have mutation in insulin receptor and have extreme insulin resistance.

5.3.3 Disease of exocrine pancreas

Injury to pancreas can cause diabetes and it include pancreatitis, trauma, infection, pancreatectomy and pancreatic carcinoma

Endocrinopathy

Excess amount of some hormone like growth hormone, cortisol, glucagon, apinephrine can cause diabetes as they are antagonize insulin action.

Drug or chemical induce diabetes

Impairinsulin secretion or insulin resistance also cause by some drugs. For example vacor (rat poison), pentamidine, nicotinic acid, glucocorticoids, thyroid hormones, diazoxide, β adrenergic agonists, dilantin,α interferon and other.

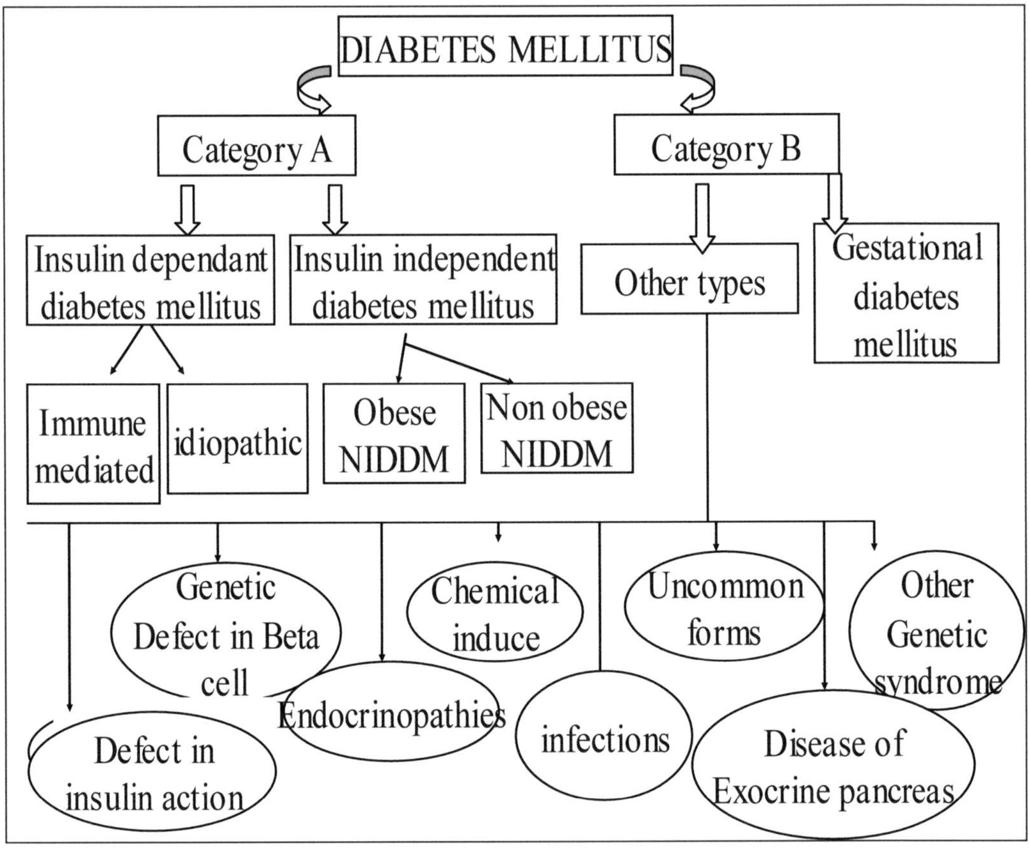

Fig. 2. Etiologic classification of diabetes mellitus

Infection

Some viruses cause the β cell destruction. They include congenital rubella, coxsackie virus B, cytomegalovirus, adenovirus and mumps.

Uncommon

Two conditions are known for it.

1. in stiffman syndrome glutamic acid decaroxylase autoantibodies are produced.
2. antiinsulin receptor antibodies bind with insulin receptor and these antibodies are present in some autoimmune disease and systemic lupus erythemoatosus.

5.3.4 Other genetic syndrome

Incidence of diabetes mellitus also increase with many genetic syndromes. For example Down syndrome, Turner's syndrome, Kline-felter's syndrome, Wolfram's syndrome, Huntington's chorea, Porphyria etc. Autopsy shows the absence of β cells.

5.4 Gestational diabetes mellitus

Impair glucose tolerance normally occur in third trimester of pregnancy. (O'Sullivan and Mahan 1964) Complications of gestational diabetes mellitus increase risk of cesarean delivery and chronic hypertension.

6. Long term complications of diabetes

Long term complications of diabetes include the:

- retinopathy (potential loss of vision)
- nephropathy (renal failure)
- peripheral neuropathy (risk of foot ulcer)
- autonomic neuropathy cause gastrointestinal, genitourinary and cardiovascular symptoms
- periodontal disease(disease of bone and tissue supporting teeth)
- and sexual dysfunction. (Report of the Expert Committee on the Diagnosis and classification of Diabetes Mellitus)

6.1 Nephropathy

Nephropathy is a damage or disease of the kidney. It may be because of several factors and diabetes is one of the major factor of nephropathy.

6.2 Diabetes and nephropathy

Diabetes nephropathy is microvascular complication that associate with diabetes it slowly deteriorate the kidney and lead to end stage renal disease that is chronic and irreversible. Diabetic nephropathy need for chronic dialysis or a kidney transplant.

Since recovery is irreversible so early detection is effective prevention tool. (American diabetes association diabetic nephropathy diabetic care 2002; 25 (supplement)

6.3 Symptoms of diabetic hypertensive nephropathy

Diabetic hypertensive nephropathy is characterized by

- polyuria (frequent urination)
- polydipsia and polyphagia (excess thirst and food intake)
- weight loss
- blurred vision
- and susceptibility to infection
- Biochemical changes in diabetic patients
- Glycation of macromolecules and tissue proteins
- Risk of cardiovascular peripheral vascular and cerebrovascular disease
- Abnormalities of lipoproteins metabolism (hypertension)
- Psychosocial dysfunction also produce because of social impact of diabetes. (Report of the Expert Committee on the Diagnosis and classification of Diabetes Mellitus)

6.4 Prevalence of diabetic hypertensive nephropthy

40% of type 1 and 20% type 2 diabetic patients develop the nephropathy. While prevalence of hypertension in type 2 diabetic patients is estimated at 50% with one estimated as high as 74%. (Riaz, S *et al.* 2009)

6.5 Sources of urinary proteins

The total urinary protein excreted

- 48% was contained in sediments
- 49% was soluble
- and the remaining 3% was in exosomes(Zhou, H., 2006)

6.5.1 Soluble proteins

6.5.1.1 Glomerular filteration of plasma proteins

From glomerular filteration urinary soluble proteins are derived. In proximal tube most of the proteins and peptides are scavenged by highly specialized apical uptake process and this process involves receptor like recognition of peptide molecules. (Christensen, E. I., and Birn, H. 2001; Christensen, E. I. 2002). So in final urine the mount of soluble proteins changes with change concentration in blood plasma, change in glomerular filteration and change in proximal tubule scavenging system.

Based on mechanism change in excretion rate of protein indicative of systemic disease, globular disease or tubular disease.

6.5.1.2 Epithelial cell secretion of soluble proteins

Some proteolytically cleaved membrane bound proteins also present in urine. One of them is Tamm-Horsfall protein. It is most abundant protein in urine and if it is not removed its presence interfare with detection of other proteins.

6.5.2 Solid phase components

Solid phase components consist of sediments that can be precipitated at low centrifugation. It mainly consist of epithelial cells. They are important for diagnostic information because increase number of these cells indicates the renal disease.

6.5.3 Exosomes

Exosomes are derived from glomerular podocytes, renal tubule cells from proximal and distal nephron segments and transitional epithelial cell lining the urinary drainage system.

Exosome are the internal vesicles of multivasculr bodies and transfer to extracellular fluid by fusion of outer membrane of multivesicular bodies with plasma membrane. (Pisitkun, T., 2004)

6.6 Urinary protein marker for diabetic nephropathy

Urinary protein profiling can reveal changes in excretion rates of specific proteins that can have predictive value in the clinical arena, for example

- In the early diagnosis of disease
- In classification of disease with regard to likely therapeutic responses
- In assessment of prognosis
- and in monitoring response to therapy

6.7 Up-regulated urinary proteins in diabetic nephropathy

6.7.1 Albumin and non-immunoreactive albumin

The molecular weight of albumin is 71,658 KDa. Clinically, diabetic nephropathy can be diagnosed when albumin is detected in the urine (albumin excretion 30–300 mg/day). The presence of albumin in the urine is considered predictive of the subsequent development and clinical progression of diabetic nephropathy. (The Microalbuminuria Collaborative Study Group) Microalbuminuria is not specific for diabetic nephropathy , since albumin can also be detected in some other pathological conditions and the prevalence of microalbuminuria in the general population is rather high. Finally, microalbuminuria is a poor predictor of diabetic nephropathy.(Riaz, S *et al.,* 2010)

6.7.2 α1B-Glycoprotein

The molecular weight of α1B-Glycoprotein is 54,239 KDa. It is homologous to the immunoglobulin supergene family and contains five Ig-like V type (immunoglobulin-like) domains. α1B-glycoprotein binds heme and transports it to the liver for breakdown and iron recovery, after which the free hemopexin returns to the circulation. α1B-Glycoprotein has possible role in the autoimmunity involved in nephropathy. Its levels have been described to be higher in type 2 diabetes, its relationship with C-reactive protein is lost in both type 1 and type 2 diabetes, and its levels are independently determined by triacylglycerol and the diabetic state (Van Campenhout, A., et al 2006). This molecule can potentially act as a toxic protease, leading in the rat to proteinuria and glomerular alterations (Bakker, W.W., et al 2005). Although there were no direct references to its possible effects in humans with diabetes or nephropathy, because diabetes is an inflammatory condition associated with iron abnormalities, it can be postulated that α1B-Glycoprotein is altered in diabetes.

6.7.3 Zinc-α2-glycoprotein

The molecular weight of Zinc-α2-glycoprotein is 34,223 KDa. . This protein stimulates lipid degradation in adipocytes and may also bind polyunsaturated fatty acids. Zinc-α2-glycoprotein was the second most abundant urinary protein in diabetic nephropathy. An earlier study of type 2 diabetes described zinc-α2-glycoprotein and three other proteins, α1-acid glycoprotein, α1- microglobulin, and IgG, as specific markers for diabetic nephropathy (Jain, S., et al 2005).

6.7.4 α2-HSglycoprotein precursor (fetuin A)

The molecular weight of α2-HSglycoprotein is 39,300KDa. α2-HSglycoprotein precursor is an inflammation-related calcium regulatory glycoprotein that acts as a systemic calcification inhibitor. Both chronic inflammation and uremia may contribute to exhausting fetuin A release in the late stages of kidney disease. Deficiencies of calcification inhibitors such as fetuin A are relevant to uncontrolled vascular calcification and may offer potential for future therapeutic approaches (Ketteler, M., 2005).

6.7.5 Vitamin D binding protein (VDBP)

The molecular weight of vitamin D binding protein is 52,964KDa. Vitamin D binding protein is a multifunctional protein found in body fluids and on the surface of many cell types. In plasma, it carries vitamin D sterols and prevents polymerization of actin by binding its monomers. VDBP also associates with membrane bound immunoglobulin on the surface of B lymphocytes and with IgG Fc receptors on the membranes of T lymphocytes, suggesting its possible role in the immunepathogenesis and progression of the disease. Vitamin D binding protein was also found in the vitreous in diabetic macular edema, along with pigment epithelium-derived factor, apoA-4, apoA-1, trip-11, and plasma retinol-binding protein (RBP). These chemical mediators in the posterior vitreous may play a role in the pathogenesis of diabetic macular edema (Ouchi, M., et al 2005).

6.7.6 Calgranulin B

The molecular weight of calgranulin is 13,234KDa. Calgranulin B is expressed by macrophages in inflamed tissues and is an inhibitor of protein kinases. Differences in the isoforms and abundance of several urine proteins, including calgranulin B, inter-α-trypsin inhibitor, prothrombin fragment 1, and CD59, were known to be associated with stone formation (Bergsland, K. J., et al 2006). There have been no previous reports on their association with diabetes or other renal diseases. A1AT is an inhibitor of serine proteases, and its primary target is elastase, but it also has a moderate affinity for plasmin and thrombin. The serum levels of A1AT and a α1-acid glycoprotein, as well as their glycosylated protein fractions, were reported to be significantly greater in sera from patients with diabetic nephropathy compared with healthy adults. Marked linear deposition of these proteins in the glomerular or dermal vascular walls was also observed in the same patients (Inoue, W., 1989), linking them to diabetic nephropathy. Whereas the association between A1AT deficiency and glomerulonephritis has been reported only sporadically. (Os, I., et al 1997).

6.7.7 Type IV collagen

The molecular weight of Type IV collagen is 500,000. Type IV collagen is the major component of the glomerular extracellular matrix and the level of type IV collagen in the urine might reflect the rate of matrix turnover in diseased kidneys. Findings indicate that type IV collagen has a specificity for diabetes nephropathy that albumin itself has not, but since urinary collagen IV is detectable only when microalbuminuria is already present.(Tomino, Y., *et al.,* 2001)

6.7.8 Podocytes and nephrin

Podocytes are key structural elements of the glomerular filtration barrier. Podocytes and podocyte-specific proteins can be potentially interesting urinary markers for the early diagnosis of an alteration of the glomerulus.(Dalla Vestra, M., et al 2003) Indeed, urinary podocytes have been detected only in the urine of diabetic patients with micro- and macroalbuminuria, whereas they were absent in healthy controls, type 2 diabetes patients without microalbuminuria or patients suffering from chronic renal failure.(Nakamura, T., et al 2000). Nephrin is one of the many podocyte-specific proteins that have been described in the last few years. nephrin was totally absent in the urine of non-diabetic patients.

6.7.9 Advanced glycation end products

Advanced glycation end products (AGEs) are a heterogeneous group of proteins and lipids to which sugar residues are covalently bound during physio-pathological processes.

Kidneys are thought to be one of the key organs for the clearance of AGEs. In type 2 diabetes serum low molecular weight advance glycation end products are usually higher than non-diabetic.(Turk, N., *et al.,* 2004)

6.7.10 Betaig-h3

The molecular weight of intact Betaig-h3 is 68KDa. Betaig-h3 is an extracellular matrix protein that is induced by transforming growth factor beta, a growth factor implicated in the pathogenesis of diabetic nephropathy. Ha *et al.*(Ha, S. W., *et al.,* 2004) first showed that the betaig-h3 to creatinine ratio is significantly higher in type 2 diabetes patients than in control subjects. In another study,(Cha, D. R., *et al.,* 2005) it was also observed that the urinary level of betaig-h3 is higher in diabetic patients (betaig-h3/creatinine ratio: 25.02 ± 8.84) than in healthy individuals (18.67 ± 6.56).

6.7.11 L1 cell adhesion molecule (CD171)

L1 cell adhesion molecule (CD171) is a potential new marker for tubular injury. It is expressed in human acute kidney injury and excreted in urine. In normal kidney L1 is located in basolateral membrane in all epithelial cells of collecting duct except for intercalated cells. In acute tubular necrosis, L1 lost its polarized distribution and induce in thick ascending limb and distal tubule cells.

6.7.12 Tamm-Horsfall protein

The molecular weight of Tamm-Horsfall protein is 95KDa. It is produced by ascending limb of loop of Henle. It is most prevalent protein and excretion rate is 25-40mg/day.(Cvoriscec, D., *et al.*, 1985). In renal disease as number of tubules decrease excretion of this protein also accordingly decrease.

6.8 Downregulated urinary proteins in diabetic nephropathy

6.8.1 Transthyretin (prealbumin)

The molecular weight of transthyretin is 15,877KDa. Transthyretin (prealbumin) is a thyroid hormone-binding protein, which transports a small part of thyroxine from the bloodstream to the brain. About 40% of plasma transthyretin circulates in a tight complex with plasma RBP. Transthyretin was reported as a better and suitable marker for nutrition assessment in patients with chronic renal failure (Saito, K., *et al.*, 2004). Elevated plasma RBP in insulin-resistant humans with obesity and type-2 diabetes was known to induce hepatic expression of the gluconeogenic enzyme phosphoenolpyruvate carboxykinase and impairs insulin signaling in muscle (Yang, Q., *et al.*, 2005). It is possible that low RBP-4 in diabetic nephropathy increases insulin sensitivity and causes spontaneous hypoglycemia, because low RBP-4 is potentially hypoglycemic. (Riaz, S *et al.*, 2010)

6.8.2 AMBP proteins

The molecular weight of AMBP is 38,974KDa. AMBP contains both α1-microglobulin and inter-α-trypsin inhibitor light chain (bikunin). Bikunin is an important anti-inflammatory substance to modulate inflammatory events. Decreases level of this protein affect immunocompetence in diabetic renal disease remains unstudied. The other component of AMBP protein, α1-microglobulin, in urine was directly related to progressive albuminuria in Chinese, Malays, and Asian Indians with type 2 diabetes (Hong, C. Y., et al 2003). This is in contrast to the decreasing levels of this protein observed in our study. Urinary α1-microglobulin indicates proximal tubular dysfunction and could be a useful biomarker for the early detection of nephropathy in diabetic subjects in addition to albuminuria, which indicates glomerular dysfunction.

6.8.3 ApoA-I

The molecular weight of ApoA-I is 30,759KDa. ApoA-I acting as a cofactor for the lecithin cholesterol acyltransferase, participates in the reverse transport of cholesterol from tissues to the liver for excretion.ApoA1, as well as apoB/A1, was included among several nontraditional cardiovascular risk factors in the progression to pediatric metabolic syndrome (Retnakaran, R., *et al.*, 2006), but there have been no reported references to its association with diabetes or nephropathy. (Riaz, S *et al.*, 2010)

6.8.4 Adiponectin

The molecular weight of adiponectin is 28KDa. Adiponectin is an adipocyte-secreted cytokine (adipokine) of human plasma. Decreased adiponectin plasma levels are linked to obesity, insulin resistance and type 2 diabetes. Koshimura *et al.* found, in the urine of type 2 diabetes patients with macroalbuminuria, a 30 kDa protein immunoreactive towards an anti-adiponectin monoclonal antibody.(Koshimura, J., et al 2004) Urinary adiponectin may result from the elevation of the serum concentration and enhanced filtration through the damaged kidney. Similar findings were more recently obtained, showing that both serum and urinary adiponectin concentrations are elevated in type 2 diabetes patients with nephropathy, as compared to patients with microalbuminuria alone.(Fujita, H., *et al.*, 2006)

7. Hypertensive nephropathy

This is a condition in which kidney damage occur due to chronic blood pressure. In diabetic patients major risk factor for cardiovascular morbidity and mortality is hypertension. (Hypertension in Diabetes Study (HDS) 1993 ; Hansson, L., et al 1998) Diabetic nephropathy develop in 40% of patients with type 1 diabetes (Krolewski, A. S., *et al.*, 1985) and 35% of patients with type 2 diabetes (Mehler, P. S., 1997) rigorous treatment of hypertension slow the rate of decrease in renal function and improve mortality (Parving, H. H., *et al.*, 1987 ; Parving, H., and Hommel, E., 1989)

7.1 Diabetes and hypertension

Blood pressure, serum lipids and several cardiovascular factors are effected by central adiposity and insulin resistance. (Niaura, R., *et al.*, 2000) Diabetes mellitus and hypertension both are associated with high urinary albumin excretion. In type 2 diabetes patients the presence of microalbuminuria is often a better predictor of cardiovascular disease than of diabetic nephropathy. (Molitch, M. E., *et al.*, 2004) Microalbuminuria is also important marker of atheromatosus and potential of coronary heart disease in diabetic patients. (Donnelly, R., (2002) Recommended target blood pressure in all diabetics is ≤130/80 and urinary albumin excretion >200mg/l the goal is 125-130/75-80. (Augustine, J., Donald, G., diabetic nephropathy (2003)

7.2 Treatment of nephropathy

Currently ACE inhibitors or ARBs are used for preventing progression of microalbuminurea to macroalbuminurea and advance stages of nephropathy. These drugs have a large amount of adverse effects such as extreme hypotension, hyperkalemia and dry cough which has in certain cases becomes sever enough to stimulate tuberculous cough resulting in wrongful antituberculous treatment being prescribed to the patient. In such a scenario it is important that another biomarker other than microalbuminurea be found for diabetic hypertensive nephropathy which would reveal the development of incipient diabetic nephropathy and a specific drug be designed for that biomarker which would have a fewer side effects as it would be biomarker specific.(Martin- Gallan, *et al.*, (2003).

Type 2 diabetic patients, and same age and sex-matched normal healthy controls were recruited from the Sheikh Zayed Hospital, Lahore, Pakistan. Total Urine and urinary proteins were estimated and analyzed initially by different protein assays and 1-D SDS polyacrylamide gel electrophoresis. The samples were purified further by passing through the high abundance protein removal and desalting columns. These serum and urine samples from control and diabetic groups before or after thiamine therapy were further analysed by 2-D liquid chromatographic system in which samples were initially fractionated by

Protein name	MW (KDa)	PI	Function	Up or down regulated
α1-Antitrypsin	46,707	5.52	Defense response	+
Serotransferrin precursor	77,000	7.19	Transport	
Ceruloplasmin Precursor	122,128	5.64	Transport	+
Hemopexin	51,643	6.96	Transport	
AMBP protein	38,974	6.21	Metabolism	-
Complement factor H	139,034	6.64	Defense response	
Serum albumin	71,658	6.79	Transport	+
Alpha1-Antichymotrypsin precursor	47,651	4.6	Defense response	
Antithrombin-III	52,658	6.41	Defense response	
Complement component C3	187,046	6.32	Defense response	
ApoA-1	30,759	5.72	Metabolism	-
Alpha2-Glycoprotein 1, zinc	34,223	5.97	Defense response	+
Ig gama 1 chain C region	51,628	8.1	Defense response	
Kininogen precursor	47,853	6.64	Signal transduction	
B-factor, properdin	68,829	6.48	Metabolism	
Alpha1B-Glycoprotein	54,239	5.82	FNA	+
ApoA-IV	45,343	5.37	Metabolism	
Haptoglobin precursor	31,362	8.65	Transport	
Clusterin	52,461	6.19	Signal transduction	
Beta 2-Glycoprotein 1 precursor	38,273	8.42	Metabolism	
Complement factor B	85,479	7.06	Defense response	

Protein name	MW (KDa)	PI	Function	Up or down regulated
Complement factor I	65,677	7.87	Defense response	
Complement component C7	93,457	6.43	Defense response	
Hepatocellular carcinoma associated protein TB6	83,232	5.69	Transport	
Sulfated glycoprotein 2	57,796	6.62	Signal transduction	
Angiotensinogen	53,121	6.22	Signal transduction	
Leucine-rich alpha 2-glycoprotein	38,154	6.88	FNA	
Transthyretin precursor	15,877	5.71	Metabolism	-
Alpha2-HS-glycoprotein precursor	39,300	5.64	Metabolism	+
Prostaglandin H2 D-isomerase precursor	21,015	8.15	Metabolism	
Calgranulin B	13,234	6.04	Defense response	+
Complement component 9 precursor	63,133	5.53	Defense response	
Ig alpha -1 chain C region	53,163	6.06	Defense response	
Inter-alpha-trypsin inhibitor heavy chain h4 precursor	101,179	6.57	Metabolism	
Plasma retinol-binding protein precursor	22,995	5.95	Signal transduction	
Epidermal growth factor–containing fibulin-like extracellular matrix protein	54,517	4.99	Signal transduction	
Hypothetical protein	52,553	7.9	FNA	

Protein name	MW (KDa)	PI	Function	Up or down regulated
Predicted immunoglobulin	23,530	7.6	FNA	
Ig k chain C region	15,170	8.65	Defense response	
Beta2-microglobulin	13,706	6.45	Defense response	
Dystroglycan precursor	97,520	8.9	Metabolism	
Hypothetical protein	70,309	7.9	FNA	
Hypothetical protein	37,651	6.4	FNA	
VDBP	52,964	5.2	Transport	+
Epididymal secretory protein E1	16,559	8.04	Defense response	
Hypothetical protein FLJ31320	67,970	8.49	FNA	
Lumican precursor	38,405	6.54	Cell Development	
Ig gama4 chain C region	35,941	8.2	Defense response	
Alpha 2-Antiplasmin precursor	54,531	6.2	Defense response	
ApoA-II precursor	11,168	6.82	Metabolism	
Fibrinogen beta chain precursor	55,892	8.66	Metabolism	
Hypothetical protein FLJ35322	18,511	6.2	FNA	
ApoD	21,262	5.11	Metabolism	
Corticosteroid-binding globulin Precursor	45,112	5.93	Transport	
Novel protein	94,331	5.47	FNA	
Vitronectin precursor	54,306	4.6	Defense response	
Fibrinogen gama chain	51,479	5.51	Metabolism	
Hypothetical protein FLJ22612	58,511	4.62	FNA	
Ig gama2 chain C region	46,032	7.88	Defense response	

Table 1. Urinary protein identified in type 2 diabetic patients with macroalbuminuria (Riaz, S. 2009, 2010, 2011)

chromatofocusing and the selected fractions were further analysed by reverse-phase high performance liquid chromatography. The proteins which showed variation between test and control samples were identified by mass spectrometry MALDI TOF/TOF and LC MS analysis. All the samples belonging to the control and diabetic groups were then analyzed by ELISA and estimated the levels of some proteins which were found to vary. (Samreen Riaz, 2009,2010, 2011)

8. References

American diabetes association diabetic nephropathy diabetic care 2002; 25 (supplement).

Atkinson, M. A., Maclaren, N. K., (1994). The pathogenesis of insulin dependent diabetes. N Engl J Med 331:1428-1436.

Atkinson, M. A., Maclaren, N.K., Riley, W.J., Winter, W.E., Fisk, D.D., Spillar, R.P., (1986). Are insulin autoantibodies markers for insulin-dependent mellitus? Diabetes 35: 894-898.

Augustine, J., Donald, G., diabetic nephropathy (2003). The Cleveland Clinic, Department of nephrology and Hypertension, The Cleveland Health Foundation, United States.

Baekkeskov, S., Neilsen, J. H., Marner, B., Bilde, T., Ludvigsson, J., Lernmark, A., (1982). Autoantibodies in newly diagnosed diabetic children with immunoprecipitate human pancreatic islet cell proteins. Nature 298: 167-169.

Banerji, M. A., Chaiken, R. L., Huey, H., Tuomi, T., Norin, A. J., Mackay, I. R., Rowley, M. J., Zimmet, P., Lebovitz, H., (1994). GAD antibody negative NIDDM in adults black subjects with diabetic ketoacidosis and increased frequency of human leukocyte antigen DR3 and DR4. Diabetes 43:741-745.

Banerji, M., Lebovitz, H., (1989). Insulin sensitive and insulin resistant variants in IDDM. Diabetes 38:784-792.

Barnett, A. H., Eff, C., Leslie, R. D. G., Pyke, D. A., (1981). Diabetes in identical twins. Diabetologia 20:87-93.

Barrett, T. G., Bundey, S. E., Macleod, A. F., (1995). Neurodegeneration and diabetes: UK nation wide study of Wolfrm (DIDMOAD) syndrome. Lancet 346:1458-1463.

Berelowitz, M., and Eugene, H.G., (1996). Non-insulin dependent diabetes mellitus secondary to other endocrine disorders. In Diabetes Mellitus. LeRoith D, Taylor SI, Olefsky JM, Eds. New York, Lippincott-Raven, p.496-502

Bergsland, K. J., Kelly, J. K., Coe, B. J., Coe, F. L., 2006. Urine protein markers distinguish stoneforming from non-stone-forming relatives of calcium stone formers. *Am J Physiol* 291:F530–F536.

Bogardus, C., Lillioja, S., Mott, D. M., Hollenbeck, C., Reaven, G., (1985). Relationship between degree of obesity and in vivo insulin action in man. Am J Physiol 248:E286-E291.

Cersosimo, E., Pister, P. W. T., Pesola, G., McDermott, K., Bajorunas, D., Brennan, M. F., (1991). Insulin secretion and action in patients with pancreatic cancer. Cancer 67:486-493.

Cha, D. R., Kim, I. S., Kang, Y.S., et al. (2005). Urinary concentration of transforming growth factor-beta-inducible gene-h3(beta ig-h3) in patients with Type 2 diabetes mellitus. Diabet Med 22:14–20.

Christensen, E. I. (2002). Pathophysiology of protein and vitamin handling in the proximal tubule. Nephrol. Dial. Transplant. 17, Suppl. 9, 57-58.

Clement, K., Pueyo, M. E., Vaxillaire, M., Raketoambinina, B., Thuillier, F., Passa, P., Froguel, P., Roberts, J., Velho, G., (1996). Assessment of insulin sensitivity in glucokinase-deficient subjects. Diabetologia 39: 82-90.

Cousins, L., 1995. Obstetric complications. In Diabetes Mellitus and Pregnancy: Principles and Practice. 2nd ed. New York, Churchill Livingstone, p. 455-468.

Dalla Vestra, M., Masiero, A., Roiter, A. M., et al (2003). Is podocyte injury relevant in diabetic nephropathy? Studies in patients with type 2 diabetes. Diabetes 52:1031–1035.

Defronzo, R., Deibert, D., Hendler, R., Felig, P., (1979). Insulin sensitivity and insulin binding to monocytes in maturity-onset diabetes. J Clin Invest 63:939-946.

Diabetes: Could vitamin 'B' the answer? Chloë Harman Comments on Original article, Naila Rabbani, Saadia Shahzad Alam, Samreen Riaz, James Larkin, M Waheed Akhtar, Tahir Shafi and Paul J Thornalley. High dose thiamine therapy for people with type 2 diabetes and microalbuminuria: a randomised, double-blind, placebo-controlled study. Diabetologia 52, 208–212 (2009). Nature Reviews Endocrinology (5), 236-236 (30 April 2009) doi:10.1038/nrneph.2009.8 Research Highlights (Impact factor 3.76). http://www.Nature.com/ review endocrinology/ htm.

Diabetes: Could vitamin 'B' the answer? Chloë Harman Comments on Original article, Naila Rabbani, Saadia Shahzad Alam, Samreen Riaz, James Larkin, M Waheed Akhtar, Tahir Shafi and Paul J Thornalley. High dose thiamine therapy for people with type 2 diabetes and microalbuminuria: a randomised, double-blind, placebo-controlled study. Diabetologia 52, 208–212 (2009). Nature Reviews Nephrology 5, 182 (April 2009) doi:10.1038/nrneph.2009.8. Research Highlights (Impact factor 4.764). http://www.Nature.com/ review enephrology/ htm.

Forrest, J.A., Menser, M.A., Burgess, J.A., (1971). High frequency of diabetes mellitus in young patients with congenital rubella; Lancet ii:332-334.

Fujita, H., Morii, T., Koshimura, J., et al. (2006). Possible relationship between adiponectin and renal tubular injury in diabetic nephropathy. Endocr J 53:745–752.

Group TMCS (the Microalbuminuria Collaborative Study Group) (1999). Predictors of the development of microalbuminuria in patients with Type 1 diabetes mellitus: a seven-year prospective study. Diabet Med 16:918–925.

Ha, S. W., Kim, H. J., Bae, J. S., et al. (2004). Elevation of urinary betaig-h3, transforming growth factor-beta-induced protein in patients with type 2 diabetes and nephropathy. Diabetes Res Clin Pract 65:167–173.

Hansson, L., Zanchetti, A., Carruthers, S. G., Dahlof, B., Elmfeldt, D., Julius, S., Menard, J., Rahn, K. H., Wedel, H., Westerling, S., 1998. Effects of intensive blood-pressure lowering and low-dose aspirin in patients with hypertension: principal results of the Hypertension Optimal Treatment (HOT) randomized trial. Lancet 351:1755-1762.

Herman, W. H., Fajans, S. S., Oritz, F. J., Smith, M. J., Sturis, J., Bell, G. I., Polonsky, K. S., Halter, J. B., (1994). Abnormal insulin secretion, not insulin resistance, is the genetic or primary defect of MODY in the RW pedigree. Diabetes 43:40-46.

Hong, C. Y., Hughes, K., Chia, K. S., Ng, V., Ling, S. L., 2003. Urinary α1-microglobulin as a marker of nephropathy in type 2 diabetic Asian subjects in Singapore. *Diabetes Care* 26: 338–342.

Hypertension in Diabetes Study (HDS) 1993. Increased risk of cardiovascular complications in hypertensive type 2 diabetic patients. J Hypertens 11:319-325.

Inoue, W., 1989. Immunopathological analysis of acute phase reactant (APR) proteins in glomeruli from patients with diabetic nephropathy. *Nippon Jinzo Gakkai Shi* 31: 211–219.

Jadresic, A., Banks, L. M., Child, D. F., Diamant, L., Doyle, F. H., Fraser, T. R., Joplin, G. F., (1982). The acromegaly syndrome. J Med202:189-204.

Jain, S., Rajput, A., Kumar, Y., Uppuluri, N., Arvind, A. S., Tatu, U., 2005. Proteomic analysis of urinary protein markers for accurate prediction of diabetic kidney disorder. *J Assoc Physicians India* 53:513–520.

Kahn, C. R., Flier, J. S., Bar, R. S., Archer, J. A., Gorden, P., Martin, M.M., Roth, J., (1976). The syndromes of insulin resistance and acanthosis nigricans. N Engl J Med 294:739-745.

King, H., Rewers, M., (1993). Global estimates for prevalence of diabetes mellitus and impair glucose tolerance in adults: WHO Ad Hoc Diabetes Report Group. Diabetes Care 16:157-177.

King, M. L., Bidwell, D., Shaikh, A., Voller, A., Banatvala, J. E., (1983). Coxsackie-B-virus-specific IgM responses in children with insulin-dependent (juvenile-onset; type 1) diabetes mellitus. Lancet i:1397-1399.

Koshimura, J., Fujita, H., Narita, T. (2004). Urinary adiponectin excretion is increased in patients with overt diabetic nephropathy. Biochem Biophys Res Commun 316:165–169.

Krolewski, A. S., Warram, J. H., Chrislieb, A., Busick, R. J., Kahn, C. R., 1985. The changing natural history of nephropathy in type 1 diabetes. Am J Med 78:785-794.

Lan, M. S., Wasserfall, C., Maclaren, N. K., Notkins, A. L., (1996). 1A-2, a transmembrane protein of the protein tyrosine phosphatase family, is a major autoantigen in insulindependent diabetes mellitus. Proc Natl Acad Sci USA 93:6367-6370.

Larsen, S., Hilsted, J., Tronier, B., Worning, H., (1987). Metabolic control and B cell function in patients with insulin-dependent diabetes mellitus secondary to chronic pancreatitis. Metabolism 36:964-967.

Lu, J., Li, Q., Xie, H., Chen, Z., Borovitskaya, A. E., Maclaren, N. K., Notkins, A.L., Lan, M. S., (1996). Identification of a second transmembrane protein tyrosine phosphatase, 1A-2β, as an autoantigen in insulin-dependent diabetes mellitus: precursor of the 37-KDa tryptic fragment. Proc Natl Acad Sci USA 93: 2307-2311.

Magee, M.S., Walden, C.E., Benedetti, T.J., 1993. Influence of diagnostic criteria on the incidence of gestational diabetes and perinatl morbidity. JAMA 269:609-615.

Mehler, P. S., Jeffers, B. W., Estacio, R., Schrier, R. W., 1997. Association of hypertension and complications in non-insulin dependent diabetes mellitus. Am J Hypertens 10:152-161.

Molitch, M. E., DeFronzo, R. A., Franz, M. J., Keane, W. F., Mogensen, C. E., Parving, H. H., Steffes, M. W., (2004). Nephropathy in diabetes (position statement). Diabetes Care 27 (Suppl 1):S79-S83.

Naila Rabbani, Saadia Shahzad Alam, Samreen Riaz, James Larkin, M Waheed Akhtar, Tahir Shafi and Paul J Thornalley. 2009. High dose thiamine therapy for people with type 2 diabetes and microalbuminuria: a randomised, double-blind, placebo-controlled study. Diabetologia. Springer Berlin / Heidelberg. Vol. 52 (2), 208-212. (Impact factor 5.822) http://www.springerlink.Journal Issue/ Diabetologia/htm. PubMed.

Samreen Riaz, "Study of Protein Biomarkers for Diabetes Mellitus Type 2 and Role of High Dose Thiamine on their Level" Advances in Medicine and Biology (2010). Editor, Leon V Berhardt. Book Hauppauge, N.Y. 11788-3619, USA. Phone (631) 231-7269 * Fax (631) 299-0165. http://www.novapublishers.com. I:\Nova publishs\Advances in Medicine and Biology_Volume 13.htm.Chapter 11. Volume 13. Nova Science Publishers, Inc. 400 Oser Avenue, Suite 1600,

Nakamura, T., Ushiyama, C., Suzuki, S., et al. (2000). Urinary excretion of podocytes in patients with diabetic nephropathy. Nephrol Dial Transplant 15:1379–1383.

Newman, B., Selby, J. V., Slemenda, C., Fabsitz, R., Friedman, G. D., (1987). Concordance for type 2 (non-insulin-dependent)diabetes mellitus in male twins. Diabetologia 30: 763-738.

Niaura, R., Banks, S. M., Ward, K. D., et al. 2000. Hostility and metabolic syndrome in older males. The normative aging study. Psych Som Med; 62:7-16

O'Byrne. S., and Feely, J., (1990). Effects of drugs on glucose tolerance in non-insulin-dependent diabetes (part 1 and 2). Drug 40: 203-219.

Olesfsky, J. M., Kolterman, O. G., Scarlett, J. A., (1982). Insulin action and resistance in obesity and noninsulin-dependent tye 2 diabetes mellitus. Am J Physiol 243:E15-E30.

Os, I., Skjorten, F., Svalander, C., Berge, E., 1997. α1-Antitrypsin deficiency associated with hepatic cirrhosis and IgA nephritis. *Nephron* 77:235–237.

O'Sullivan, J. B., Mahan, C. M., (1994). Criteria for the oral glucose tolerance test in pregnancy. Diabetes 13:278.

Ouchi, M., West, K., Crabb, J. W., Kinoshita, S., Kamei, M., 2005. Proteomic analysis of vitreous from diabetic macular edema. *Exp Eye Res* 81:176 –182.

Pak, C.Y., Eun, H., McArthur, R.G., Yoon, J., (1988). Assocition of cytomegalovirus-infection with autoimmune type 1 diabetes. Lancet ii:1-4.

Pandit, M. K., Burke, J., Gustafson, A. B., Minocha, A., Peiris, A. N., (1993). Drug-induced disorders of glucose tolerance. Ann Int Med 118:529-540.

Parving, H. H., Andersen, A. R., Smidt, U. M., Hommel, E., Mathiesen, E. R., Svendsen, P. A., 1987. Effect of antihypertensive treatment on kidney function in diabetic nephropathy. BMJ 294:1443-1452.

Parving, H., Hommel, E., 1989. Prognosis in diabetic nephropathy. BMJ 299:230-233.

Pisitkun, T., Shen, R. F., and Knepper, M. A. (2004) Identification and proteomic profiling of exosomes in human urine. Proc. Natl. Acad. Sci. U. S. A. 101, 13368-13373.

Rabbani, N., Shahzad Alam, S., Riaz, S., Larkin, J.R., Akhtar, M.W., Shafi, T. and Thornalley, P.J. Response to comment on Rabbani *et al.*, (2009) High dose thiamine therapy for patients with type 2 diabetes and microalbuminuria: a pilot randomised, double-blind, placebo-controlled study. Diabetologia, 52(2): 208 - 212, 2009. Diabetologia. 52 (6): 1214-1216. (Impact factor 5.822) http://www.springerlink.Journal Issue/ Diabetologia/htm. PubMed.

Reaven, G. M., Bernstein, R., Davis, B., Olefsky, J. M., (1976). Nonketotic diabetes mellitus: insulin deficiency or insulin resistnce? Am J Med 60:80-88.

Retnakaran, R., Zinman, B., Connelly, P. W., Harris, S. B., Hanley, A. J., 2006. Nontraditional cardiovascular risk factors in pediatric metabolic syndrome. *J Pediatr* 148:176–182.

Rimoin, D. L., (1976). Genetic syndromes associated with glucose intolerance. In The Genetics of Diabetes Mellitus. Berlin Springer-Verlag.

Saito, K., Shimizu, A., Inoue, S., Hamada, C., Fukui, M., Tomino, Y., 2004. Effective usage of nutrition assessment proteins in patients with diabetic nephropathy. *Nippon Jinzo Gakkai Shi* 46:73–78.

Samreen Riaz, Saadia Shahzad Alam and M. Waheed Akhtar. (2010). Proteomic Identification of human serum biomarkers in diabetes mellitus type-2. Journal of Pharmaceutical and Biomedical Analysis. Volume 51 issue 5, 1103-1107.

Samreen Riaz, Diabetes mellitus (Review article) Scientific Research and Essay. Vol. 4 (5) pp. 367-373, May, 2009.

Samreen Riaz, Mehreen Raza, Saadia Shhazad Alam, Shahida Hasnain and M. Waheed Akhtar. 2009. Obesity as risk factor and study of obesity related proteins in diabetes mellitus. African Journal of Biotechnology Vol. 8 (5), pp. 737-744, 6 March, 2009. (Impact factor 0.456)

Samreen Riaz, Saadia Shahzad Alam, Surjit Kaila Srai, Vernon Skinner, Aasma Riaz and M. Waheed Akhtar. (2010). Proteomic Identification of human urine biomarkers in diabetes mellitus type-2. Journal of Diabetes technology & Therapeutics. 2010. 12 (12): 979- 988. (Impact factor 2.620).

Samreen Riaz, Vernon Skinner and Surjit Kaila Srai. (2011). Effect of high dose thiamine on levels of human urine protein biomarkers in diabetes mellitus type 2. Journal of Pharmaceutical and Biomedical Analysis. JPBA-D-10-01119. Volume / issue. . (Impact factor 2.453).

Samreen Riaz and Ansa Butt (2010). Study of Protein profiling of human urine in diabetic hypertensive nephropathy versus normal healthy controls. Diabetes technology & Therapeutics.. 12 (5): 379-386

World Health Organization: Diabetes Mellitus: Report of a WHO Study Group. Geneva, World Health Org., 1985 (Tech Rep Ser, no. 727)